An Atlas of Hair Pathology with Clinical Correlations

An Atlas of Hair Pathology with Clinical Correlations

Second Edition

Leonard C. Sperling, MD
Professor of Dermatology and Pathology
Chair of Dermatology at the Uniformed Services University
Bethesda, Maryland, USA

Shawn E. Cowper, MD
Associate Professor of Dermatology and Pathology
Yale University
New Haven, Connecticut, USA

Eleanor A. Knopp, MD
Fellow in Dermatopathology and Clinical Dermatologist
Yale University
New Haven, Connecticut, USA

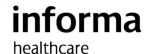

A CIP record for this book is available from the British Library.

Library of Congress Cataloging-in-Publication Data available on application

ISBN-13: 978-1-84184-733-7
eISBN: 978-1-84184-734-4

Orders may be sent to: Informa Healthcare, Sheepen Place, Colchester, Essex CO3 3LP, UK
Telephone: +44 (0)20 7017 6682
Email: Books@Informa.com
Informa Healthcare Website: http://informahealthcarebooks.com
Informa website: www.informa.com

For corporate sales please contact: CorporateBooksIHC@informa.com
For foreign rights please contact: RightsIHC@informa.com
For reprint permissions please contact: PermissionsIHC@informa.com

Typeset by Exeter Premedia Services Private Ltd., Chennai, India
Printed and bound in the United Kingdom

Contents

Preface

This second edition differs from the first in several ways. There are now three authors, instead of one, which has allowed for new approaches and a more critical and synergistic presentation of the material. Every section has been a group effort, with careful editorial inputs from all three of us. In this way, poor-quality images and confusing or nebulous text have been excluded (we hope), and innovative ideas have had a chance to take root and undergo refinement. The images, which are truly the heart and soul of the text, are a dramatic improvement from the first edition, thanks to improved cameras and technology. Several additional sections have been added to capture the latest thinking in nomenclature as well as some of the less common diseases that are entering the mainstream of clinical and pathological practice.

What has not changed is the purpose of the book, which is intended to serve as a primer, an atlas, and a reference text. As a primer, the book reviews very basic information, including hair anatomy and the "nuts and bolts" of processing and evaluating specimens. The authors assume that the reader knows very little about hair disease or hair pathology, and so a step-by-step approach is utilized. As an atlas, the book is rich in photographs demonstrating both basic and advanced histological features of hair disease. As a reference, the book includes the most up-to-date information about the pathology of hair disease, presented with a synopsis format. Basic clinical features are reviewed to provide clinicopathological correlation.

We expect that dermatopathologists will be the most enthusiastic audience for this book. However, many general pathologists and dermatologists were avid users of the first edition, and we expect the same to be true of the second.

LEN

The science of hair pathology has come a long way since Dr. Headington's seminal article on the subject (Headington J. Transverse microscopic anatomy of the human scalp. *Arch Dermatol* 1984;120:449–56). We still owe Dr. Headington a debt of gratitude; and many of his keen observations are utilized in this text. I have been fortunate to follow the footsteps of many pioneers in the field of hair disease, such as David Whiting, Vera Price, Wilma Bergfeld, Al Solomon, and Rodney Dawber. David Whiting, in particular, has been a selfless mentor and "cheerleader" for much of my work. I have also received support and encouragement from many other leaders in the field of hair disease, such as Jerry Shapiro, George Cotsarelis, Kurt Stenn, Elise Olsen, Amy McMichael, Rodney Sinclair, Lynne Goldberg, Antonella Tosti, Catherine Stefanato, Laila El Shabrawi-Caelen, and Jeffrey Miller.

The confidence to move forward with an ambitious project such as this text is due, in part, to the encouragement I have received from my academic idols and mentors: William D. James, Stephen I. Katz, John Stanley, Kim Yancey, George Lupton, Jeffrey Callen, Jennifer McNiff, and Larry Laughlin, among others.

My co-authors, Shawn Cowper and Eleanor Knopp, are simply brilliant and have brought so much to this endeavor. And of course Joanne and Laura are always there for me. They make the effort worthwhile.

SHAWN

My interest in alopecia comes from "hands on" experience in the alopecia clinic at UCSF, where I worked with Vera Price and her fellow, Paradi Mirmarani. This was bolstered by the excellent dermatopathology training I received from my fellowship mentors Tim McCalmont and Phil Leboit.

Besides these early influences in my academic career, I would like to thank Len, whose work I admired long before I finally got to work with him in 2006. He is a patient and unflappable teacher, and a pragmatic practitioner of evidence-based medicine. I want to thank him not only for his instruction and example, but also for inviting me to be a part of this project—a true team effort created over many months of authoring, imaging, editing, revising, and re-revising.

Our coauthor, Eleanor, is among the kindest and smartest people I have ever met, and I know she will have a truly great career. It has been a pleasure working with her as she made her way through Yale over the years, culminating in the successful completion of her fellowship in dermatopathology virtually coincident with her co-authorship of this second edition.

My wife Carolyn, and our children Nathaniel, Benjamin, and Emma all deserve medals for their patience while this edition came together. I love you all.

I would like to thank our dermatopathology fellow, Ashley Mason, for taking on the proofreading of this text in addition to her many other duties. In addition, thanks to Carol Hribko, whose expertise with image editing and careful proofreading brought this edition to a new standard of excellence. Lastly, I thank my partners at Yale for their support of this effort.

ELEANOR

There are many minds, eyes, and hands that helped create this work. To all who contributed ideas, research, images, and time: thank you.

Len has a knack for making difficult things simple. His knowledge is profound, his thinking is clear, and lucky for the rest of us, he is open and generous with his insights. He has been an incomparable teacher, mentor, and friend, and I am grateful to him for inviting me to contribute to this project.

Shawn is a remarkable physician, an innovator with expertise in diverse areas of dermatopathology, and a phenomenal teacher. Our collaborative "hair service" was a highlight of my dermatopathology education. I feel incredibly fortunate to have trained with Shawn, to count him as a friend, and to have worked together on this project.

I would like to offer my heartfelt gratitude to Jennifer McNiff, Earl Glusac, and the whole team of amazing dermatopathologists at Yale: Rossitza Lazova, Tony Subtil, Christine Ko, Anjela Galan, and Marcus Bosenberg—each has had a profound impact on me. I am enormously thankful for the instruction, guidance, and mentorship from Richard Edelson, Robert Tigelaar, and my Yale Dermatology family.

I am grateful to the North American Hair Research Society and the Women's Dermatologic Society for facilitating my earliest experiences studying under and learning from Len through their mentorship programs. They worked!

I send my love and deepest appreciation to my family, including my father, Robert Knopp, MD, who is missed every moment.

My copy of the first edition of the atlas is well worn and coming apart at the seams—may this edition fare as well in your hands!

1   Using this book

THE "TRICHOPATHOLOGIST'S" FIELD GUIDE

Within the medical subspecialty of dermatopathology, there is yet another smaller world inhabited by those who specialize in (and struggle with) the challenge of diagnosing alopecia. These ultraspecialists lack an official label. One might consider calling them "alopecists" but according to the Oxford English Dictionary (OED), that label has already been taken to describe those who "undertake to cure or prevent baldness." "Trichologist" might be a better term, and the OED informs us that a trichologist is one "who is versed in the study of the structure, functions, and diseases of the hair." Indeed this is a broader, more inclusive term, but appears to be already in use. The term also tends to describe a nonphysician paramedical expert who completes a two-year certification course and is subsequently recognized as a trichologist after passing a certifying exam.

Practitioners (both novice and expert) of the histopathologic evaluation of alopecia need their own custom label. For the expediency of this introductory chapter, we will use the term "trichopathologist." Trichopathologists are engaged in the first steps necessary for the successful work of the alopecist, namely, ensuring an accurate diagnosis. Successful trichopathologists need to understand the three-dimensional anatomy of the hair follicular unit and associated supporting structures. They should understand something of the clinical presentation of various alopecias, as well as have a thorough understanding of the nature of the hair follicle cycle, the impact of alopecic states on the shape of the hair shaft, and on the results of some easily performed clinical tests. Also, trichopathologists should understand the use of ancillary testing and something about the appropriate treatment of various alopecias to provide guidance to their alopecist colleagues.

Our intent is that this book will serve not only as a field guide to the "budding" trichopathologists, but also as a framework for the seasoned trichopathologists who may be encountering an unusual feature or alopecia variant for the first time. Whether our readers ultimately come to *refer* to themselves as "trichopathologists" is yet to be determined. We do hope, however, that the following chapters will inspire a new generation of dermatopathologists to take the next step and *think* of themselves as trichopathologists.

USING THE GUIDE

This book is organized into several sections (each comprising one or more chapters) meant to systematically lead the diagnostician to a specific diagnosis. Sections I–IV provide the fundamental skills needed to tackle the evaluation of any sort of alopecia. Section V provides a detailed discussion of many specific diagnoses, as well as a quick reference box at the end of the chapter with the most salient features and critical facts. Section VI is an atlas of hair shaft disorders. The last section, Section VII, is a comprehensive glossary of terminology and an in-depth index of the entire work.

Section I: Acquisition

Before the study of biopsy specimens, one must understand how to sample and process the biopsy in order to maximize the diagnostic yield. This is the focus of chapter 2.

Section II: Context

Before beginning an evaluation of what is *abnormal* about a specimen, one must first understand *normal* cycling and hair follicular anatomy. Chapters 3 and 4 cover this in detail, including a discussion and rationale for our advocacy of horizontal (transverse) sectioning of scalp biopsies.

Section III: Walking

We must "walk before we can run." Chapter 5 sketches out a broad concept of classes of alopecia that will allow the student of trichopathology to establish a foundation of important concepts. Chapter 6 discusses a specific methodology that walks the student through the first steps of identifying salient (and sometimes specific) histologic features, and narrowing the broad field of alopecia into several clear and smaller groups that one can study in more specific detail.

Section IV: Correlation

The student of trichopathology will quickly learn that the number of histologic features one may encounter in a case of alopecia is not broad. Making sense of these features often requires clinical input. If the clinician provides no better information than "alopecia" on the requisition form, the pathologist and the clinician will probably find the diagnostic endeavor less than satisfactory. Good clinical input may provide enough information to render a specific diagnosis when histologic features are borderline, or favor a diagnosis when histologic features are nonspecific. Chapter 7 includes a discussion about specific clinical features that can provide the correlation needed for a fruitful diagnostic collaboration.

Section V: Running

After walking through the basics of Section III and embracing any clinical input provided, the trichopathologist should be able to "run" to one of several diagnoses. Section V constitutes chapters 8–35. The chapters in this section are focused on a specific diagnosis. Each diagnosis has a paragraph of introduction, sometimes containing information about the known or presumed cause of the disease. This is followed by paragraphs detailing the clinical findings (including a brief summary of treatment options) and the histological findings. Special diagnostic techniques (e.g., direct immunofluorescence, special stains) are also discussed in this section. A boxed summary (toward the end of each diagnosis chapter) contains critical and salient clinical features, followed by histologic findings. The first set of histologic findings (denoted by ❖) is considered the minimal criteria needed to establish a particular diagnosis. These are followed by round bullets (●) that denote

additional supporting features that might be helpful in secur-
ing a firm diagnosis but are not required to establish the diagnosis. The boxed summary also lists reasonable differential
diagnostic considerations along with information helpful in
excluding or including the differential, as well as avoiding
potential diagnostic pitfalls. Of course, there are numerous
supporting illustrations to accompany the text.

Section VI: An Atlas of Hair Shaft Disorders

Chapter 36 is a unique section in this book, constituting a
photographic gallery of various hair shaft disorders with
discussion regarding known causes and associated disease
states. Not all hair specimens are punch biopsies. Clinicians
sometimes submit hair shafts for evaluation, and this section
can serve as a starting point for proper interpretation.

Section VII: Glossary and Index

All good field guides should have guideposts and a means of
internal navigation. This text contains a comprehensive glossary

of terms from the text. Many of these are unique to our specialty.
If you, the reader, encounter a term you wish defined, please
check the glossary. Chances are it can be found there.

ADDENDUM

The authors are sensitive to concerns about racial labels. The
labels included in this text are used only when there are clear
distinctions to be made in incidence of disease and for clarity
of discussion. The authors have chosen to use the term "Caucasian" to describe persons with light colored skin who are
non-Asian. The term is interchangeable with "White" in this
context. "African-American," while admittedly an imprecise
term, is used in this book to denote persons of African heritage, whether American or not. The term is interchangeable
with "Black" or "persons of color" in this context.

2   Specimen acquisition, handling and processing

ACQUISITION

Selecting the biopsy site is the most difficult and important part of the acquisition process. The most fruitful site will vary depending on the disease, and often the clinician is uncertain of the diagnosis. Sampling the center of a lesion of alopecia areata or trichotillomania would be appropriate. Sampling the bald center of a lesion of cicatricial alopecia is seldom useful. In such cases, the "active" peripheral margin is a more suitable target. Compounding the difficulty of site selection is sampling error. Clinicians cannot see below the surface of the skin, and even the most experienced physician may choose an unrewarding spot. If a recently involved area of scalp showing early clinical changes is selected, the diagnostic yield will be higher. Highly inflamed sites (pustules or papules) are often very advanced lesions and are frequently nondiagnostic. Multiple separate specimens chosen from several sites in or around the lesion will increase the diagnostic yield. However, clinicians may not have the luxury of obtaining multiple specimens.

In some cases the patient's normal-appearing scalp can serve as a basis for comparison with the abnormal scalp. For example, a specimen from the mid-occiput can help establish a diagnosis of common balding in a patient with hair loss on the crown and is especially helpful diagnostically when telogen effluvium is also on the differential diagnosis.

Once the site is selected, it should be anesthetized with lidocaine with epinephrine. A generous amount of anesthetic (1–3 ml) should be injected into the deep dermis and superficial fat and allowed to act for 15–30 min before the biopsy is performed. This will minimize bleeding. The blade of the punch biopsy tool should extend through the dermis down into the fat so that intact bulbs of deeply rooted terminal hairs can be removed.

A 4 mm biopsy wound can be easily closed with 3–0 suture because the needle can traverse the wound in a single pass. A suture color that contrasts with the patient's hair will assist in suture removal one week after the biopsy is performed. Slightly longer than average suture tails can also assist in locating the suture at the time of removal.

HANDLING

Once obtained, the scalp biopsy specimen should be allowed to fix in formalin for at least 24 hours before sectioning. Biopsy specimens obtained for direct immunofluorescence testing should be placed in an appropriate transport solution.

PROCESSING

The authors prefer horizontally-oriented (transverse) sections for the evaluation of alopecia. The rationale is discussed further in Chapter 4. Transverse sectioning was recently adopted as the recommended standard in the consensus statement from a working group of alopecia experts (1). Processing specimens for transverse sections requires a sharp blade, a blade holder, a pair of fine-toothed forceps, marking ink, a cotton-tipped applicator, and a standard plastic specimen cassette. Sponges should be used inside the cassette to prevent the thin slices of tissue from escaping. The sharpest blade for the job is a disposable, flexible shaving blade (Fig. 2.1). The authors prefer to use red marking ink, but any color will do. A specially colored cassette will alert the histology technician that embedding must be performed in a particular way.

There are several ways to slice the tissue into transverse sections. The technique used by Headington (2) and Whiting (3) involves a single transverse slice about 1 mm below the epidermal surface. Both *cut* sides of the specimen are embedded *down* in the cassette. As the microtome cuts deeper into the tissue block, the sections become progressively more superficial in one half of the specimen and deeper in the other. Simply sectioning deeper into the block allows one to obtain sections as superficial or as deep as required.

An alternative method is that of Frishberg and Sperling (4). Using this technique, the biopsy specimen is sliced like a cylindrical loaf of bread into two to four slices (Figs. 2.2 and 2.3). The "slices" are about 1 mm thick. The *deep* surface of each slice is inked (Fig. 2.4) and the inked sides are placed *down* in the cassette. Once the ink has been removed by the microtome, a single section is taken. In this way, the specimen is sampled at several different depths (Fig. 2.5). Because only a single section is needed to view multiple levels on a single slide, the remainder of the tissue in the block is available for "recuts" and special stains.

A more tedious method, best suited to research purposes, involves embedding either the epidermal or fat end down in the cassette, and taking multiple horizontal sections through the entire specimen. Dozens of sections may be required to section through the entire block, and the block is exhausted in the process. However, every possible level of every follicle in the specimen can be carefully studied.

Other means of processing scalp biopsies have been proposed in order to allow for the evaluation of both horizontal and vertical specimens simultaneously. This is typically easier when two specimens are available. One such method involves sectioning one entire specimen horizontally, while splitting the other specimen vertically, submitting half for immunofluorescence (if desired) and embedding the other half for vertical sections in the same block as the specimen for horizontal sections (5). There are a number of approaches that have been advocated if only one specimen is available. The "HoVert" technique involves removing the epidermis (via a horizontal section through the papillary dermis), bisecting it and embedding these two pieces to achieve vertical sections through the epidermis. The remaining deeper portion of the specimen is embedded for horizontal sections (6). Another method involves bisecting the punch specimen longitudinally, cutting several vertical sections for review, then approximating the two halves back together so that the remainder can be sectioned horizontally. While the authors prefer the simplicity of

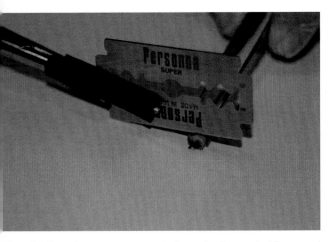

Figure 2.1 Preparing to cut transverse sections using fine-toothed forceps and a flexible blade with a blade holder.

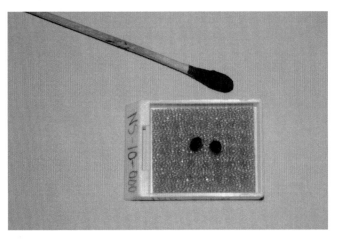

Figure 2.4 The inked slices are placed in a cassette, packed between sponges. They will be paraffin-embedded, ink side down.

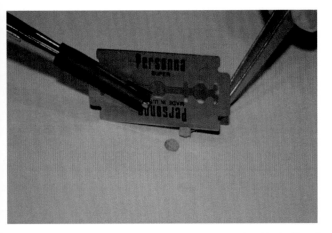

Figure 2.2 The specimen is placed on its side like a cylindrical loaf of bread, and is gently stabilized with the forceps. A flexible, disposable shaving blade is ideal for taking the slices.

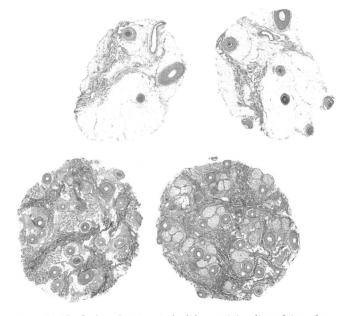

Figure 2.5 The final product is a single slide containing discs of tissue from multiple levels.

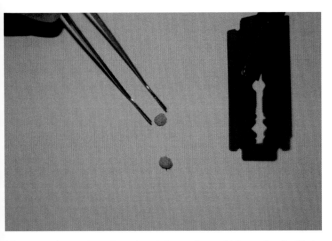

Figure 2.3 The specimen is cut into 2, 3 or 4 slices, which are placed with the cut surfaces "up" so that they are ready for inking.

a single embedding for horizontal sections, the ultimate choice and method of processing should facilitate the comfort and maximal ability of the pathologist to render a diagnosis. Our clinician and pathologist colleague, Dirk Elston has stated, "I do not hesitate to choose the method that will make my job easiest," (7) and with this statement we wholeheartedly agree.

REFERENCES

1. Olsen EA, Bergfeld WF, Cotsarelis G. Summary of North American Hair Research Society (NAHRS)-sponsored Workshop on Cicatricial Alopecia, Duke University Medical Center, February 10 and 11, 2001. J Am Acad Dermatol, 2003; 48: 103–10.
2. Headington J. Transverse microscopic anatomy of the human scalp. Arch Dermatol, 1984; 120: 449–56.
3. Whiting D. Diagnostic and predictive value of horizontal sections of scalp biopsies in male pattern androgenetic alopecia. J Am Acad Dermatol, 1993; 28: 755–63.
4. Frishberg DP, Sperling LC, Guthrie, VM. Transverse scalp sections: a proposed method for laboratory processing. J Am Acad Dermatol, 1996; 35(2 Pt 1): 220–2.
5. Elston D, McCollough M. Angeloni V. Vertical and transverse sections of alopecia biopsy specimens: combining the two techniques to maximize diagnostic yield. J Am Acad Dermatol, 1995; 32: 454–7.
6. Nguyen JV, Hudacek K, Whitten JA, Rubin AI, Seykora JT. The HoVert technique: a novel method for the sectioning of alopecia biopsies. J Cutan Pathol, 2001; 38: 401–6.
7. Elston DM. Vertical vs. transverse sections: both are valuable in the evaluation of alopecia. Am J Dermatopathol, 2005; 27: 353–6.

3 Normal hair anatomy and architecture

The histological findings in many forms of hair loss are subtle, and an accurate diagnosis depends on distinguishing abnormal from normal follicular architecture (1). "Architecture" refers to the anatomy of individual hair follicles as well as the number, size, and distribution of follicles within a biopsy specimen.

SIZE: TERMINAL, INDETERMINATE, AND VELLUS

Terminal hairs are large caliber hairs with bulbs rooted deeply in the fat. *Vellus* hairs have thin shafts with bulbs located in the upper portion of the dermis (they are therefore shorter in length than terminal hairs), and are often hypopigmented with respect to the baseline hair color. *Indeterminate* hairs are intermediate in size between terminal and vellus hairs. Hair shaft diameters can be readily measured in transverse section; terminal hairs are thicker than 0.06 mm and vellus hairs are less than 0.03 mm. Indeterminate hairs, which some authors call *small terminal hairs*, are 0.03–0.06 mm in diameter. A vellus hair can be readily identified by simple inspection since its inner root sheath will be as thick as, or thicker than, the shaft itself (Figs. 3.1 and 3.2).

HAIR CYCLE PHASES: ANAGEN, CATAGEN, AND TELOGEN

Every follicle, regardless of size, can be found in one of three phases of the hair cycle. The *anagen* phase is the active growing period and lasts weeks to years depending on the size and site of the hair. For human terminal scalp hair, anagen lasts between 2 and 7 years. *Catagen* is a brief transitional phase between anagen and telogen, and lasts about 2–3 weeks. The *telogen* phase lasts about 100 days, at the end of which the shaft is shed (2). Depending on the individual, at any given time 85%–100% of terminal scalp hair is in the anagen phase, 0%–15% is in the telogen phase, and only about 1% is in the catagen phase (2). The percentage of terminal telogen hairs present (original data based on locks of hairs forcibly plucked from the scalp (3)) is called the *telogen count*. This figure also can be calculated from a scalp biopsy evaluated in horizontal sections. "Average" telogen counts are in the range of 6%–13% (4–6), and a count greater than 20% is abnormal. Counts of 15%–20% are "suspicious" for an abnormally high count; specimens in this range may be normal for some individuals but elevated in others.

ANAGEN HAIR ANATOMY

Anagen, catagen, and telogen hairs differ considerably in their appearance (7). From deep to superficial, the 4 zones of the anagen hair are the *hair bulb*, the *suprabulbar zone* (called the *stem* by some authors), the *isthmus*, and the *infundibulum*.

The Hair Bulb

The hair bulb, usually located in the fat, comprises the basophilic germinative layer known as the hair *matrix*, and the hair *papilla*, a mesenchymal structure derived from the dermis. Inferiorly, the stalk of the papilla merges with the fibrous root sheath, which surrounds the entire follicle and blends into the overlying dermis (Figs. 3.3 and 3.4).

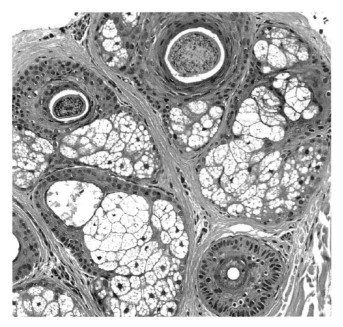

Figure 3.1 Terminal, indeterminate, and vellus hairs. An example of each type of hair is present: terminal is top center, indeterminate upper left, and vellus lower right. Note that the diameter of the vellus hair is comparable to the width of its inner root sheath. This specimen was obtained from a normal adult scalp.

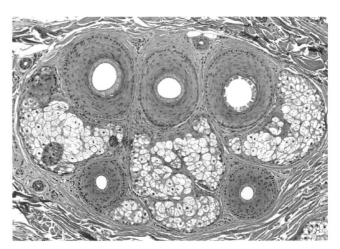

Figure 3.2 Terminal *versus* vellus hairs. This follicular unit contains three terminal hairs (top) and two vellus hairs (bottom). Three sweat ducts at the periphery are present for comparison.

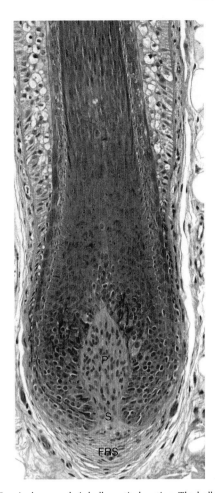

Figure 3.3 Terminal anagen hair bulb, vertical section. The bulbs of terminal hairs are usually located in the superficial fat or deep dermis. The basophilic (and often pigmented) hair matrix surrounds the follicular papilla (P) like a claw; at the center, the inferior portion of the papilla connects via its stalk (S) with the fibrous root sheath (FRS), inferiorly. The FRS sweeps up and around the matrix investing the entire lower portion of the follicle.

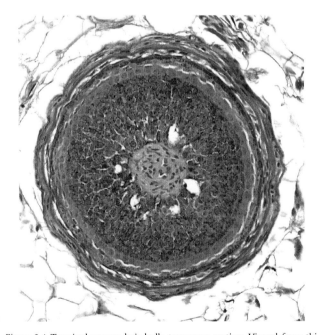

Figure 3.4 Terminal anagen hair bulb, transverse section. Viewed from this perspective, the basophilic matrix epithelium surrounds the follicular papilla like a doughnut. The pigmented dendrites of melanocytes are visible within the bulbar epithelium. The pigmented central zone will form the cortex at a more superficial level.

The Suprabulbar Zone

Just superficial to the hair bulb is the suprabulbar zone (or stem), at which point the various layers of the anagen follicle begin to differentiate (Fig. 3.5). Transverse sectioning allows all the layers of the anagen follicle to be easily identified at this level. Starting from the center of the follicle and moving outward, the layers are (*i*) the hair shaft medulla (may not always be visible), (*ii*) the hair shaft cortex, (*iii*) the cuticular layer, (*iv*) Huxley's layer of the inner root sheath, (*v*) Henle's layer of the inner root sheath, (*vi*) the outer root sheath, (*vii*) the glassy (vitreous) layer, and (*viii*) the fibrous root sheath. The cuticular layer comprises the interlocking flattened cells of the hair shaft cuticle and the inner root sheath cuticle. These cells are so tightly interlocked that they appear to form a single anatomical layer (Figs. 3.6 and 3.7).

The Isthmus

Moving toward the skin surface, the next zone is the isthmus. The inferior border of the isthmus is marked by the insertion of the arrector pili muscle into the fibrous root sheath of the follicle. The superior border of the isthmus is the entrance of the sebaceous duct into the follicular canal. The isthmus is an

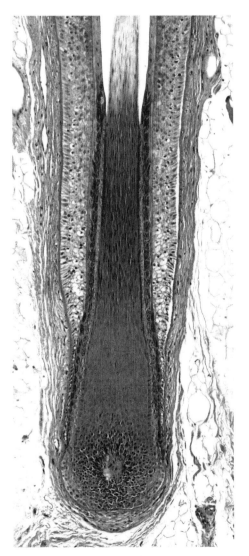

Figure 3.5 Terminal anagen hair, bulbar and suprabulbar zones, vertical section. The development of the inner and outer root sheaths (shown at higher magnification in Fig. 3.6) can be seen just above the bulb.

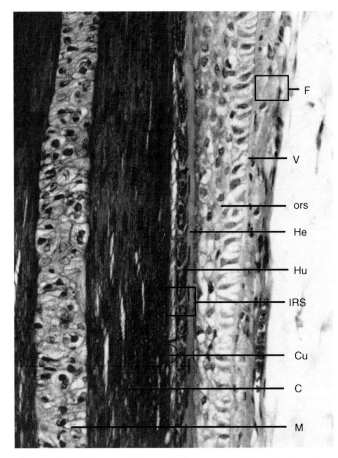

Figure 3.6 Terminal anagen hair, suprabulbar zone, vertical section. Just above the bulb, the various layers of the anagen hair can be identified. *Abbreviations*: M, medulla; C, cortex; Cu, cuticular layer; IRS, inner root sheath; Hu, Huxley's layer; He, Henle's layer; ors, outer root sheath; V, vitreous/glassy layer; F, fibrous root sheath.

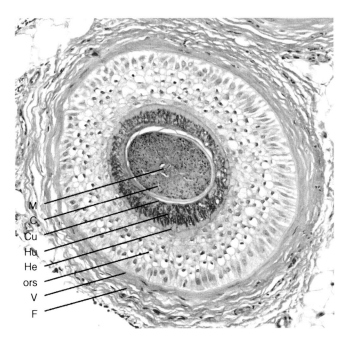

Figure 3.7 Terminal anagen hair, suprabulbar zone, transverse section. All of the same layers identified in Figure 3.6 are visible in this section, forming concentric rings starting around the small medulla in the innermost aspect of the shaft. *Abbreviations*: M, medulla; C, cortex; Cu, cuticular layer; Hu, Huxley's layer of the inner root sheath; He, Henle's layer of the inner root sheath; ors, outer root sheath; V, vitreous/glassy layer; F, fibrous root sheath.

important transitional zone of follicular keratinization. In the midportion of the isthmus, the inner root sheath desquamates, resulting in a separation between the hair shaft and the follicular wall. At this point, the cells of the outer root sheath begin to cornify without the formation of a granular layer. This is called trichilemmal keratinization (Figs. 3.8 and 3.9).

The Infundibulum

The most superficial zone of the follicle is the infundibulum, bounded inferiorly by the entry of the sebaceous duct. Within this zone, cornification of the outer root sheath occurs with the formation of a granular layer similar to the epidermal surface (Figs. 3.10–3.12).

Follicular

The follicular stem cells localize to a pocket of epithelium adjacent to the insertion of the arrector pili muscle known as *the bulge* (Fig. 3.13) (8). While an actual anatomic bulge is evident in rodent follicles, human follicles do not usually have an obvious protuberance of epithelium at this site. Special histochemical stains directed against antigens such as cytokeratin 15 facilitate identification of the stem cells (Fig. 3.14) (9).

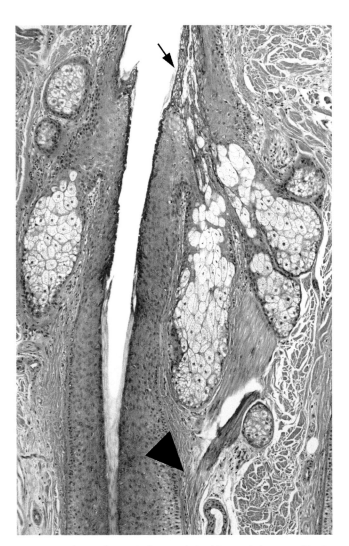

Figure 3.8 Isthmus of a terminal anagen hair. This zone is demarcated by the insertion of the arrector pili muscle below (large arrowhead) and the opening of the sebaceous duct above (arrow).

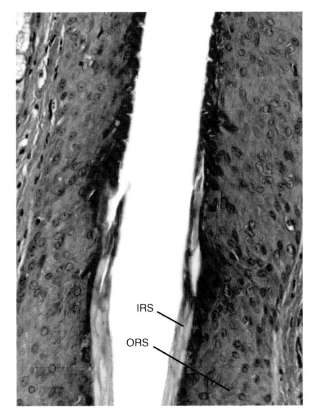

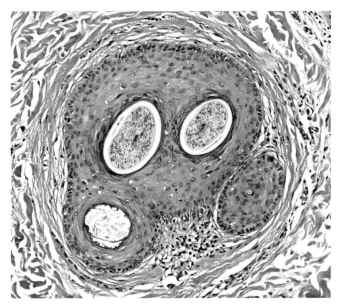

Figure 3.11 Terminal anagen hair, lower infundibulum, transverse section. A section through the lower infundibulum shows cornification with a granular layer. The infundibula of two normal, separate follicles are in the process of merging into a common infundibulum containing two hair shafts. This is often a normal finding, especially in African-American patients.

Figure 3.9 Desquamation of the inner root sheath. The inner root sheath (IRS) abruptly desquamates in the midportion of the isthmus. Above this, the outer root sheath (ORS) cornifies without the formation of a granular layer (trichilemmal cornification).

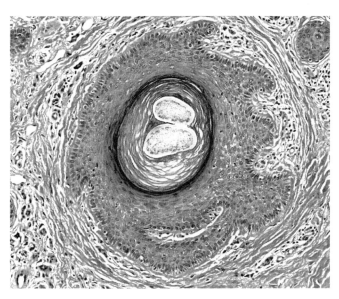

Figure 3.12 Terminal anagen hair, upper infundibulum, transverse section. The two follicles are now fully merged and the shafts share a common ostium.

Hair shaft size and shape differs between racial groups. The hair shafts of African-Americans tend to be elliptical or kidney bean–shaped (Fig. 3.15) and are situated eccentrically within the epithelium of the follicle. Caucasian hair shafts tend to be circular or slightly oval (Fig. 3.16) and are usually located directly in the center of the follicle.

CATAGEN HAIR ANATOMY

Each terminal anagen hair on the scalp grows for a period between 2–7 years, depending on the individual. At the end of that time, the hair shaft ceases active growth and enters a brief catagen phase. Within 1–2 weeks, the entire anatomy of the follicle changes. At the beginning of catagen (Figs. 3.17–3.20), the hair matrix disappears and is replaced by a thin rim of epithelial

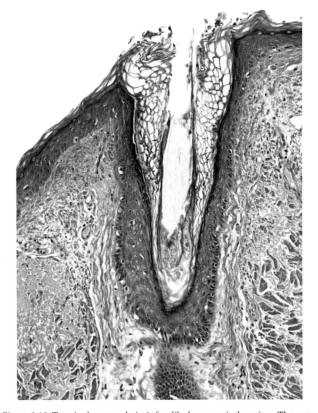

Figure 3.10 Terminal anagen hair, infundibulum, vertical section. The outer root sheath cornifies with the formation of a granular layer. The space between the hair shaft and follicular wall is filled with desquamated keratinocytes, sebum, bacteria, *pityrosporum* yeast, and cosmetics. Much of this debris is removed during processing.

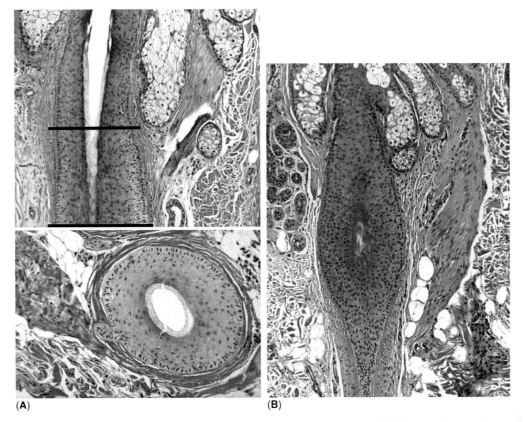

(A) (B)

Figure 3.13 (**A**) Insertion of the arrector pili muscle into the bulge zone of a follicle in the anagen phase. Two black lines in the vertical section (top panel) delimit the bulge zone. A horizontal section through the same region is shown in the bottom panel. This portion of the follicle is home to the follicular stem cells and is a landmark demarcating the lower portion of the isthmus. Unlike in the rodent follicle, a bulge of epithelium is not typically visualized in human follicles. (**B**) Insertion of the arrector pili muscle into the bulge zone of a follicle in the catagen/telogen phase. The location of the bulge zone remains constant throughout the follicular cycle.

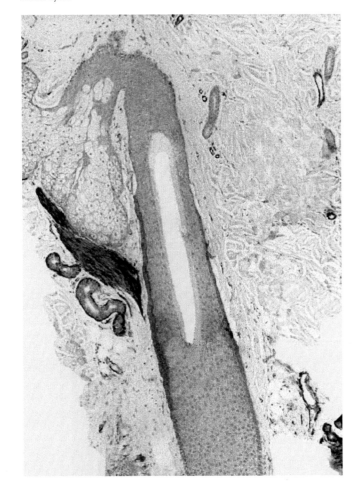

Figure 3.14 The bulge zone, as seen with immunohistochemical markers for cytokeratin 15 and smooth muscle actin. Cytokeratin 15 is a marker of the bulge zone. The presence of cytokeratin 15 is indicated by dark red staining of the peripheral layers of the outer root sheath in the vicinity of the attachment of the arrector pili muscle. The brown staining of the arrector pili muscle indicates the presence of smooth muscle actin. *Source*: Photo courtesy of George Cotsarelis, M.D.

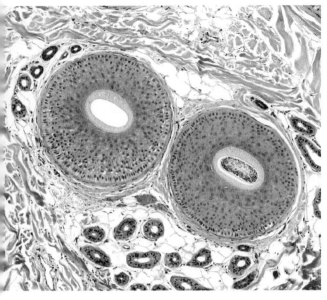

Figure 3.15 Transverse section of terminal anagen hairs from an African-American person. The hair shaft is elliptical or kidney bean-shaped and is often eccentrically placed within the surrounding epithelium.

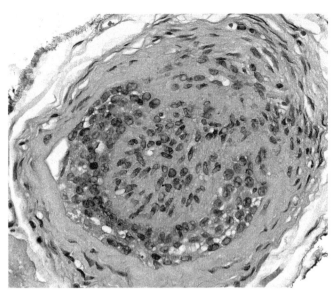

Figure 3.17 Terminal catagen hair, bulb, oblique section. This terminal bulb is recognizable as catagen because of the pale, thin epithelial rim (the residual hair matrix) surrounding the hair papilla. This follicle is clearly a terminal hair (and not vellus) given its location at the dermal/subcutaneous junction.

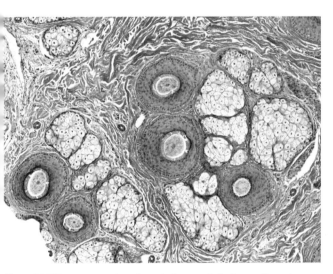

Figure 3.16 Transverse section of terminal anagen hairs from a Caucasian person. Most hair shafts are round or oval and centrally placed within the follicular epithelium.

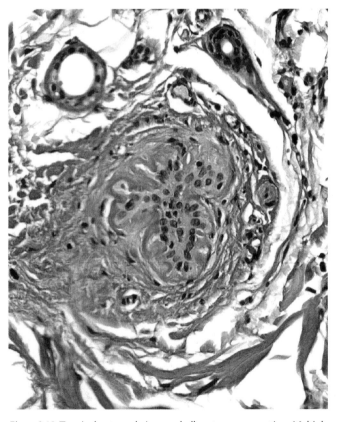

Figure 3.18 Terminal catagen hair, suprabulbar, transverse section. Multiple pyknotic nuclei are present, the epithelial layer is thinned significantly, and the markedly thickened vitreous layer is clearly visible. The collapsed, involuting epithelium can result in a floral- or asterisk-like pattern. The fibrous root sheath is beginning to thicken.

cells surrounding the hair papilla. These epithelial cells, along with an overlying homogenous column of epithelial cells, demonstrate nuclear pyknosis. The epithelium of the lower follicle undergoes disintegration via cellular apoptosis. As these epithelial changes occur, the vitreous (or glassy) layer thickens markedly, becoming a prominent structure. The fibrous root sheath also thickens. As the catagen phase evolves over a 2- to 3-week period, the hair papilla follows the disintegrating epithelial column superficially into the dermis, and the papilla eventually comes to rest just below the bulge zone (near the attachment of the arrector pili muscle).

As the epithelial column moves superficially, a collapsed fibrous root sheath is left behind. This collapsed structure is called the *stela* (or stele; plural, stelae), d erived from the Greek word for *pillar* (Figs. 3.21 and 3.22). The stela is also referred to as the follicular "streamer." In this text, the terms *stela* and *streamer* are considered to be synonymous.

Just superficial to the epithelial column of the catagen hair, an expanded mass of epithelium forms the *presumptive club hair*. In early catagen the cells of the presumptive club are still

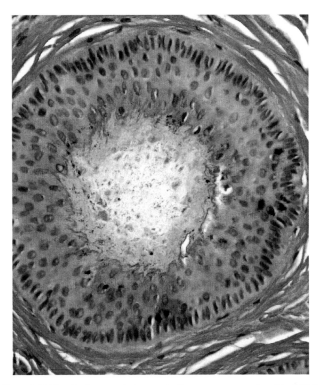

Figure 3.19 Terminal catagen hair, suprabulbar, transverse section. The follicle is sectioned through the presumptive club, which is beginning to cornify. There are still apoptotic cells demonstrating pyknosis, identifying the stage as catagen.

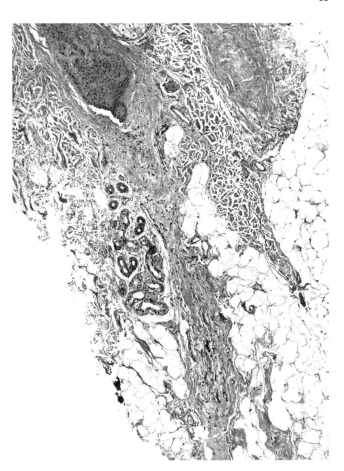

Figure 3.21 Vertical section of the stela (or "streamer") below the bulb of a telogen hair. The stela is the collapsed fibrous root sheath found below hairs in the catagen/telogen phase or hairs that have miniaturized.

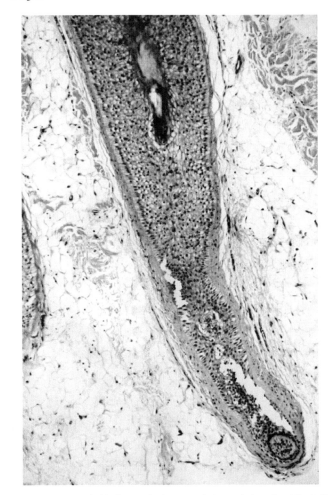

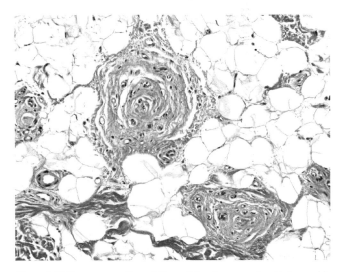

Figure 3.22 Transverse section of three stelae demonstrating their roughly circular shape and numerous small vascular spaces.

Figure 3.20 Lower half of a terminal catagen hair, vertical section. The bulb (corresponding to Fig. 3.17), disintegrating epithelial column (corresponding to Fig. 3.18) and presumptive club (corresponding to Fig. 3.19) can be seen.

nucleated, but the nuclei disappear as the club begins to cornify from the center outward.

TELOGEN HAIR ANATOMY

At the end of catagen and the beginning of telogen, the hair papilla is a condensed ball of spindle-shaped nuclei within a scanty stroma. The papilla lies just deep to a nipple of epithelium called the secondary hair germ (Fig. 3.23). When sectioned transversely, the secondary hair germ has an asterisk-like appearance (Fig. 3.24). After the club hair has been shed from the follicle, the secondary hair germ is sometimes referred to as the telogen germ unit.

The secondary hair germ is adjacent to the bulge zone and the cornifying presumptive club. This places the hair papilla cells in close proximity to the stem cells residing in the bulge zone. Just superficial to the secondary hair germ the telogen club progressively cornifies, expanding in a centrifugal fashion. Several layers of noncornified epithelium surround and tightly adhere to the cornifying club. As telogen progresses, the cornified club expands to occupy the full width of the follicle. This progressive cornification occurs over about a three-month period, at the end of which the hair shaft, with its clubbed root, is shed from the follicle (Figs. 3.25 and 3.26). Similar to terminal hairs, vellus hairs also progress through anagen, catagen, and telogen phases (Fig. 3.27). Vellus hairs cycle in a more accelerated fashion, however, spending significantly less time in anagen but similar amounts of time in catagen and telogen compared with terminal hairs.

At the end of the telogen phase, around the time the club hair is shed, the transition into anagen phase begins: the hair germ (having arisen from the stem cells of the bulge) is activated and expands to form the matrix of transit-amplifying cells that eventually form the new hair shaft (10,11). The newly growing hair extends down from the bulge zone (Fig. 3.28). The new anagen hair will continue to produce a hair shaft for the next 2–7 years.

PULLED, PLUCKED, AND SPONTANEOUSLY SHED HAIRS

Hairs that are shed or extracted from the scalp can be examined directly under the microscope without any special processing. Covering the hairs with a few drops of immersion oil and a second glass slide facilitates the examination. Normally, the only hairs that can be gently and easily pulled from the scalp are telogen hairs. Any other type of hair that is easily removed from the scalp can be regarded as abnormal. Examples of abnormal findings are the tapered "pencil point" hairs seen in those who underwent chemotherapy, radiation therapy, or in those with alopecia areata (see chap 36); and these hairs are easily extracted because of "anagen arrest." Fragile hair shafts will fracture when gently pulled, and the fracture can be identified at the proximal end of the shaft. In some highly inflammatory scalp diseases, entire anagen hairs, including their root sheaths, can sometimes be extracted. This can occasionally be seen in lichen planopilaris, for example.

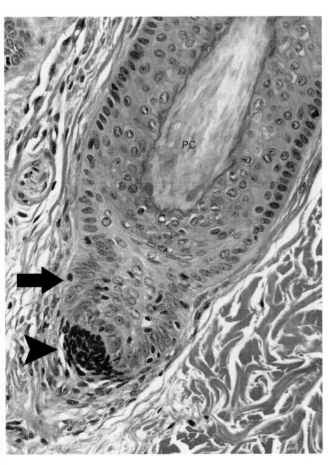

Figure 3.23 Bulb of early telogen hair, vertical section. The hair papilla (arrowhead) is seen as a tight cluster of nuclei lying just below the nipple-like secondary hair germ (arrow), also called the telogen germ unit (Fig. 3.24). Just above the secondary hair germ lies the presumptive club (PC).

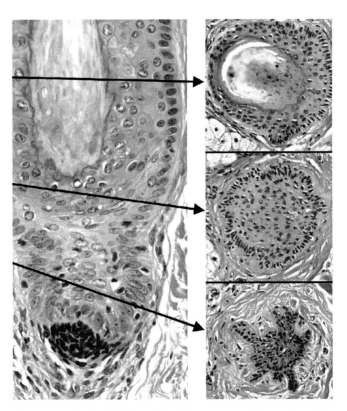

Figure 3.24 Bulb of early telogen hair with transverse section correlates. The top right panel shows a section through the cornifying "club" of a telogen hair; below this is a representative section through the telogen epithelium just under the club, demonstrating its slightly irregular contour. Finally, the secondary hair germ (telogen germ unit) is sectioned transversely to reveal an asterisk-like structure in the bottom right panel.

Hairs can also be obtained from the scalp by forcibly plucking the shafts. In this case a mixture of anagen and telogen hairs will usually be found. The process of plucking normal anagen hairs often leads to considerable artifactual distortion. Often anagen hairs are extracted with one or both of the root sheaths missing from the bulb. This sort of artifactual distortion should not be confused with a pathologic abnormality. A forcible hair pluck (the *trichogram*) can be performed to determine the percentage of terminal telogen hairs, described in further detail in the following sections.

Anagen Pull/Pluck Findings
Normally, anagen hairs cannot be gently pulled from the scalp. They must be forcibly plucked. It is abnormal for anagen hairs to be easily and painlessly extracted. This abnormality can occur in loose anagen hair syndrome, anagen arrest, and lichen planopilaris.

A plucked anagen hair is characterized by a pigmented bulb that is often expanded into a triangular, "delta" shape as it tears free from the hair papilla (Fig. 3.29). The hair papilla is usually (but not always) left behind in the dermis. Because the hair

bulb is not cornified, it is soft and can acquire a bent, or "hockey stick" configuration (Fig. 3.30). Just above the bulb, portions of both an inner and an outer root sheath can often be identified (Fig. 3.31). Unfortunately, the outer root sheath or both root sheaths are frequently left behind in the dermis (Fig. 3.30), an artifact of plucking. This gives the hair a "dysmorphic" (*not* dystrophic) appearance.

Catagen Pull/Pluck Findings
Like anagen hairs, catagen hairs are seldom gently pulled from the scalp. They are sometimes found when a lock of hair is forcibly plucked from the scalp. Plucked catagen hairs closely resemble telogen hairs, except that a clear, noncornified sac surrounds the "club," and a "tail" of soft, clear tissue lies below the bulb. This "tail" represents the degenerating epithelial column that lies between the hair papilla and the cornifying "club" (Fig. 3.32).

Telogen Pull/Pluck Findings
Telogen hair shafts are easily pulled or plucked from the normal scalp. It is estimated that the average person loses about 50–100 such hairs during the course of the day. Pulled or plucked telogen hairs have an expanded, depigmented, or hypopigmented, club-shaped bulb. Because the entire telogen hair is cornified, the bulb is not "bent" relative to the long axis of the shaft (Figs. 3.33 and 3.34).

TRICHOGRAM FINDINGS
The forcible hair pluck, or trichogram, is a useful tool employed by some clinicians who evaluate hair loss. A small

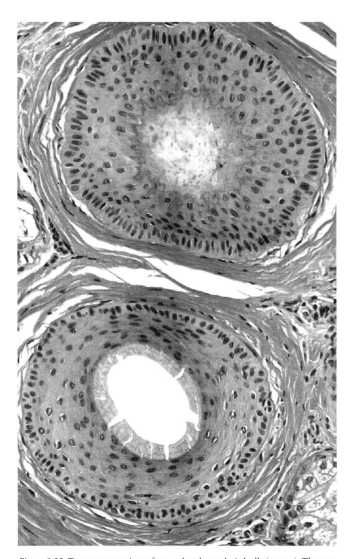

Figure 3.25 Transverse section of an early telogen hair bulb (upper). The cornifying club's serrated rim interdigitates with the surrounding envelope of outer root sheath epithelium. This should be contrasted with the terminal anagen follicle (lower).

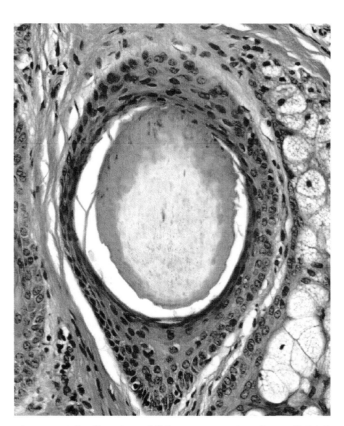

Figure 3.26 Bulb of late telogen follicle, transverse section. The cornified club now fills much of the width of the follicle and is only partially attached to the surrounding rim of noncornified outer root sheath. The club hair is now ready to be shed.

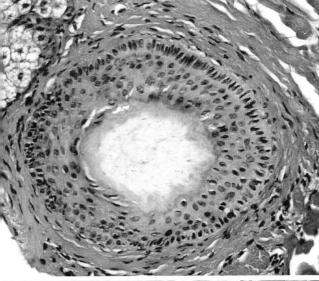

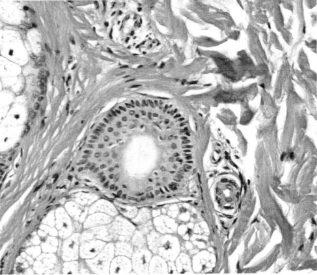

Figure 3.27 Terminal *versus* Vellus telogen hairs. Sections through the clubs of a terminal telogen hair (upper panel) and a vellus telogen hair (lower panel) at the same magnification.

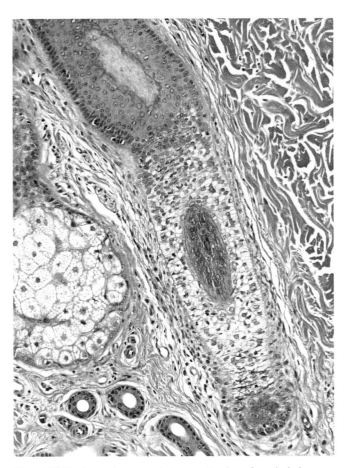

Figure 3.28 Newly growing anagen hair, extending down from the bulge zone. The overlying telogen club hair has not yet been shed.

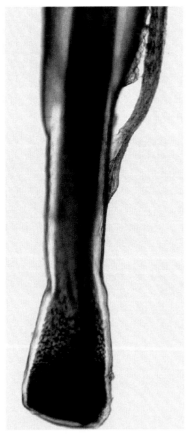

Figure 3.29 Bulb of forcibly plucked, terminal anagen hair.

lock of approximately 50 hairs is grasped in a rubber-tipped surgical clamp, and the lock is quickly jerked out of the scalp. The shafts are taped down to a glass slide, with the bulbs placed in the center, and the clamp is released. A few drops of immersion oil are placed on the slide over the bulbs, and a second glass slide or cover slip is placed on top. If the hair is curly, the slides may need to be taped together at the ends so that the hairs lie flat.

In theory, interpretation of the trichogram should be simple. The goal is to obtain a telogen count, the percentage of telogen hairs represented in the sample (Fig. 3.35). However, considerable artifact may be introduced by the act of plucking, and the anatomy of anagen hair bulbs may be badly distorted, making some of them *dysmorphic*, with incomplete anatomical features. Hairs with bulbs that have cleanly snapped off (as if cut) are counted as anagen hairs (Fig. 3.36), as are bulbs that show remnants of an outer or inner root sheath. A pigmented and "bent" bulb in the absence of root sheaths can also be counted as an anagen hair. In this case, the cuticle above the bulb will be ruffled (Fig. 3.37).

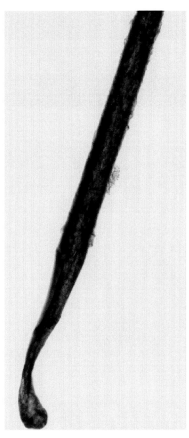

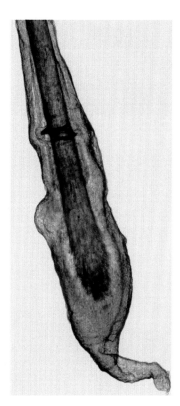

Figure 3.32 Forcibly plucked catagen hair. The tail-like remnant of the degenerating epithelial column is found just below the presumptive club.

Figure 3.30 "Dysmorphic," plucked terminal anagen hair. Here the term dystrophic should not be applied because the loss of the root sheaths is not a growth defect but merely an artifact of plucking.

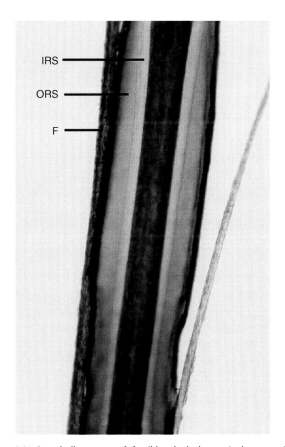

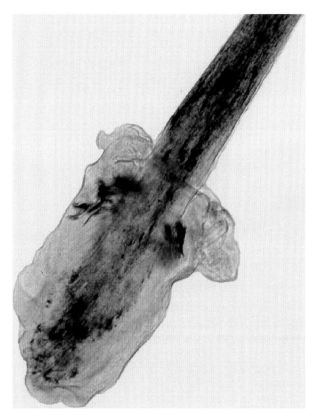

Figure 3.33 Forcibly plucked early telogen hair. A noncornified epithelial sac surrounds the cornifying club.

Figure 3.31 Suprabulbar zone of forcibly plucked, terminal anagen hair. *Abbreviations*: ORS, outer root sheath; IRS, inner root sheath; F, fibrous root sheath.

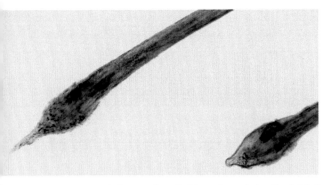

Figure 3.34 Forcibly plucked or gently pulled late telogen hairs. The "clubs" are completely cornified and the epithelial sac is gone.

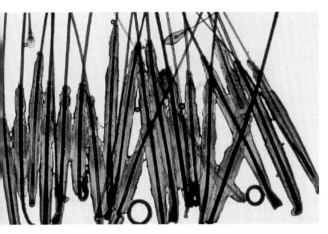

Figure 3.35 Forcibly plucked lock of hairs—the trichogram. In this field 23 terminal hairs, 21 anagen hairs, and 2 telogen hairs are present. The telogen count is therefore 2/23, or about 9%.

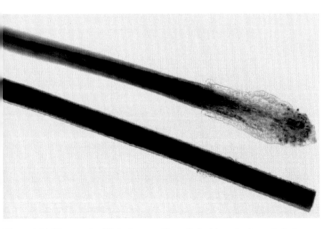

Figure 3.36 "Snapped-off" shaft, an artifact of plucking. A telogen hair (upper hair) and a "snapped-off" shaft are found in this field. When deeply rooted terminal anagen hairs are plucked, a clean transverse break in the shaft, as seen here, is sometimes the result. Shafts such as these can be counted as anagen hairs.

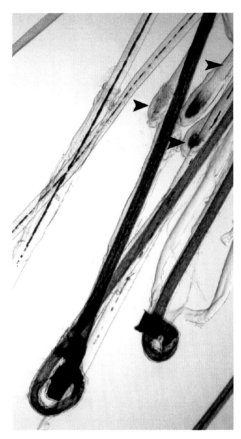

Figure 3.37 "Dysmorphic" terminal anagen hairs, an artifact of plucking. Sometimes when a terminal anagen hair is plucked, the entire shaft is removed but the root sheaths are left behind in the scalp. The bent root (sometimes resembling a hockey stick) and the ruffling of the cuticle of the proximal shaft identify it as an anagen hair. A similar hair is seen in Figure 3.30. Telogen hair bulbs (arrowheads) can be seen proximal to the dysmorphic roots of the anagen hairs.

REFERENCES

1. Sperling LC. Hair anatomy for the clinician. J Am Acad Dermatol. 1991; 25(1 Pt 1): 1–17.
2. Sperling LC, Lupton GP. Histopathology of non-scarring alopecia. J Cutan Pathol. 1995; 22: 97–114.
3. Maguire H, Kligman A. Hair plucking as a diagnostic tool. J Invest Dermatol 1964; 43: 77–9.
4. Whiting DA. Chronic telogen effluvium: increased scalp hair shedding in middle-aged women. J Am Acad Dermatol. 1996; 35: 899–906.
5. Whiting D. Diagnostic and predictive value of horizontal sections of scalp biopsies in male pattern androgenetic alopecia. J Am Acad Dermatol 1993; 28: 755–63.
6. Kligman A. Pathologic dynamics of human hair loss: I, Telogen effluvium. Arch Dermatol. 1961; 83: 175–98.
7. Headington J. Transverse microscopic anatomy of the human scalp. Arch Dermatol 1984; 120: 449–56.
8. Cotsarelis G, Sun TT, Lavker RM. Label-retaining cells reside in the bulge area of pilosebaceous unit: implications for follicular stem cells, hair cycle, and skin carcinogenesis. Cell 1990; 61: 1329–37.
9. Lyle S, Christofidou-Solomidou M, Liu Y, et al. The C8/144B monoclonal antibody recognizes cytokeratin 15 and defines the location of human hair follicle stem cells. J Cell Sci 1998; 111(Pt 21): 3179–88.
10. Greco V, Chen T, Rendl M, et al. A two-step mechanism for stem cell activation during hair regeneration. Cell Stem Cell. 2009; 4: 155–69.
11. Fuchs E. The tortoise and the hair: slow-cycling cells in the stem cell race. Cell. 2009; 137: 811–9.

4 Evaluating and describing transverse (horizontal) sections

THE RATIONALE OF TRANSVERSE/HORIZONTAL SECTIONING

There are many advantages to horizontal sectioning, but the technique of performing and interpreting transverse sections is unfamiliar to many pathologists. Although routine vertical sections have their role in the diagnosis of hair loss (1,2), most specimens should be sectioned transversely (horizontally). A few vertical sections are of limited value in the study of hair disease because the number and type of hairs found on any given section are subject to considerable sampling error (3). Those who wish to use vertical sections can overcome this obstacle by performing multiple serial sections. One group of authors took a mean of 53 sections to achieve success (3)!

The information obtained from a small sample of vertical sections is often incomplete and misleading, as demonstrated in Figure 4.1. A vertical section bisecting the specimen through plane "X" would only sample four follicles out of a total of 25 contained in the specimen. A section through plane "Y" would not sample *any* follicles. In many examples of alopecia, the diagnosis hinges on just a few follicles. The chance of "hitting" these follicles on a routine vertical section is slim.

In addition, counting follicles accurately using vertical sections is difficult, requiring an exhaustive sampling of dozens of sections through the entire tissue block. Therefore, quantitative data cannot be easily obtained with vertical sections. Even obtaining qualitative information is "hit or miss."

A perceived disadvantage of transverse sectioning is that the epidermis may not be visualized on initial sections (4). This can usually be overcome by obtaining additional sections from the tissue block. While the dermoepidermal junction will be visualized tangentially, the utility of the specimen to yield diagnostic information regarding alopecia will not be impacted.

Transverse/horizontal sectioning ensures that all follicles in the specimen are counted and examined, at multiple levels, with just a few sections required. Pathologists and dermatologists who have been disappointed with the results of vertically sectioned scalp biopsy specimens are gratified with the increased diagnostic yield once transverse sectioning is used. Contrary to popular belief, transverse sectioning for alopecia biopsies was not "invented" by Dr. John T. Headington, although he should be given credit for popularizing and refining the technique (5).

THE PATHOLOGIST'S CHECKLIST

A simplified, stepwise approach to interpreting scalp biopsies is discussed in chapter 5. In this chapter, we discuss all the various bits of information that can be extracted from transverse sections. The pathologist can use a checklist to avoid missing important information. The order of the checklist is a matter of personal preference, but the pertinent items that must be addressed before arriving at a diagnosis include the following:

1. What is the specimen diameter (e.g., 4 mm)? This information is required to determine whether the number of follicles is normal or decreased (Fig. 4.2).
2. Are follicular units evenly spaced, or are there "blank spots" with an absence of follicles (suggesting scarring or severe miniaturization; Fig. 4.3)?
3. Do most follicular units contain 2–6 follicles, with large follicles outnumbering small follicles (Fig. 4.4)?

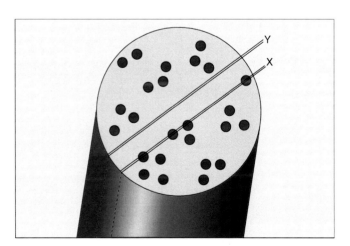

Figure 4.1 A vertical section bisecting the specimen through plane "X" would only sample four follicles out of a total of 25 contained in the specimen. A section through plane "Y" would not sample any hairs.

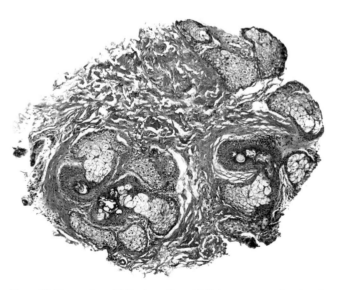

Figure 4.2 The number of follicular units and follicles appear greatly reduced, but the explanation is the size of the specimen—2 mm!

17

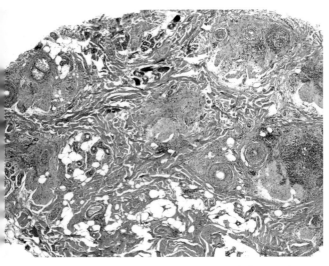

Figure 4.3 In this example of inflammatory cicatricial alopecia, there are "blank spots" with residual inflammation representing the sites of former follicles and follicular units. The sebaceous glands have disappeared with the follicles.

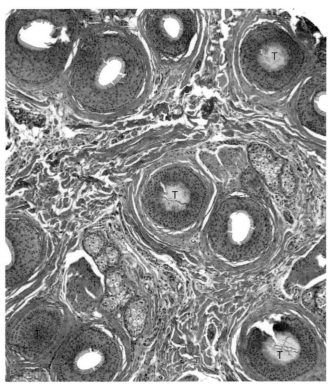

Figure 4.5 In this field, 4 of 11 of terminal hairs are in the catagen/telogen (T) phase; therefore, if this field were representative of the entire specimen, the telogen count would be 36%.

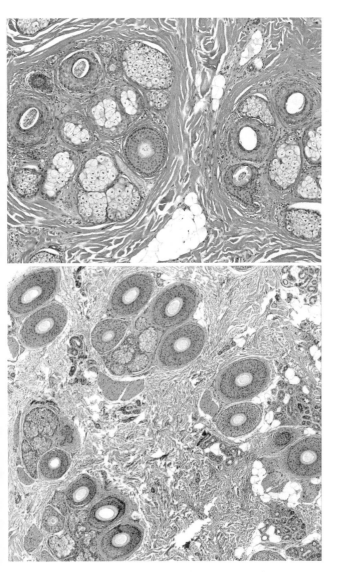

Figure 4.4 Normal follicular units in an African-American (*top*; two units shown) and a Caucasian (*bottom*; four units shown). In both cases, terminal anagen hairs are more numerous.

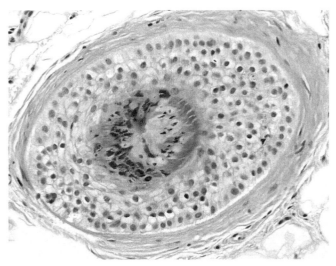

Figure 4.6 A follicle (from a patient with trichotillomania) showing the absence of hair shaft and collapse of the inner root sheath—an incomplete and distorted follicle.

4. Are a normal number (>85%) of the terminal follicles in the anagen phase? What is the telogen count (the percentage of terminal catagen/telogen hairs; Fig. 4.5)?

5. Do any follicles show incomplete or distorted anatomical features (Fig. 4.6)?

6. Is inflammation present, and at what level of the follicle (bulb, suprabulbar, isthmus, infundibulum; Fig. 4.7)?

7. Is there vacuolar interface alteration of the follicular epithelium (Fig. 4.8)?

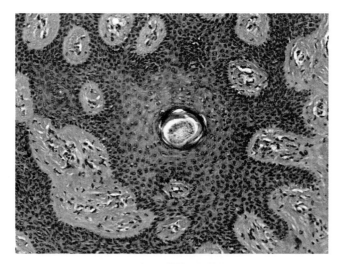

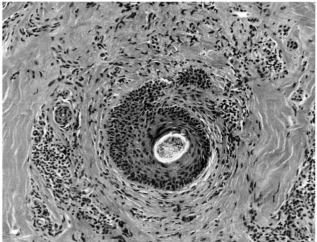

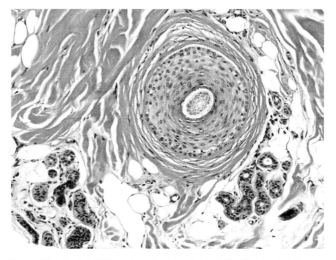

Figure 4.7 A single follicle sectioned at three levels: infundibulum (*top*), upper isthmus (*middle*), and suprabulbar (*bottom*). Inflammation is clearly most intense at the level of the upper isthmus.

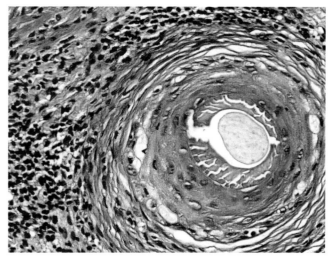

Figure 4.8 Specimen (from a patient with discoid lupus erythematosus) demonstrating obvious vacuolar interface change of the follicular epithelium.

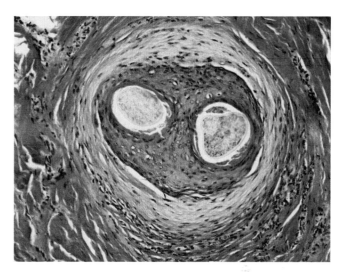

Figure 4.9 Perifollicular fibrosis (or fibroplasia) in a patient with central, centrifugal, cicatricial alopecia. The inner zone of fibrosis shows mucin deposition as well as concentric layers of collagen deposition. The presence or absence of mucin is probably related to the chronicity of the process.

The information gleaned from this evaluation will be used to compose the microscopic description. Interpreting the data and arriving at a final diagnosis is more challenging, and the major purpose of this text is to assist in this process. With few exceptions, the diagnosis of alopecia hinges on a constellation of features and not on a single finding. The constellation of findings typical of each disorder is described in each disease-specific chapter.

THE NORMAL SCALP IN TRANSVERSE SECTION

The architecture of a transversely sectioned biopsy specimen is quite predictable, and numerical data from the study of normal scalp specimens are available. Most data are based on 4 mm punch biopsy specimens, which can be considered the standard. A 4 mm diameter specimen samples a surface area of 12.6 mm² = πr^2, where "r" is the radius of the specimen. This formula can be used to compare data from larger or smaller diameter punch biopsies with those of a 4 mm punch.

8. Is perifollicular fibroplasia present (Fig. 4.9)?
9. Have individual follicles been entirely replaced by connective tissue (true follicular scars; Fig. 4.10)?
10. What is the total number of viable follicles in the specimen? The total number of terminal anagen and terminal telogen hairs? The total number of vellus hairs?

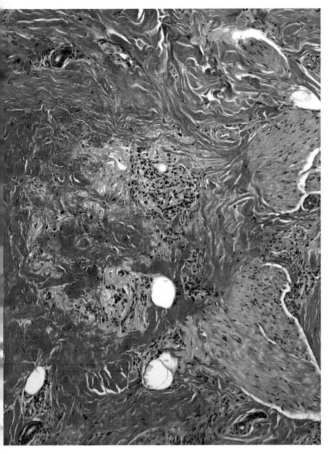

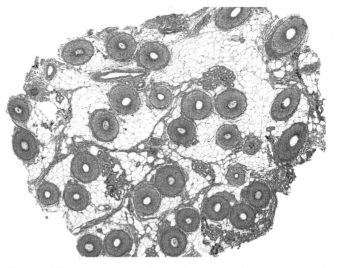

Figure 4.11 Biopsy from a normal Caucasian scalp, sectioned at the level of the fat.

Figure 4.10 Two arrector pili muscles terminate at a follicular scar. This particular scar represents the combined fibroplasia of all the terminal hairs within this follicular unit.

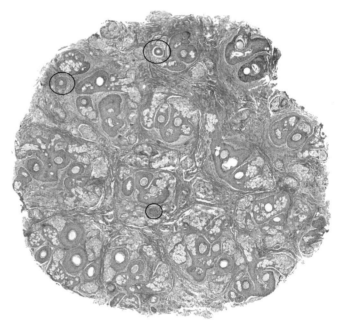

Figure 4.12 Same specimen as in Figure 4.11, but sectioned at a more superficial level, revealing three additional vellus hairs (*circled*).

For example, a 3-mm punch biopsy specimen has a surface area of $7.07\,mm^2$ and a 2 mm specimen has only $3.14\,mm^2$.

In a 4-mm punch biopsy specimen from a Caucasian, there should be about 25–30 terminal hairs in a transverse section through the deep dermis (Fig. 4.11). Sectioning through the upper dermis will reveal about five additional vellus hairs (Fig. 4.12). The average 4 mm Caucasian scalp biopsy specimen will contain about 38 follicles. Considerable individual variation exists and the range of normal is quite broad. Total hair counts as low as 19 and as high as 59 have been recorded (6). On average, two of the terminal hairs will be in the telogen phase, and 31 will be in the anagen phase. The *telogen count* (number of terminal telogen hairs divided by the total number of terminal hairs) will therefore be about $2 \div 33 = 6\%$ (6,7). Considerable individual variation exists for telogen counts among normal individuals, and figures within a range of 0%–15% (based on histologic sections) can be considered normal.

On average, African-American patients have fewer, although larger, follicles than Caucasian patients (Fig. 4.13). The average number of follicles for African-Americans, based on 4 mm biopsy specimens, is 21 (18 terminal and 3 vellus follicles) with an average telogen count of 7% (7). In Koreans (and presumably in related ethnic groups), the average number of follicles is 16 (15 terminal and 1 vellus follicles) with an average telogen count of 6% (8).

The percentage of catagen and/or telogen hairs can prove to be an important diagnostic feature in many forms of hair loss. Catagen and telogen hairs have the *same diagnostic significance* since all catagen hairs become telogen hairs within a few weeks. For the sake of simplicity, these two phases can be grouped together as the *catagen/telogen phase*. In this textbook, the term *catagen/telogen phase* will be used to refer to hairs either in the catagen *or* telogen phases. For diagnostic purposes, it is not important to differentiate between catagen and telogen hairs, but just to recognize a follicle as being in either phase. Terminal catagen hairs should be included with the terminal telogen hairs when determining the *telogen count* (Fig. 4.14).

In the superficial fat and lower dermis, home to the bulbs and suprabulbar zones of terminal anagen hairs, the follicles are spaced apart fairly evenly. However, in the mid and upper dermis, groups of follicles are arranged in *follicular units*

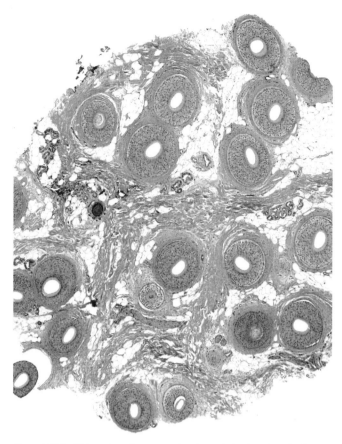

Figure 4.13 In African-Americans, a section through the deep dermis of a normal scalp biopsy specimen will usually reveal about 16–20 terminal hairs, a number that seems diminished if compared with a normal Caucasian scalp specimen.

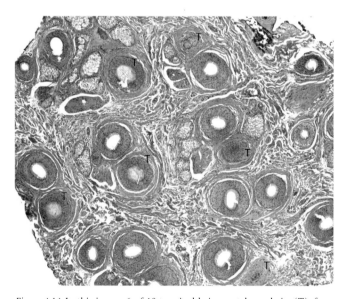

Figure 4.14 In this image, 6 of 18 terminal hairs are telogen hairs (T), for a telogen count of 33%.

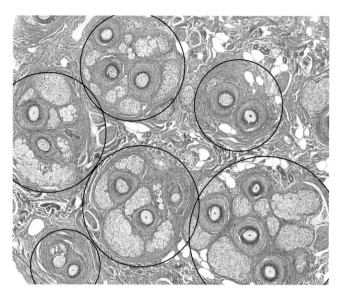

Figure 4.15 Several follicular units are circled.

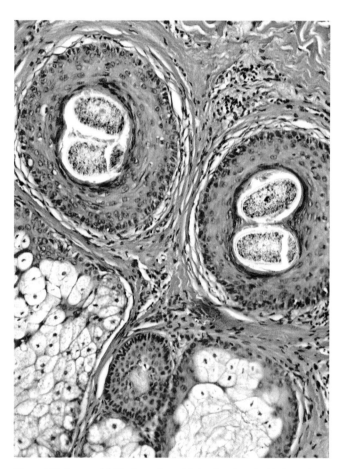

Figure 4.16 A normal follicular unit containing four terminal hairs and one vellus hair.

(Fig. 4.15). Discrete follicular units are best seen in sections taken at the level of upper isthmus or lower infundibulum (4). Each follicular unit contains 2–5 terminal hairs and 0–2 vellus hairs (Fig. 4.16). A shortcut for assessing numerical "normality" can be performed by looking at individual follicular units. If each unit contains 2–5 terminal hairs (outnumbering vellus hairs), and most units are similar, then the number and size of hairs is probably normal (Fig. 4.17). As would be expected, the number of terminal hairs per follicular unit may be smaller in patients of African descent than in Caucasians. The average density of follicular units is about one per square millimeter of surface area. Therefore, a 4 mm diameter horizontal section (12.6 mm²) will contain about 12 follicular units.

In the normal scalp, the terminal:vellus (T:V) hair ratio should be *at least* 2:1 or greater. Whiting reported a ratio of 7:1 in a group of 22 normal subjects *versus* 1.7:1 in 106 patients with common balding (6). Sperling reported a ratio of 6:1 in a group of 32 normal subjects (7). The T:V ratio varies somewhat from author to author. This can be largely accounted for by the lack of consensus on how to count medium-sized (indeterminate) hairs. Assigning these medium-sized hairs to either the terminal or vellus group will alter the calculated ratio.

The widely used nomenclature for hair size was defined by Dr. J.T. Headington in 1984 (5). Follicles with shafts less than or equal to the thickness of the adjacent inner root sheath, *or* less than 0.03 mm in diameter, are labeled *vellus* hairs. Those between 0.03 and 0.06 mm in diameter are called *indeterminate* hairs, and shafts larger than 0.06 mm are called *terminal* hairs. Some authors have simplified this system by referring only to vellus hairs (less than 0.03 mm) and terminal hairs (greater than 0.03 mm). For hair shafts that are circular in cross section, the size of the hair is simply the diameter of the shaft. For elliptical follicles, the size of the hairs is the average of the widest and the narrowest portion (Fig. 4.18).

Actually measuring numerous hair shaft diameters with a micrometer is clearly a tedious exercise, but with only a little experience, it becomes simple to identify most hair shafts as clearly terminal (greater than 0.06 mm) or clearly vellus (smaller than 0.03 mm). The major difficulty lies with the "medium-sized" or indeterminate hairs, which can be difficult to precisely gauge without a micrometer, and are often found in sizeable numbers. For purposes of this text, we have established some conventions that allow for rapid measurement, and yet allow for the accumulated data to be diagnostically valid. We discourage pathologists from agonizing over the actual nomenclature for a medium-sized hair. When the data is tallied, one or two extra vellus or terminal follicles will seldom change the ultimate diagnosis.

We also discourage pathologists from struggling to label small hair shafts as vellus *versus* miniaturized. Officially, they are quite different, because we are born with a complement of vellus hairs, but acquire miniaturized hairs from pathological processes. True vellus and miniaturized hairs can often be differentiated with careful serial sectioning, as might be performed for a research study. For purposes of the pathologist, however, vellus hairs and miniaturized hairs can be pooled together, resulting in diagnostically valid information. This information can be expressed as the *terminal:vellus ratio*, a datum important for the diagnosis of several forms of alopecia.

We will now describe the method that we use to determine hair size. It has not been validated in a formal study, and there are certainly other ways than ours to arrive at a valid hair count. But our experience in the examination room and at the microscope suggests that the method results in good clinical/pathological correlation and strikes a good balance between efficiency and precision.

Throughout this text, we used the following conventions:

1. The terms *vellus* and *miniaturized* may be used synonymously, both based simply on the diameter of the hair shafts (not the diameter of the follicular epithelium).
2. Vellus hairs can be identified by their small diameter and often superficial location (mid-dermis or higher). A deeply rooted follicle with a very small shaft is probably miniaturized, but can be counted as vellus to determine the T:V ratio.
3. Terminal hairs in the same biopsy specimen will vary slightly in diameter. However, a shaft that is less than half the diameter of the majority of larger hairs can be considered to be an indeterminate hair, and less than a third can be labeled as vellus (Fig. 4.19). For example, in Figure 4.20, even without micrometer confirmation, the hair shaft on the upper right is clearly less than one-third the diameter of the larger follicles, and is therefore a vellus hair.

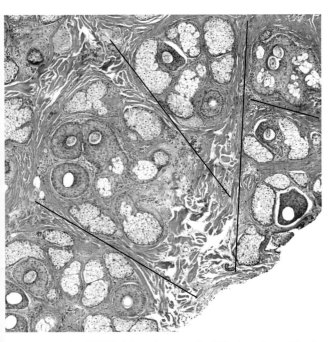

Figure 4.17 In this field, black lines demarcate five follicular units. 4 of 5 units are normal; the fifth (in *top center*) contains one large and one medium-sized hair. Therefore, overall the specimen looks normal.

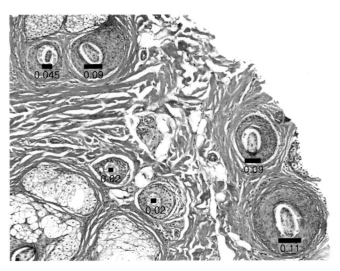

Figure 4.18 The bars used to label the size of the elliptical hair shafts in this image are the average of the length and width of the ellipses. An indeterminate hair (*top left*, 0.045 mm) and two vellus hairs (bottom left, both 0.02 mm) are present, along with three terminal hair shafts.

4. In Figure 4.21, the shaft on the upper left is greater than half the diameter of the largest shaft, and so is also a terminal hair. The shaft on the lower left is less than half the diameter of the largest shaft, but is larger than one-third. Thus it could be counted as an indeterminate follicle.

5. A fairly large (total epithelium) or deeply seated follicle with a small hair shaft (about 0.03 mm, *or* less than one-third the diameter of the largest shaft) is considered to be a vellus hair.

6. Some hair shafts appear too small to be terminal and too large to be vellus. It is most convenient to label such hairs as indeterminate. After all hairs are counted, a half of all indeterminate hairs are assigned to the terminal hair group, and the other half of the indeterminate hairs are assigned to the vellus hair group. This distribution of indeterminate hairs allows for simple calculation of a T:V ratio. For example, if there are nine terminal hairs, six indeterminate hairs, and three vellus hairs, the T:V is 12:6 or 2:1.

If biopsy specimens from the crown and occiput of the same person are compared, they should be similar in terms of follicular size, number, and percentage of anagen/telogen hairs. The architecture of scalp biopsy specimens should be uniform over the entire scalp, with the possible exception of the fringes.

Mild *upper* dermal perifollicular inflammation may be present in normal scalp specimens. This is especially true for African-American patients (Fig. 4.22).

"COUNTING HAIRS"—PERFORMING A FOLLICULAR CENSUS ON A TRANSVERSELY SECTIONED BIOPSY

The ideal candidate specimen consists of transverse sections cut at multiple levels—superficial, mid-dermal, and deep-dermal.

1. Draw a circle to begin the diagram.
2. Decide on symbols that make sense to you. We use the following:
   - A = terminal anagen hair
   - a = vellus or miniaturized anagen hair
   - T = terminal telogen or catagen hair
   - t = vellus or miniaturized telogen or catagen hair
   - N = "naked" hair shaft free in dermis
   - n = nanogen hair
   - s = stele

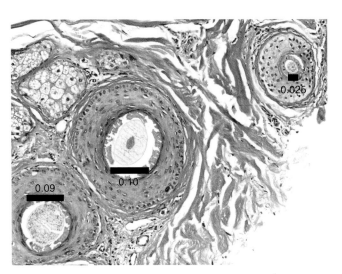

Figure 4.20 The vellus hair (on the right) is clearly less than one-third the diameter of the two terminal hairs on the left.

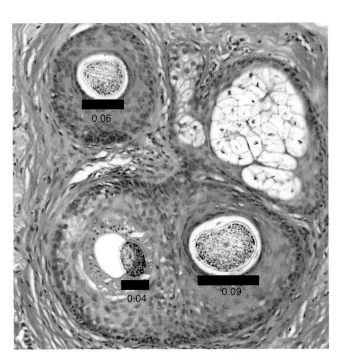

Figure 4.21 An indeterminate or medium-sized hair (lower left) and two terminal hairs.

Figure 4.19 In this cartoon of a transversely sectioned follicular unit, the three largest hair shafts can be labeled as terminal hairs (T). A medium-sized hair, less than half of the average diameter of the largest shafts, is labeled as an indeterminate hair (i). The remaining hair shaft, less than one-third the diameter of the largest hairs, is labeled as vellus.

3. Begin at the level of the deep dermis where follicles are evenly spaced (without follicular unit grouping). Record symbols on the diagram at this level, as shown in Figure 4.23, top panel. It can often be helpful to draw ovals around follicular units to maintain organization as new follicles are added (follicular units can be easily identified at the level of the sebaceous glands). Deeper levels allow for visualization of features that might be missed at higher levels. Such features include follicular stele, the bulbs of deeply situated catagen/telogen hairs, and peribulbar inflammation, to name a few.

4. Repeat at the level of the mid-dermis, adding follicles not seen at lower levels (usually because they are miniaturized or are in the telogen phase; see Fig. 4.23, bottom panel).

5. Repeat at the level of the upper dermis, adding follicles not seen at lower levels. These will include the remaining vellus and miniaturized follicles.

6. At the level of the upper dermis—the level of the upper infundibula of most follicles—all follicles should

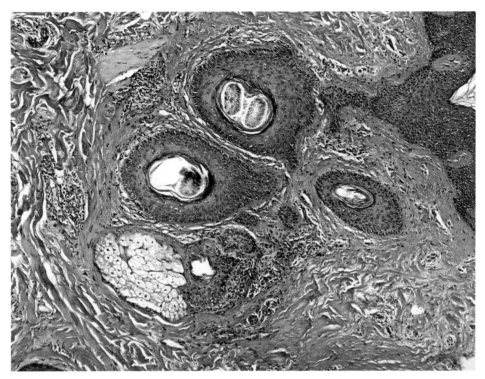

Figure 4.22 Nonspecific, chronic inflammation surrounding the infundibula of follicles in an African-American patient.

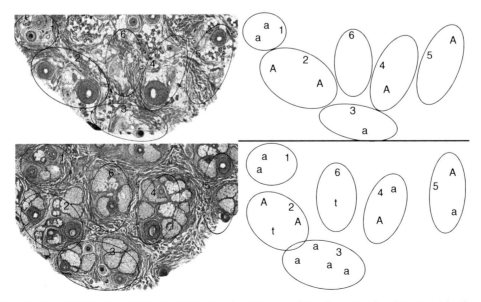

Figure 4.23 Six follicular units (labeled 1–6) sectioned at the level of the deep dermis (upper left) are diagrammed on the *upper right*. The same six follicular units sectioned at the level of the mid-to-upper dermis (*lower left*) are diagrammed on the lower right. As the epidermal surface is approached, seven additional follicles (all vellus hairs) are identified.

be "present and accounted for." At this level, one often begins to see a peripheral rim of epidermis, which can be evaluated for pathological changes (Figure 4.22).

REPORTING HISTOLOGICAL FINDINGS—THE BIOPSY REPORT

Transverse sectioning allows the pathologist to gather a considerable amount of data about the specimen. This can be summarized in a microscopic description (e.g., "A reduced number of hairs are present, and most are miniaturized"). Alternatively, detailed data can be presented in tabular form. A template for a report is shown in Table 4.1.

Table 4.1 Template for a "Scalp Biopsy Report"

Accession number:
Date:
Patient name/age/sex/race:
Submitting physician:
Clinical impression:
Macroscopic description: biopsy diameter/location on scalp:
  e.g., 4 mm punch biopsy, vertex of scalp
Microscopic description of vertical sections:
Microscopic description of horizontal sections:
Terminal anagen hairs:
Terminal catagen/telogen hairs:
Vellus hairs:
TOTAL hairs (terminal plus vellus, all phases):
Telogen count (terminal telogen hairs÷total terminal hairs):
Terminal : vellus ratio: *e.g., 3:1*
Inflammatory infiltrate (type and location): *e.g. upper follicle vs. lower follicle/bulb; lymphohistiocytic vs. neutrophilic; vacuolar interface type vs. no significant interface change; mild vs. dense*
Fibrosis or follicular scars (columns of connective tissue at the site of former follicles):
Additional features noted: *e.g., stelae, solar elastosis, follicular distortion, pigment incontinence, naked hair shafts*
Comments:
DIAGNOSIS:
Consultants:
Pathologist's signature _____

REFERENCES

1. Elston DM. Vertical vs. transverse sections: both are valuable in the evaluation of alopecia. Am J Dermatopathol 2005; 27: 353–6.
2. Elston DM, Ferringer T, Dalton S, Fillman E, Tyler W. A comparison of vertical versus transverse sections in the evaluation of alopecia biopsy specimens. J Am Acad Dermatol 2005; 53: 267–72.
3. Bathish N, Ben Izhak O, Shemer A, Bergman R. A study of serial vertical sectioning of scalp biopsies to increase the histological diagnostic yield in alopecias. J Eur Acad Dermatol Venereol 2010; 24: 709–15.
4. Solomon A. The transversely sectioned scalp biopsy specimen: the technique and an algorithm for its use in the diagnosis of alopecia. Adv Dermatol 1994; 9: 127–57.
5. Headington J. Transverse microscopic anatomy of the human scalp. Arch Dermatol 1984; 120: 449–56.
6. Whiting D. Diagnostic and predictive value of horizontal sections of scalp biopsies in male pattern androgenetic alopecia. J Am Acad Dermatol 1993; 28: 755–63.
7. Sperling L. Hair density in African Americans. Arch Dermatol 1999; 135: 656–8.
8. Lee HJ, Ha SJ, Lee JH, et al. Hair counts from scalp biopsy specimens in Asians. J Am Acad Dermatol 2002; 46: 218–21.

5 Classification of hair disease

For researchers, classification may offer insight into the pathogenesis of disease. For clinicians, classification (i.e., diagnosis) is the best way to arrive at an appropriate targeted therapy. Pathologists share both of these interests. Most pathologists use a classification scheme (i.e., grouping disease entities based on one or more shared characteristics) as a useful way of narrowing down a large number of potential diagnostic entities into a smaller number of possibilities. Using a systematic and iterative approach that weighs features and groups of features one against the other, pathologists can develop an expertise in alopecia biopsy interpretation that ultimately yields either a single, confident diagnosis or a narrow differential that can be further refined with clinical input or ancillary testing.

The purpose of this book is to provide assistance to researchers, clinicians, and especially pathologists endeavoring to understand histopathological findings observable by light microscopy. A classification system based on easily identifiable and objective histopathological clues would be ideal. Unfortunately, most forms of alopecia demonstrate at least some overlapping clinical and histological features. It would make more sense to segregate diseases by etiology, but the causes of many forms of hair loss are unknown, making it difficult to group diseases with confidence.

Hair loss (alopecia) can occur through a variety of mechanisms. If hair shafts are defective or traumatized, they can be prone to breakage or premature loss. These hair shaft disorders are further examined in the final chapter of this text (chap. 36).

Intentionally or unintentionally, people may subject their hair follicles to physical trauma that can result in alopecia. Traction alopecia, postoperative pressure–induced alopecia, and trichotillomania are a few examples. The remaining types of alopecia are due to failure of the follicular epithelium itself. This can be due to inflammation, infection, senescence, hormonal influences, medications, genetics, combinations of these, and other unknown causes. As one might imagine, mechanistic classification schemes can become complex. And, as will be seen in the following pages, the histopathological features of many of these mechanisms of alopecia are shared and therefore nonspecific.

CICATRICIAL (SCARRING) VS. NONCICATRICIAL ALOPECIA

The most common classification system divides the diseases into cicatricial (scarring) *versus* noncicatricial (nonscarring) forms of alopecia. In this book, the terms *cicatricial* and *scarring* are considered synonymous and used interchangeably. *Cicatricial* or *scarring* implies that follicular epithelium has been replaced by connective tissue. However, in some cases of alopecia, the follicles seem to simply "disappear" without any noticeable alteration in the supporting tissue architecture. The broadest definition of cicatricial alopecia might include all forms of alopecia in which hair follicles are permanently lost. In contrast, noncicatricial forms of alopecia preserve the follicular epithelial apparatus (in particular the bulge zone harboring the follicular stem cells) and are potentially reversible (1,2).

Interestingly, some hair diseases demonstrate a *biphasic* pattern, where noncicatricial hair loss is seen *early* in the course of the disease, and permanent hair loss becomes apparent in the *later* stages of the disease (2). Examples of diseases demonstrating this biphasic pattern include androgenetic alopecia, alopecia areata, and traction alopecia. These forms of alopecia are generally considered to be noncicatricial. However, after many years or decades of active disease, permanent dropout of follicles occurs (3). These biphasic alopecias have in common a persistent underlying process that promotes accelerated and unremitting follicular cycling that could, one might surmise, hasten follicular senescence, perhaps through exhaustion of the follicular stem cells.

THE CLASSIFICATION OF CICATRICIAL (SCARRING) ALOPECIA

The classification of this group of diseases is especially confusing and controversial. There are no characteristic biological markers for most forms of cicatricial alopecia. In many cases, we do not know whether the clinical and histological features found in a given patient are manifestations of a distinct disease, or just individual host responses. Any classification of cicatricial alopecia should be considered provisional and subject to change as new information becomes available (3).

Clinically, cicatricial alopecia is defined by the loss of follicular ostia, although a retained ostium does not always guarantee the presence of a viable follicle (1–4). Histologically, cicatricial alopecia can be subdivided into two categories. The first is *primary* cicatricial alopecia, where the target of inflammation appears to be the follicle, more specifically, the noncycling portion of the follicle and/or the bulge zone (the location of follicular stem cells) (3,5). Most of the primary cicatricial alopecias do not have a well-defined cause. However, they usually present a sufficiently distinct clinicopathological picture (6) to allow for a confident diagnosis. That said, a combination of inadequate clinical history, an unfortunate choice of biopsy site, and the presence of overlapping histological features can stymie the most expert of pathologists.

In *secondary* cicatricial alopecia, the follicle is an "innocent bystander" in the disease process, and is destroyed in a nonspecific manner (2,6). Examples of secondary cicatricial alopecia include deep burns, radiation dermatitis, cutaneous malignancies, cutaneous sarcoidosis, sclerosing dermatoses, such as morphea and necrobiosis lipoidica, and certain chronic infections, such as cutaneous tuberculosis. The various forms of secondary cicatricial alopecia should have distinctive histological features typical of the underlying disease. For example, alopecia caused by cutaneous sarcoidosis should reveal sarcoidal granulomas in the dermis. A discussion of the various forms of secondary cicatricial alopecia is beyond the scope of this text.

All forms of cicatricial alopecia share the loss of follicular and sebaceous epithelium. The primary cicatricial alopecias

Table 5.1 North American Hair Research Society (2001) Proposed Working Classification of Primary Cicatricial Alopecia

Lymphocytic
  Chronic cutaneous lupus erythematosus
  LPP
    Classic LPP
    Frontal fibrosing alopecia
    Graham–Little syndrome
  Classic pseudopelade (Brocq)*
  Central centrifugal cicatricial alopecia*
  Alopecia mucinosa
  Keratosis follicularis spinulosa decalvans
Neutrophilic
  Folliculitis decalvans
  Dissecting cellulitis/folliculitis (perifolliculitis abscedens et suffodiens)
Mixed
  Folliculitis (acne) keloidalis
  Folliculitis (acne) necrotica
  Erosive pustular dermatosis
Nonspecific*

Please refer to the original reference regarding strict definitions of entities marked with an asterisk (*) (6).
Abbreviation: LPP, lichen planopilaris.

Table 5.2 A Simplified Classification Scheme for Primary Cicatricial Alopecia

Central, centrifugal, cicatricial alopecia
Lichen planopilaris
Chronic, cutaneous lupus erythematosus (discoid lupus erythematosus)
Folliculitis keloidalis (folliculitis nuchae, acne keloidalis nuchae)
Dissecting cellulitis (perifolliculitis abscedens et suffodiens)
Cicatricial alopecia, not otherwise classified

often result in "naked" hair shafts in the dermis, suggesting that the follicular epithelium is quickly destroyed around terminal anagen shafts. This, in contrast to the biphasic mechanism suggested above, would be a rapid and fulminant process. Sebaceous lobules are typically lost along with the follicles in primary cicatricial alopecia. It is easy to imagine that any inflammatory process brisk enough to destroy the follicular stem cells in the bulge zone could also destroy the delicate sebaceous glands residing in close proximity. The exception to this observation would be dissecting cellulitis, which, owing to the epicenter of the inflammation in the deep dermis and subcutis, tends to maintain normal sebaceous lobules until late in the disease course.

In 2001, members of the North American Hair Research Society (NAHRS) convened to discuss cicatricial alopecia. Attendees developed a series of mechanistic hypotheses for primary cicatricial alopecias, and, from these, future research targets were established (2,6). In addition, a proposed working classification of primary cicatricial alopecias was formulated. The group ultimately developed a classification system based on the primary inflammatory cell present in the biopsy specimen, subdivided as follows: lymphocytic, neutrophilic, mixed, and nonspecific (Table 5.1).

One challenge with this classification scheme (in the opinion of the authors of this text) stems from determining how many of the included diagnoses actually represent distinct and reproducible clinical and histopathological entities (as will be seen in the discussion of diagnoses that appear in the following chapters) (2). One example is folliculitis decalvans (FD), which we favor as a pattern of cicatricial alopecia and not as a distinct diagnosis *sui generis*. If considered a distinct diagnosis, FD is placed in the neutrophilic category. If FD is a pattern that can be seen in a variety of conditions, it could represent a variant pattern of central, centrifugal, cicatricial alopecia (classified

in the NAHRS schematic as a lymphocytic alopecia), or as indistinguishable from some examples of bacterial or fungal folliculitis (secondary infectious alopecias).

Our experience, is that classification using the dominant inflammatory cell lumps together several clinically disparate entities (7). This approach has not always been useful in our hands, and time will tell whether this classification scheme significantly clarifies the future diagnosis and treatment of primary cicatricial alopecias.

An alternative approach to the classification of primary cicatricial alopecia that does not rely primarily on the constituent inflammatory cells is outlined in Table 5.2. In this approach, primary cicatricial alopecia can be divided into six diagnostic groups. This short list is a simplification of a long list of confusing, vague, and poorly defined diagnostic terms, many of which have also been abandoned by the NAHRS in their 2001 classification. Notably absent from the list are terms, such as pseudopelade, pseudopelade of Brocq, and folliculitis decalvans, which we feel are poorly defined, lack unique histopathological correlates, and are used nonspecifically by authors and clinicians. Historically, these terms have arisen to match clinical patterns of disease, often end-stage, many of which are shared by the well-defined cicatricial alopecias listed in Table 5.2 (3). We favor the use of specific diagnostic terms and the abandonment of poorly defined descriptive categories. Nevertheless, many of the older terms (such as *folliculitis decalvans*) will be discussed in this text for the sake of clarity and historical context.

In summary, the classification of the various forms of alopecia can be considered a work in progress. A definitive classification schema will depend on further research efforts and the elucidation of the underlying etiologies of these diseases.

REFERENCES

1. Sperling LC, Mezebish DS. Hair diseases. Med Clin North Am. 1998; 82: 1155–69.
2. Ross EK, Tan E, Shapiro J. Update on primary cicatricial alopecias. J Am Acad Dermatol. 2005; 53: 1–37; quiz 38–40.
3. Sperling LC, Solomon AR, Whiting DA. A new look at scarring alopecia. Arch Dermatol. 2000; 136: 235–42.
4. Sullivan JR, Kossard S. Acquired scalp alopecia. Part I: a review. Australas J Dermatol. 1998; 39: 207–19; quiz 220–201.
5. Olsen E, Stenn K, Bergfeld W, et al. Update on cicatricial alopecia. J Investig Dermatol Symp Proc. 2003; 8: 18–19.
6. Olsen EA, Bergfeld WF, Cotsarelis G, et al. Summary of North American Hair Research Society (NAHRS)-sponsored Workshop on Cicatricial Alopecia, Duke University Medical Center, February 10 and 11, 2001. J Am Acad Dermatol. 2003; 48: 103–10.
7. Pincus LB, Price VH, McCalmont TH. The amount counts: distinguishing neutrophil-mediated and lymphocyte-mediated cicatricial alopecia by compound follicles. J Cutan Pathol. 2011; 38: 1–4.

6 Distinctive or critical histological features and associated diseases

Classification schemes are of little value to pathologists trying to extract the diagnosis from a glass slide. The histological features, in conjunction with a brief clinical description, must somehow guide the pathologist to the correct diagnosis. To assist in this process, some especially important histological features can help to segregate the diagnostic entities. Identifying additional specific histological features can then make it easier to establish the diagnosis. Frequently, different diseases may share two or more histological features. When this occurs, separating such diseases may rest on good clinical correlation or subtle histological clues.

THE FOUR-STEP METHOD
Attempts have been made to create algorithms for arriving at a diagnosis, and sometimes pathologists may find them useful. However, as a starting point we use a four-step technique based on the answers to four histological questions:

1. Is the total number of hairs normal or reduced?
2. Is the overall size of hairs (on average) normal or reduced?
3. Is the telogen count (percentage of total terminal telogen hairs) normal or increased?
4. Is there a significant amount of inflammation present?

Arriving at an answer to these four questions can narrow the histological differential diagnosis considerably, and sometimes the exact diagnosis may be obvious at this point. One of the four features (number, size, telogen count, or inflammation) may be a dominant finding, which also helps to narrow the differential diagnosis.

Unfortunately, no *single* histological feature is sufficient to establish a definitive diagnosis in *any* form of hair loss. However, a differential diagnosis based on one or two histological abnormalities will help to create a "short list" of possible diagnoses. Additional histological features characteristic of the entities on the "short" list can then be used to narrow the field of possibilities. Clinical information will often help to decide the issue. We will start by discussing the four-step method in more detail, with a differential diagnosis listed for each critical feature.

STEP 1: IS THE *TOTAL NUMBER OF HAIRS* NORMAL OR REDUCED?
Determining this with confidence requires transverse sections at the levels of both lower and upper dermis (Figs. 6.1 and 6.2). In most cases, it is *not* necessary to count all the follicles, but an overall impression is sufficient to determine "normal or nearly normal" or "reduced in number" (Fig. 6.3). One must take into consideration the ethnic background of the patient, which will put the total number of hairs seen in the proper context. Hair density for most people of Asian descent and in African-Americans is lower, on average, than in Caucasians.

Conditions with decreased hair density (*total* viable follicles per mm²)

- Cicatricial alopecia (all forms)
- Congenital hypotrichosis (various syndromes)
- "End-stage" traction alopecia (an example of biphasic hair loss)
- Androgenetic alopecia or hereditary balding (long-standing disease; an example of biphasic hair loss)
- Alopecia areata (longstanding disease; an example of biphasic hair loss)
- Aplasia cutis congenita

STEP 2: IS THE OVERALL *SIZE OF HAIRS* (ON AVERAGE) NORMAL OR REDUCED?
The size of hairs refers to the diameter of the hair shafts not the overall diameter of the follicular epithelia. Determining the size of hairs is discussed in chapter 3. As a rule of thumb, the largest shafts are usually the normal terminal hairs. In the lower half of the dermis, almost all shafts should be terminal hairs, and in the upper half of the dermis, the terminal hairs should outnumber vellus (or miniaturized) shafts by at least a margin of 2:1. When it is obvious at first inspection (or with more careful hair counts) that this is not the case, the average size of hairs is reduced (Figs. 6.4 and 6.5).

Conditions with miniaturization of hairs (diminished shaft diameter)

- Androgenetic alopecia/hereditary balding
- Temporal triangular alopecia
- Alopecia areata
- Patchy hair loss in systemic lupus erythematosus
- Patchy or diffuse hair loss in secondary syphilis
- Psoriatic alopecia
- Medication-related psoriasiform alopecias
- Chemotherapy-induced alopecia

STEP 3: IS THE *TELOGEN COUNT* (PERCENTAGE OF TOTAL TERMINAL CATAGEN/TELOGEN HAIRS) NORMAL OR INCREASED?
As previously noted, the diagnostic significance of catagen and telogen hairs is the same, since all catagen hairs become telogen hairs within a few weeks. Therefore, follicles in either of these two phases can be referred to as catagen/telogen hairs. A normal telogen count (total terminal catagen/telogen hairs ÷ total terminal hairs) should be between 0% and 15%. Although an increased percentage may be evident from a single section (Fig. 6.6), multiple levels are often required to determine the total number of terminal catagen/telogen hairs. In most cases, vellus or miniaturized telogen hairs can be ignored when determining the telogen count. However, when the majority of follicles are miniaturized, as often occurs in alopecia areata, the presence of a very high percentage (>50%) of telogen hairs of all sizes cannot be ignored. As a rule of thumb, if most hairs

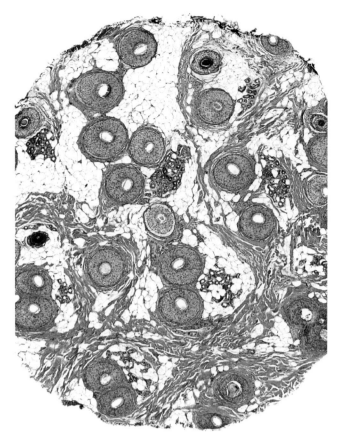

Figure 6.1 An example of normal hair density. A transverse section at the level of the deep dermis/superficial fat, taken from the normal (uninvolved) scalp of an African-American woman. The section contains 26 follicles, slightly greater than average.

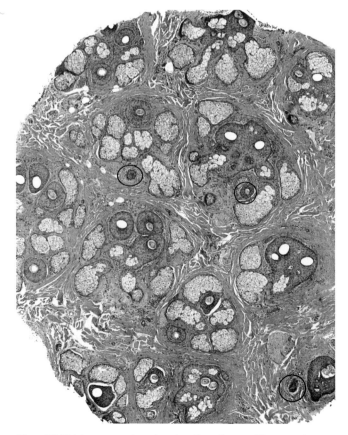

Figure 6.2 This is an upper dermal section (from the same biopsy specimen as in Fig. 6.1) containing three additional vellus follicles (circled).

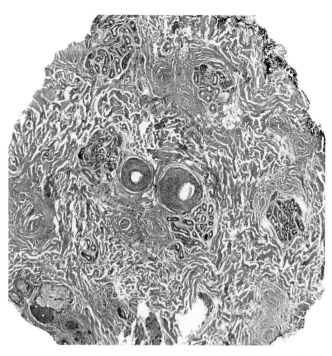

Figure 6.3 An example of significantly decreased hair density in an African-American woman with cicatricial alopecia. This section is at the level of the mid-dermis, where all terminal hairs should be evident.

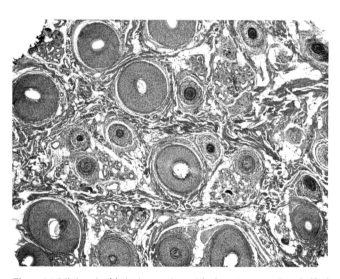

Figure 6.4 Miniaturized hairs in a patient with alopecia areata. Over half of all follicles are small, which is always abnormal, regardless of the level of the section.

in a specimen are miniaturized and most of these are in the catagen/telogen phase, this finding has diagnostic significance and must be taken into consideration (Fig. 6.7).

Conditions with an increased percentage of catagen/telogen hairs

- Trichotillomania
- Traction alopecia (acute)
- Postoperative (pressure induced) alopecia
- Telogen effluvium
- Alopecia areata
- Androgenetic alopecia/hereditary balding
- Psoriatic alopecia
- Medication-induced psoriasiform alopecias
- Patchy hair loss in systemic lupus erythematosus

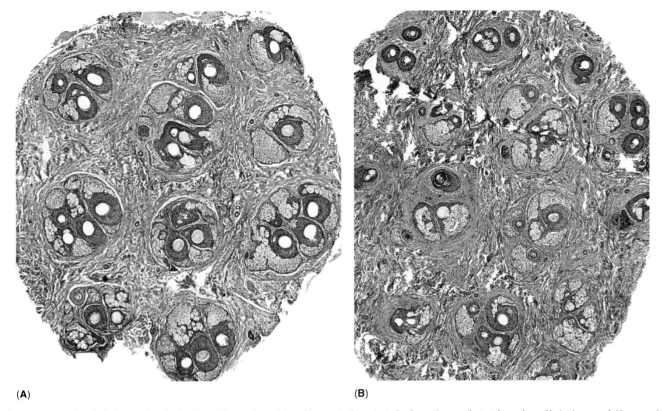

(A)   (B)

Figure 6.5 Normal scalp (**A**) *versus* involved scalp (**B**) in a patient with androgenetic alopecia. In both specimens, the total number of hairs is normal. However, in the involved scalp, the average size of hairs is greatly reduced in the involved area as compared with normal appearing scalp.

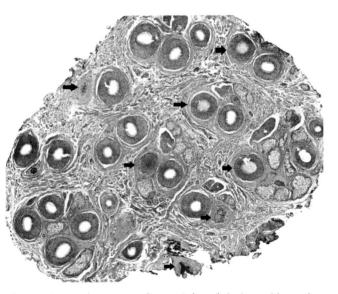

Figure 6.6 Increased percentage of catagen/telogen hairs (arrows) in a patient with telogen effluvium. The majority of hairs are terminal (big) hairs, but when all follicles are counted, 25% are in the catagen/telogen phase.

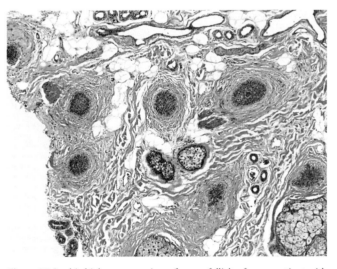

Figure 6.7 In this higher power view of seven follicles from a patient with alopecia areata, all hairs are miniaturized (producing little if any shaft) but 100% are in the catagen/telogen phase; such a high percentage of catagen/telogen follicles, regardless of their size, is almost always of diagnostic significance.

- Patchy hair loss in secondary syphilis
- Inflammatory, cicatricial alopecia
- Chemotherapy-induced alopecia

STEP 4: IS THERE A SIGNIFICANT AMOUNT OF INFLAMMATION PRESENT?

By significant, we mean, "is there a degree of inflammation that would be unexpected or unusual in a biopsy from normal scalp skin?" Mild, peri-infundibular chronic inflammation is very common in normal scalp specimens (Fig. 6.8) and even more common when mild seborrheic dermatitis is present. It can

usually be regarded as "background noise" of no diagnostic significance. However, dense or deep inflammation (Fig. 6.9) should always be regarded as abnormal and characterized further. Three special patterns of inflammation (followed by a list of associated diseases) are described below.

Pattern 1: Inflammation predominantly involving the lower half of the follicles (Fig. 6.10)

- Alopecia areata (predominantly lymphocytic)
- Patchy hair loss in systemic lupus erythematosus (predominantly lymphocytic)

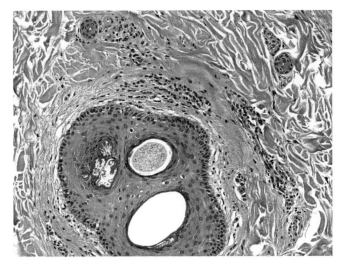

Figure 6.8 Mild peri-infundibular chronic inflammation in a specimen taken from normal scalp skin.

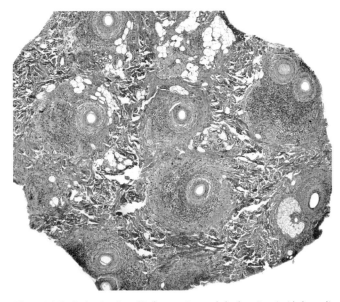

Figure 6.9 Both the density of inflammation and the location (mid-dermal) are abnormal. This is a specimen from a patient with lichen planopilaris.

- Patchy hair loss in secondary syphilis (predominantly lymphocytic with occasional plasma cells)
- Dissecting cellulitis/perifolliculitis capitis abscedens et suffodiens (dense, mixed, acute, and chronic inflammation)

Pattern 2: Inflammation predominantly involving the upper half of the follicles, *with* vacuolar interface alteration (Fig. 6.11)

- Lichen planopilaris
- Frontal, fibrosing alopecia
- Chronic, cutaneous (discoid) lupus erythematosus (foci of deep inflammation may often be present)

Pattern 3: Inflammation predominantly involving the upper half of the follicles, *without* vacuolar interface alteration (Fig. 6.12)

- Acne keloidalis
- Central, centrifugal cicatricial alopecia

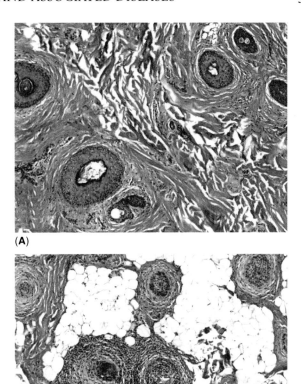

Figure 6.10 In this patient with alopecia areata, the upper follicles (**A**) are spared while the lower halves, specifically the bulbs (**B**) are surrounded by lymphocytic inflammation.

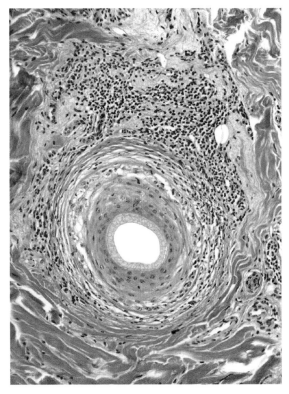

Figure 6.11 In this example of lichen planopilaris, lymphocytic inflammation is concentrated around the mid- and upper half of the follicle. Basal vacuolar degeneration is present.

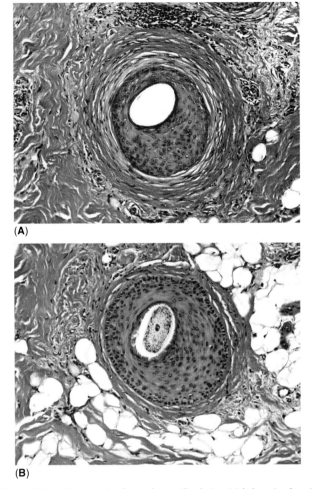

(A)

(B)

Figure 6.12 In this example of central, centrifugal cicatricial alopecia, chronic inflammation is concentrated at the level of the isthmus and lower infundibulum (**A**). There is perifollicular fibroplasia but not vacuolar interface alteration. The lower panel (**B**) shows a section through the same follicle but at the level of the dermal/subcutaneous junction. Inflammation spares the lower half of the hair follicle. Of note, premature desquamation of the inner root sheath as is sometimes seen in CCCA is well-demonstrated in this section.

Pattern 4: Inflammation of both the superficial and deep halves of the follicles

- Chronic, cutaneous (discoid) lupus erythematosus
- Medication-induced psoriasiform alopecias (predominantly lymphocytes, plasma cells, and eosinophils)

FINAL FOCUSING

The four-step method may lead to a specific diagnosis, but in some cases only a narrowed differential will result. The final focus is used to narrow the differential by seeking additional specific histological features that will support one diagnosis above others. Listed are diseases that often demonstrate a specific histological feature that may be useful in cinching a specific diagnosis.

Conditions with decreased hair density at the level of the lower dermis (if counted *only* at this level; Fig. 6.13)

- Telogen effluvium
- Androgenetic alopecia
- Temporal triangular alopecia
- Traction alopecia
- All forms of cicatricial alopecia

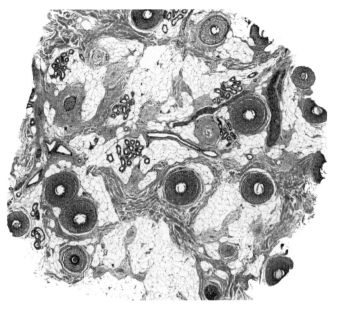

Figure 6.13 In this specimen from a patient with androgenetic alopecia, an abnormally low number of hairs is found at the dermal/subcutaneous junction. However, more superficial levels reveal additional vellus/miniaturized hairs and a few terminal telogen follicles, bringing the total number of hairs into the normal range. In this example, the presence of several streamers and the marked variation in hair shaft diameters offer a clue to the correct diagnosis. However, accurate hair counts cannot be performed at a single level!

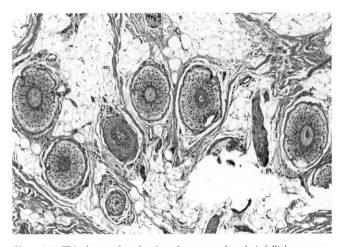

Figure 6.14 This cluster of predominantly anagen-phase hair follicles seems to contradict the clinical reality—a totally bald patch in a patient with alopecia areata. The explanation in this case is that all of these hairs are miniaturized, nanogen follicles producing little if any shaft.

- Alopecia areata (longstanding disease)
- Psoriatic alopecia
- Psoriasiform medication-induced alopecias

Conditions with normal hair density if counted at all levels (total viable follicles per mm²) despite a *clinical* reduction in the amount of hair. Note: In these cases, there is a discrepancy between the clinical impression of marked hair loss and the histological finding of numerous hairs (Figs. 6.14–6.16).

- Telogen effluvium (increased catagen/telogen)
- Trichotillomania (increased catagen/telogen)
- Androgenetic alopecia/hereditary balding (increased miniaturized hairs)
- Alopecia areata (increased miniaturized/telogen hairs)

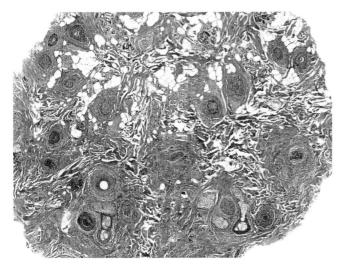

Figure 6.15 In this specimen from a patient with alopecia totalis, a normal or nearly normal number of follicles is present despite the clinical absence of hair. The explanation is a massive conversion to the catagen/telogen phase and miniaturization of most follicles regardless of phase.

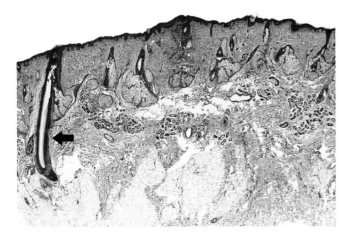

Figure 6.16 Even with vertical sectioning, it is clear that numerous follicles are present in the bald zone of a patient with temporal triangular alopecia. The explanation is that almost all hairs are greatly miniaturized. A terminal hair (*arrow*) is present for comparison.

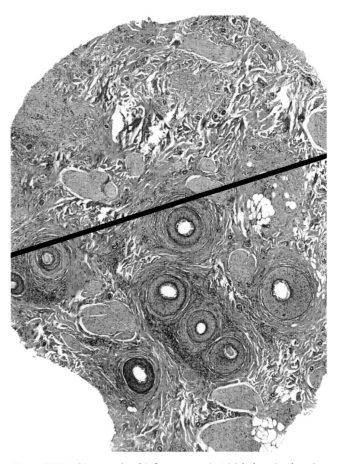

Figure 6.17 In this example of inflammatory cicatricial alopecia, there is a large "blank spot above the black line" (*top*) representing the sites of former follicles and follicular units. The sebaceous glands have disappeared with the follicles.

- Psoriatic alopecia (increased miniaturized/telogen hairs)
- Psoriasiform medication-induced alopecias (increased miniaturized/telogen hairs)
- Temporal triangular alopecia (increased miniaturized hairs)
- Loose anagen hair syndrome (increased catagen/telogen)
- Most hair shaft disorders (increased shaft fragility)

Conditions with follicular dropout (replacement of follicles by connective tissue)

With loss of associated sebaceous glands (Fig. 6.17)

- Cicatricial alopecia: all forms

Without loss of associated sebaceous glands (Fig. 6.18)

- Traction alopecia (end-stage)
- Androgenetic alopecia (advanced and longstanding)
- Alopecia areata (very advanced and longstanding)

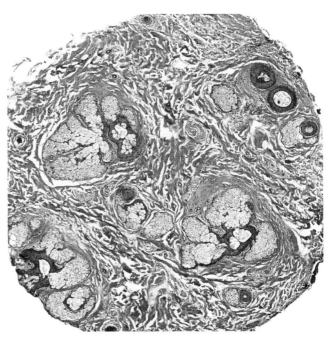

Figure 6.18 In this example of end-stage traction alopecia, many terminal hairs have disappeared but sebaceous glands are spared.

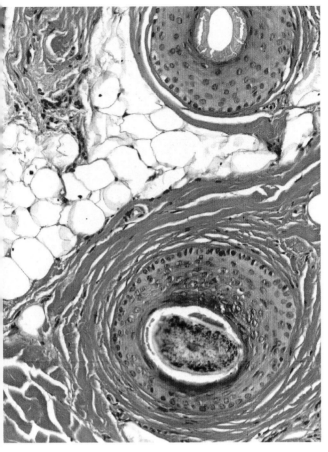

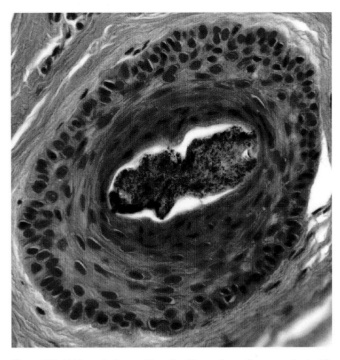

Figure 6.20 Trichomalacia is evident in this specimen from a patient with trichotillomania. The hair shaft is distorted in shape, irregularly pigmented and incompletely cornified.

Figure 6.19 In this specimen from a patient with central, centrifugal, cicatricial alopecia, there is a follicle whose inner root sheath has desquamated well below the isthmus (follicle on *bottom*). A normal follicle with an intact inner root sheath (*top*) is present for comparison.

Conditions with premature desquamation of the inner root sheath (Fig. 6.19)

- Central, centrifugal, cicatricial alopecia
- Acne keloidalis (occasionally)
- Any highly inflammatory alopecia eventuating in secondary follicular destruction

Conditions with trichomalacia (Fig. 6.20)

- Trichotillomania
- Acute traction alopecia
- Pressure-induced alopecia
- Alopecia areata

7   Clinical correlation

Clinicians who contribute even a brief clinical description and differential diagnosis are of considerable assistance to the pathologist and increase diagnostic accuracy. Some clinical features that may be described include the following:

- Age and race of patient
- Diffuse *versus* patterned hair loss
- Evidence of hair breakage (hairs of uneven length)
- Evidence of inflammation
- Evidence of permanent hair loss
- Obliteration of follicular ostia
- Normal *versus* abnormal hair density
- Precise location of biopsy site

DIFFUSE VS. PATTERNED HAIR LOSS

The most important feature is the *pattern* of hair loss (1,2). Hair loss can be diffuse or patterned, favoring one or more portions of the scalp over others. Truly diffuse hair loss suggests a uniform reduction in hair density over all portions of the scalp (3). Telogen effluvium (Fig. 7.1) is an example of truly diffuse alopecia with all areas of the scalp showing some thinning of the hair. Patterned hair loss implies that the area of alopecia is confined to one or several portions of the scalp, leaving at least a portion of the scalp uninvolved. For example, this is usually the case for alopecia areata and trichotillomania.

The various patterns of hair loss are listed at the end of this chapter.

Androgenetic alopecia has been described as being both diffuse and patterned. Although on rare occasion the balding process seems to affect the entire scalp, including the occiput, in the vast majority of cases, the crown of the scalp (including frontal region and posterior vertex region) is predominantly involved. Therefore, the condition has a distinctive pattern of thinning (Fig. 7.2).

EVIDENCE OF HAIR BREAKAGE (HAIRS OF UNEVEN LENGTH)

Hair shaft disorders associated with hair fragility, such as trichorrhexis nodosa, tend to cause localized zones of alopecia containing hairs of uneven length (Fig. 7.3). When the hair is particularly fragile, as is true in monilethrix, patches of hair stubble will be found. In disorders caused by hair shaft fragility, the shaft defect is usually readily apparent under the light microscope. In trichotillomania, the patches of alopecia are seldom totally "bald." Usually there are short hairs of varying lengths scattered within the involved area.

EVIDENCE OF INFLAMMATION

Clinicians should examine the scalp surface in all cases of hair loss. Abnormalities may or may not be related to the hair loss

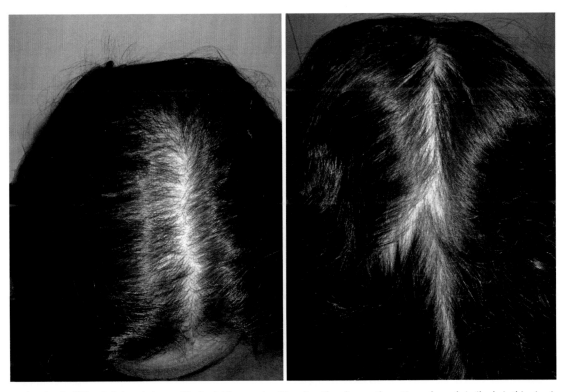

Figure 7.1 Example of truly diffuse hair loss (*telogen effluvium*). The part is widened uniformly over the entire scalp, and similar hair thinning is noted on the crown/vertex (*left panel*), occiput (*right panel*), and sides of the head.

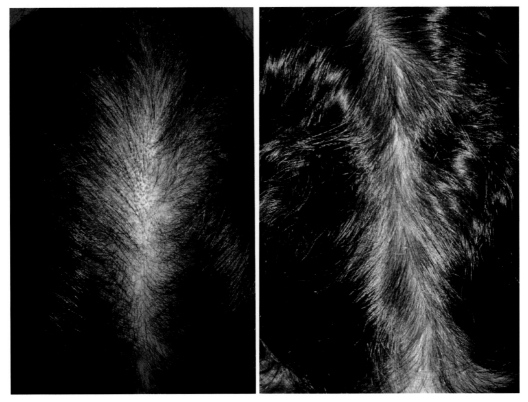

Figure 7.2 Example of patterned hair loss in a woman with *androgenetic alopecia*. The crown/vertex (*left panel*) is symmetrically affected with relative sparing of the occiput (*right panel*), as evidenced by the width of the part.

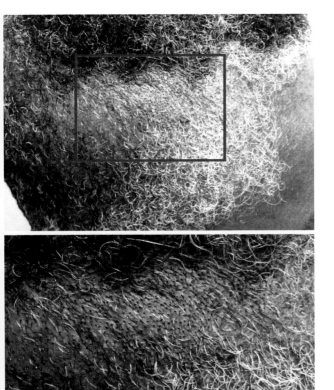

Figure 7.3 Dramatic hair thinning in a patient with severe *trichorrhexis nodosa* and hair fragility secondary to intractable scalp pruritus. Residual stubble (*lower panel*, a magnified view of boxed area in *upper panel*) shows that hair density remains normal.

but need to be documented. Erythema, pustules, follicular papules, and perifollicular scaling or hyperpigmentation suggest an inflammatory form of alopecia.

EVIDENCE OF PERMANENT HAIR LOSS AND OBLITERATION OF FOLLICULAR OSTIA

Wide spacing between follicles, clusters of shafts exiting single follicular ostia (polytrichia, "tufting," or "doll's hairs") and the obliteration of follicular openings are all signs of cicatricial alopecia. Follicular "plugging," with keratinaceous material filling dilated ostia devoid of hair shafts, can be another indication of follicular destruction, as seen in chronic cutaneous lupus erythematosus.

NORMAL *VS.* ABNORMAL HAIR DENSITY

Some patients have normal-appearing hair density (by all objective evidence) and yet complain of thinning or shedding. This can either represent mild or early telogen effluvium or, in some cases, the hair loss is more perceived than real. Marked erythema and scaling or numerous papular lesions *without* a loss of follicular density suggest a primary scalp (as opposed to hair) disorder. Seborrheic dermatitis, psoriasis, and Langerhans cell histiocytosis (histiocytosis X) of the scalp can cause dramatic scalp disease with little effect on hair density, although the latter two conditions can certainly cause hair loss in some cases.

Not uncommonly, the pathologist must render a diagnosis of "normal scalp," although the patient is being evaluated for hair loss. Some possible explanations for this discrepancy are as follows:

1. The area that was sampled may be in the recovery phase of a preexisting form of alopecia, such as a

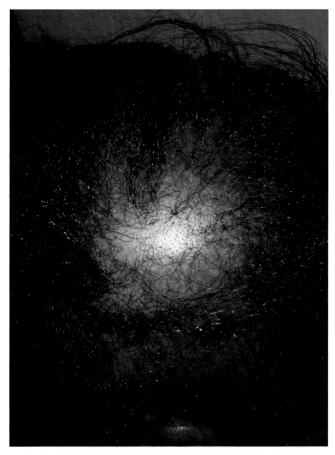

Figure 7.4 Truly diffuse hair loss in a patient with alopecia areata. Other causes include telogen effluvium, chemotherapy/radiation therapy, and congenital alopecia.

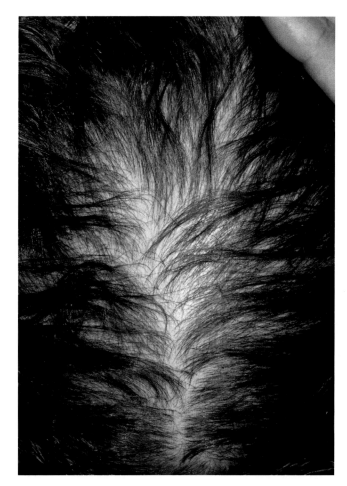

Figure 7.5 Androgenetic alopecia: diminished density over the crown/posterior vertex with relative sparing of parietal/occipital areas.

telogen effluvium or a patch of alopecia areata that is in the early stages of remission.

2. The findings may be so subtle as to be at or just below a diagnostic threshold, as might be found in very early androgenetic alopecia.
3. The problem may be a hair shaft disorder with external hair breakage.
4. The patient's concern about hair loss may be more perceived than real.
5. The clinician inadvertently biopsied normal scalp adjacent to a zone of alopecia.

Patterns of Hair Loss (examples in italics)

Truly diffuse hair loss—*telogen effluvium, alopecia totalis in evolution, alopecia areata incognita, chemotherapy/radiation therapy, and congenital alopecia* (Fig. 7.4)

Diminished density over crown/posterior vertex with relative sparing of parietal/occipital—*androgenetic alopecia* (Fig. 7.5)

Nearly total hair loss centrally with obliteration of follicular ostia, centered on the central crown or posterior vertex—*central centrifugal cicatricial alopecia* (Fig. 7.6)

Patches of hair loss with bizarre or geometric shapes—*trichotillomania* (Fig. 7.7)

Randomly scattered, roughly oval, or polycyclic patches of nearly complete hair loss (with little or no inflammation)—*alopecia areata* (Fig. 7.8)

"Moth-eaten": Randomly scattered oval or circular patches of *incomplete* hair loss (with little or no inflammation)—*secondary syphilis* (Fig. 7.9)

Zones of partial or complete hair loss with loss of follicular openings and shiny skin surface—*cicatricial alopecia, all types* (Fig. 7.10)

Randomly scattered, irregularly shaped patches of partial or complete hair loss (with inflammation)—*lichen planopilaris* (Fig. 7.11)

Marked thinning of both frontotemporal regions—*burnt-out traction alopecia* (Fig. 7.12)

Small, geometric patches of diminished hair density of the anterior margin of the temple (unilateral or bilateral)—*temporal triangular alopecia* (Fig. 7.13)

Irregularly or geometrically shaped, variably atrophic and hypopigmented, well-demarcated plaques of hairless skin which may be clustered—*Brocq's alopecia pattern* (Fig. 7.14)

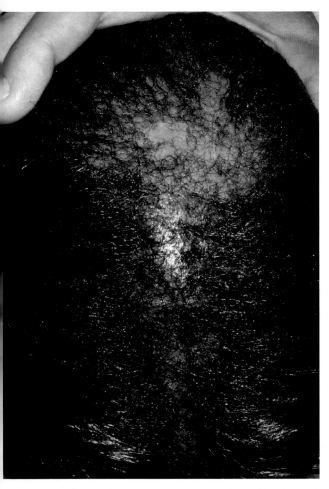

Figure 7.6 Central, centrifugal, cicatricial alopecia: nearly total hair loss with obliteration of follicular ostia, centered on the central crown or posterior vertex.

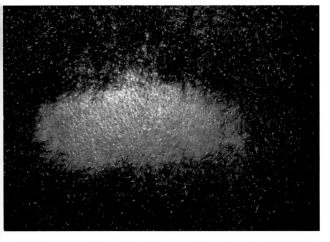

Figure 7.7 Trichotillomania: patches of hair loss with "bizarre" or geometric shapes.

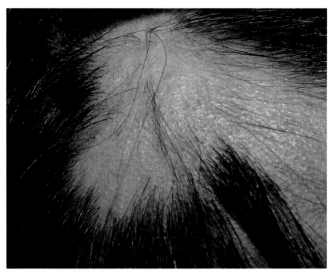

Figure 7.8 Alopecia areata: randomly scattered, roughly oval, or polycyclic patches of nearly complete hair loss with little or no inflammation.

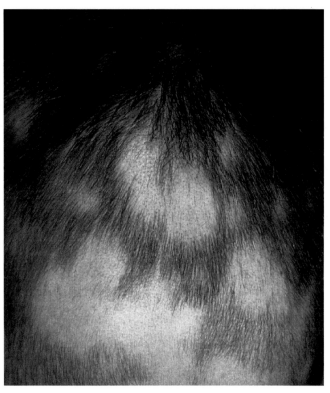

Figure 7.9 Secondary syphilis: "moth-eaten," randomly scattered oval or circular patches of *incomplete* hair loss with little or no inflammation.

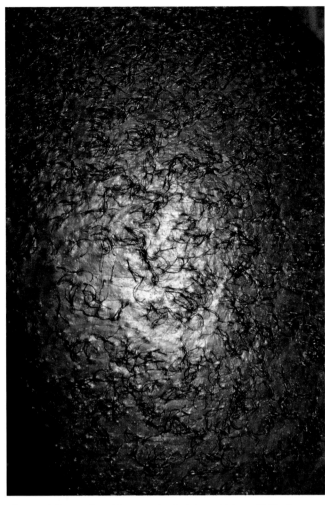

Figure 7.10 Zones of partial or complete hair loss with loss of follicular openings and a shiny skin surface can be seen in cicatricial alopecias of all types. This example is a case of *central, centrifugal, cicatricial alopecia*.

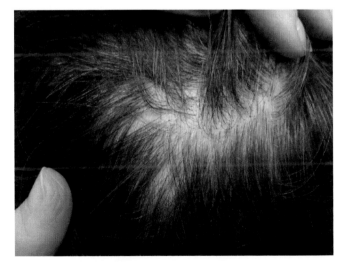

Figure 7.11 *Lichen planopilaris*: randomly scattered, irregularly shaped patches of partial or complete hair loss (with inflammation).

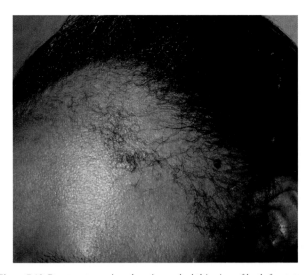

Figure 7.12 Burnt-out *traction alopecia*: marked thinning of both frontotemporal regions.

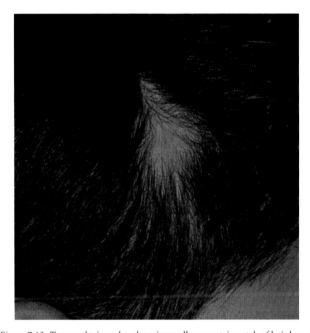

Figure 7.13 *Temporal triangular alopecia*: small, geometric patch of hair loss of anterior margin of temple (unilateral or bilateral).

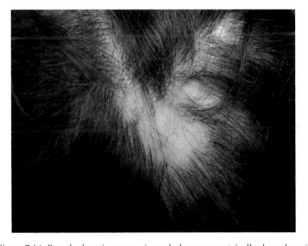

Figure 7.14 *Brocq's alopecia pattern*: irregularly or geometrically shaped, variably atrophic and hypopigmented, clustered, and well-demarcated plaques of hairless skin.

REFERENCES

1. Rietschel RL. A simplified approach to the diagnosis of alopecia. Dermatol Clin. 1996; 14: 691–5.
2. Sperling L. Evaluation of hair loss. Curr Probl Dermatol 1996; 8: 97–136.
3. Sperling LC. Hair and systemic disease. Dermatol Clin 2001; 19: 711–26, ix.

8   Senescent alopecia ("senile alopecia" or "senescent balding")

The diagnostic criteria for senescent balding, as enumerated by Kligman, are "(i) no family history of male pattern balding and (ii) decreased hair density that does not become apparent until after about age 50 years" (1).

CLINICAL FINDINGS

The typical person with senescent alopecia has normal-appearing hair density well into middle age and denies a family history of balding. Patients with senescent alopecia note a very slow but steady, diffuse, decreased density of scalp hair starting at age 50 years or more. The vast majority of such people attribute their hair loss to the aging process and do not seek medical care. Women who complain of a marked degree of decreased hair density in the few years following menopause probably have a component of androgenetic alopecia. Many (and perhaps most) patients with senescent alopecia also have mild concomitant androgenetic alopecia, and the superimposed clinical and histological features of common balding and senescent alopecia may be impossible to separate.

Several authors have assessed the effect of aging on hair density by studying the scalp surface (i.e., clinical rather than histological evaluation). The results of these studies suggest that the density of hair follicles and the average diameter of individual follicles decrease steadily with aging (2–6). There are no recent data (within the past 40 years) to confirm this, and in particular there have been no studies based on the histological evaluation of scalp biopsy specimens taken from a sufficiently large population of "normal" individuals of various ages. However, Whiting (7) has presented data on 852 patients (almost all female) with "diffuse alopecia," that is, without clinical evidence of androgenetic alopecia. When divided into age groups by decades (from 20–29 to 90–99), there was only a modest reduction in total hair numbers with time, with a 10% reduction (as compared with the youngest group) in the 70–79 group, and a 21% reduction in the 80–89 group. The data suggest that decreased hair density is not an inevitable consequence of aging, and noticeable hair loss should only be expected in the very elderly. However, the data were pooled and did not exclude the possibility of outliers, namely, those few patients whose decreased hair density occurred prematurely, for example, in the 6th or 7th decade of life.

It is this group of patients with prematurely decreased hair density that we label as having "senescent alopecia." The criteria listed by Kligman (see above) still apply. Other forms of alopecia must first be excluded before the diagnosis of senescent alopecia can be rendered.

HISTOLOGICAL FINDINGS

The global impression when studying transverse sections is that there is only a slight reduction in the overall number of otherwise normal follicles. Compared with normal (or youthful) scalp, more follicles are in the telogen phase, but the telogen count may still be within the normal range. Inflammation is uncommon, and fibrous streamers, such as those found in androgenetic alopecia, are absent or few in number. The follicles may not appear to be as long or as wide as expected, but miniaturization as seen in androgenetic alopecia is absent. All of these subtle findings are uniform over the scalp surface.

The following combination of histological findings (based on 4 mm punch biopsy specimens) is typical of senescent alopecia (8) (Figs. 8.1 and 8.2): (*i*) a slight decrease in the total

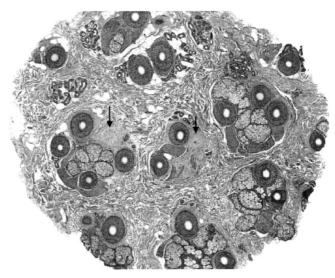

Figure 8.1 Senescent alopecia. The specimen is from a 65-year-old Caucasian woman with mild, diffuse, decreased density of hair. She described gradual hair loss over several years. The total hair count is at the lower end of the range of normal, and the size and follicular phase of hairs is normal. Two columns of connective tissue (*arrows*) indicate that there has been permanent dropout of at least a few terminal hairs.

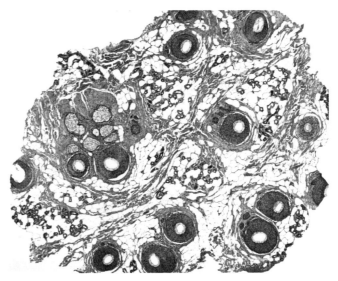

Figure 8.2 Senescent alopecia. The specimen is from a 70-year-old African-American woman with mild, diffuse, decreased density of hair with gradual hair loss over several years. The uniformity of terminal hair size, low telogen count, and absence of stelae exclude androgenetic alopecia and telogen effluvium. The lower end of the range of normal total hair count is typical of senescent alopecia.

number of hairs (20–35 as opposed to the normal 30–45 in a Caucasian individual); (*ii*) numbers of telogen hairs within the range of normal (less than 15%); (*iii*) a normal percentage of terminal hairs, with terminal hairs outnumbering vellus hairs by at least 2:1; and (*iv*) an absence of deep, perifollicular inflammation. With these findings, androgenetic alopecia can be excluded because of the relative preponderance of terminal hairs, and telogen effluvium is excluded by the normal number of telogen follicles. If crown/vertex and mid-occipital biopsy specimens from patients with senescent alopecia are compared, the histological findings will be similar at both sites. This contrasts with androgenetic alopecia, where any evidence of miniaturization of hairs will always be less dramatic on the occiput than at the vertex or crown.

Senescent Alopecia in Summary

Clinical correlation: an elderly person who admits to very gradual decreased hair density; on examination, hair density appears normal (for age) or diminished diffusely over the entire scalp. There is not a patterned distribution to the hair loss.

Histological findings
- ❖ Findings from the crown/vertex resemble those found on the occipital scalp
- ❖ In advanced disease, the *total* number of hairs is reduced
- ❖ Terminal: vellus hair ratio and telogen count remain normal

Histological differential diagnosis:
- **Normal scalp**: the specimen may appear entirely normal, and so a definitive diagnosis of senescent alopecia is impossible to make on a purely histological basis. Clinical correlation is required.
- **External hair breakage**: as can be seen with hair shaft disorders or weathering
- **Androgenetic alopecia**: in its earliest prediagnostic stage

REFERENCES

1. Kligman AM. The comparative histopathology of male-pattern baldness and senescent baldness. Clin Dermatol. 1988; 6: 108–18.
2. Pecoraro V, Astore I, Barman JM. Growth rate and hair density of the human axilla. A. Comparative study of normal males and females and pregnant and post-partum females. J Invest Dermatol 1971; 56: 362–5.
3. Barman J, Astore I, Pecoraro B. The normal trichogram of people over 50 years but apparently not bald. In: Montagna W, Dobson R, eds. Advances in Biology of the Skin. Vol. 9. New York: Pergamon Press; 1967: 211–20.
4. Giacometti L. The anatomy of the human scalp. In: Montagna M, ed. Advances in Biology of Skin. Vol. 6. New York: Appleton-Century-Crofts; 1965: 97–110.
5. Barman J, Astore I, Pecoraro V. The normal trichogram of the adult. J Invest Dermatol. 1965; 44: 233–6.
6. Hordinsky M, Sawaya M, Roberts JL. Hair loss and hirsutism in the elderly. Clin Geriatr Med. 2002; 18: 121–33, vii.
7. Whiting DA. How real is senescent alopecia? A histopathologic approach. Clin Dermatol. 2010; 29: 49–53.
8. Sperling LC, Lupton GP. Histopathology of non-scarring alopecia. J Cutan Pathol. 1995; 22: 97–114.

9 Androgenetic alopecia

Androgenetic alopecia (AGA) is an encompassing term for hair loss that typically begins in adult life, gradually assumes a characteristic "male" or "female" pattern, and is mediated by the action of androgens on genetically susceptible hair follicles (1,2). The term "androgenetic," introduced by Orentreich in 1960 and championed by Ludwig, is an etymological hybrid of the last two qualities noted above (3). Through the years AGA has been known as common balding, hereditary balding, and male pattern balding. Some authors advocate the use of the term "female pattern hair loss" (FPHL) in women (1,4–6). Because the histopathology of the male and female conditions is identical, the term AGA has been used in this chapter.

AGA is the most common cause of human hair loss (7–9). Many authors believe the process to be a normal biological phenomenon rather than a disease (2). Regardless of how it is classified, some individuals with AGA perceive it as abnormal or psychosocially unacceptable and consequently seek a definitive diagnosis and therapeutic intervention (10).

In 400 BC, Hippocrates first noted that neither eunuchs nor children became bald (8). Others noted that males castrated before puberty did not develop AGA unless administered testosterone (11). In a seminal work in 1942, Hamilton was the first to make the definitive link between androgens and AGA (2,12). The work that followed focused on the conversion of testosterone to dihydrotestosterone (DHT) by the enzyme 5α-reductase type II (5αR-II) (13). Hair follicles of men and women with AGA have increased levels of 5αR-II (6). DHT formed from the action of 5αR-II on testosterone binds to the androgen receptor (AR) located in the outer root sheath and follicular papillae of hair follicles (14,15). The hormone–receptor complex then activates genes responsible for the gradual transformation of large, terminal follicles to small, miniaturized ones (6).

Besides this mechanism, women harbor an additional enzyme that may modulate the effects of androgens on the hair follicle (14). Cytochrome p450 aromatase (AROM) acts by converting androgens to estrogens (14). This enzyme, which is present in trivial amounts in men, may contribute to the differing propensities and patterns of AGA observed in women (6).

The pattern observed in AGA is thought to be dictated by the distribution of enzymes and enzyme receptors within the hair follicles of the scalp (6,11,16). It is known that the dermis of the frontal/parietal scalp is of neural crest origin, whereas the dermis of the occipital scalp is of mesodermal origin (6). These differing embryologic origins may be the key to understanding why follicles in one part of the scalp are particularly susceptible to androgen effects, and others seem to be immune to them. Both young men and women have more 5αR (types I and II) and AR in frontal hair follicles than in occipital follicles, with levels in women being about half those seen in men (6,15). The "protective" enzyme AROM is much higher in the frontal follicles of women than men, and even higher in the occipital follicles of women (6).

Ultimately, the signaling described above leads to the activation of genes. Several lines of inquiry have proved that the propensity to develop AGA is polygenic and not Mendelian (6,17). In general, sons of fathers who have no alopecia are at a low risk for hair loss themselves (18). Risk increases in men with a positive maternal grandfather history and even more so in men with a history of paternal alopecia (18). Twenty percent of males with AGA have no family history of balding (19). Women with AGA are less likely than men with AGA to have a history of first-degree relatives with male pattern hair loss (19). Twin studies identified heredity as accounting for an estimated 80% of the predisposition to baldness (20).

Besides the gender and genetic risk factors noted above, disorders that lead to the overproduction of androgens, or the exogenous administration of androgens, may also trigger or worsen AGA. Some of the described scenarios include polycystic ovary syndrome (21), postmenopausal ovarian hyperthecosis (22), and administration of adrenocorticotropic hormone (23).

CLINICAL FINDINGS

AGA is extremely common. By age 30 years, 30% of men are affected (24). By age 50 years, 50% of men and 40% of women have signs of AGA (6,24–27). The hair thinning begins between the ages of 12 and 40 years in both sexes (6). The frequency and severity of AGA increase with age in both sexes, with females lagging behind males by a decade (19). In females, AGA reaches its peak after age 50 years or perimenopausally (16,28). AGA in females is less severe than in males, and never progresses to full baldness (6,11,15,16). Racial differences can also be detected in AGA. Caucasian men are four times more likely than African-American men to develop premature balding (24). Asian and Native American populations also have a decreased propensity for AGA compared with caucasians (7,19).

The typical "male" pattern of AGA begins with recession of the frontal hairline. This is followed by thinning over the vertex of the scalp leading to a bald spot that gradually enlarges, eventually merging with the frontal recession (Fig. 9.1). In time only the marginal parietal and occipital hair remains (19,29,30). Sparse hairs below (anterior to) the frontal hairline are an early sign of AGA in men (31).

The "female" pattern also demonstrates thinning throughout the frontoparietal scalp, but typically without frontal hairline recession (Figs. 9.2 and 9.3) (6,11,16,19,32). Typically, there is widening of the central part at the frontal scalp, creating the so-called Christmas tree pattern (6,16,19,32). The "tree" is broadest anteriorly, tapering toward the vertex of the scalp. In this zone the hair is miniaturized (and therefore of finer caliber) and will not grow as long (16). The part width of the occipital scalp is unaffected and serves as a "normal control" for the patient's baseline part width.

There is considerable overlap between the male and female patterns. Infrequently males will present with the female pattern

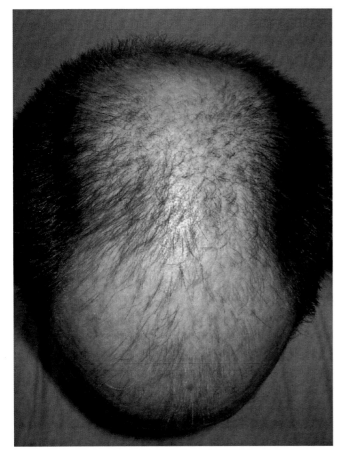

Figure 9.1 The typical "male" pattern of AGA begins with recession of the frontal hairline and continues with thinning over the vertex of the scalp leading to a bald spot that gradually enlarges to merge with the frontal recession.

Table 9.1 Test Recommendations in the Workup of Female AGA

Total testosterone
Free testosterone
Dehydroepiandrosterone sulfate
Prolactin
When indicated, other assays for androgen excess (1,9,10)

unremarkable, especially early in the course. Follicular ostia may become smaller with time, and eventually may not be clinically detectable (30).

In men, the clinical pattern of typical AGA is characteristic, and no further testing needs to be done unless the history seems incompatible with the physical findings. In women, a careful history is recommended. Any history of menstrual irregularity, infertility, galactorrhea, or physical findings suggesting hirsutism, severe cystic acne, virilization, or acanthosis nigricans should be further evaluated with laboratory studies (1,10). While specific test recommendations vary from author to author, the most commonly used in the workup of female AGA are listed in Table 9.1 (1,9). Most women with AGA have normal menses and pregnancies and normal androgen levels (6,16,19). In adolescents and young girls, assessment for hyperandrogenemia is worthwhile. In adolescent and young boys with FPHL and/or with aberrant pubertal development, laboratory evaluation is also recommended (1).

The clinical differential for AGA includes many causes of noncicatricial alopecia and early manifestations of some cicatricial alopecias (19). The most challenging, chronic telogen effluvium, manifests as sudden hair shedding without evidence of miniaturization or widening of the central part (32). A positive hair pull test in areas not typically affected by AGA is characteristic (34). Other diagnoses are generally resolvable via biopsy and a focused clinical history.

Specific therapy aims to promote hair regrowth and slow further thinning. All medical therapies may need to be used indefinitely to maintain their effects. The therapeutic response is slow and a minimum 6- to 12-month trial should be anticipated. The maximal treatment benefit might take years (11). A comparison between specific therapies is hampered by the difficulties in achieving a completely objective method for measurement of therapeutic response (38). In addition, large scale, randomized, double-blinded, placebo-controlled studies are difficult to conduct in this setting.

While an exhaustive discussion of available therapies is beyond the scope of this chapter, several commonly used strategies are briefly discussed in the following sections.

Finasteride

Finasteride is an orally administered inhibitor of 5αR-II, and thus reduces the conversion of testosterone to the more potent DHT (11). Large clinical studies in men with mild-to-moderate AGA demonstrated increased hair growth and slowing of progression of hair loss. The response was most efficacious at the vertex (11,27). It has not shown efficacy in postmenopausal women (27) and is not recommended for use in women who may become pregnant. It has not been tested in the adolescent population (9).

(24) and females will present with the male pattern (16,19). The latter scenario is more common in postmenopausal women (16). A third, rarely described pattern of AGA diffusely involves the scalp (including hairs of the occiput) (33). In these cases, histologic confirmation may be required to establish the diagnosis with certainty, as there can be overlap with telogen effluvium. The possibility of superimposed telogen effluvium may be suspected with a patient history of recent increased shedding, a complaint not typically ascribed to AGA (6).

A hair pull test may be useful in delineating the areas of active disease. To do this, the examiner grasps about 20 hairs in the affected area between the thumb and forefinger and tugs with gentle but firm pressure from their proximal to distal ends. Some authors feel that removal of more than six hairs indicates a "positive" pull test (9). Our experience with AGA suggests that pull tests are usually "negative" (0–3 hairs extracted per pull), but if positive, should only be so on the top of the scalp (34). If positive diffusely (including the occipital scalp), superimposed telogen effluvium should be considered (19).

Variably sized hairs with evidence of miniaturization are the hallmark of AGA in both males and females (6). Dermoscopy has been advocated as a noninvasive method for detecting hair diameter diversity (35), termed "anisotrichosis" (36). One group identified anisotrichosis as the most accurate early clinical sign of AGA (37). The presence of short and fine (miniaturized) hairs aside, the appearance of the scalp is typically

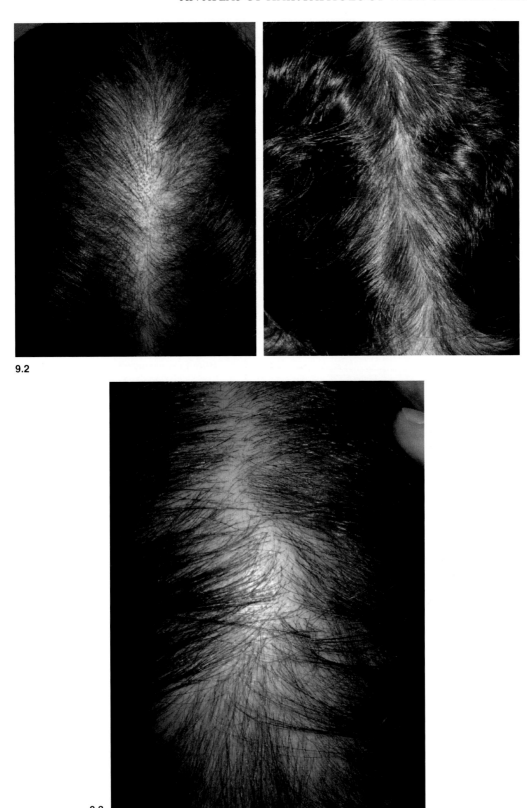

Figures 9.2 and 9.3 The "female" pattern of AGA is characterized by widening of the frontal part width, creating the so-called Christmas tree pattern. The "tree" (the part) is broadest anteriorly, tapering toward the vertex scalp. The part width of the occipital scalp (Fig. 9.2, right panel) is unaffected and serves as a "normal control" for the patient's baseline part width.

Minoxidil (topical)

The mechanism of action of minoxidil is not known (11). Minoxidil has its greatest effect in less severe early presentations of AGA primarily involving the crown and parietal regions. The frontotemporal region usually responds poorly to treatment (11). Cosmetically acceptable hair growth is noted in 20% of cases at 4 months, but all beneficial effects disappear within months of discontinuing therapy (11). In general, women respond better than men to minoxidil. A retrospective review of adolescents treated with minoxidil revealed favorable responses in 95% (9). Patients should be warned of a limited effluvium that frequently occurs due to the initiation or discontinuation of minoxidil (see chap. 10 for further information).

Systemic Hormonal Therapy
Cyclic estrogens combined with low androgenic progestins could be considered in women with AGA already on or considering oral contraceptives (11). Minoxidil may be combined with hormonal therapy (11).

Antiandrogen Therapy
Agents such as cyproterone acetate, flutamide, and spironolactone cause unacceptable feminization in men, but may be useful in selected cases of female AGA (39).

Dutasteride
Dutasteride is an orally administered inhibitor of $5\alpha R$ types I and II currently approved by the US FDA for benign prostatic hypertrophy. A phase II study has shown efficacy in AGA (40).

Surgical Micrografting
Hair transplantation involves removal of hair from the occipital scalp and re-implantation into the balding vertex and frontal scalp. After relocation, the follicle retains characteristics of its native site; hence, occipital follicles relocated to the vertex tend to be resistant to the effects of AGA (2). In the hands of an experienced surgeon, this technique may yield excellent results. Prerequisites for the procedure are stabilization of the hair loss with medical treatment prior to surgery and a suitable donor hair population on the occiput (39).

Camouflage
There are a variety of techniques and products that hide or obscure clinical hair loss. In many cases, these may be appropriate options (10).

It is important to explain to patients what they may expect in terms of continuing hair loss and response to any considered therapy. Foregoing medical treatment may be an appropriate strategy for some patients (10).

HISTOLOGICAL FINDINGS
The diagnosis of AGA is usually made from the history and clinical findings alone (1,10). In males, a biopsy is helpful when the pattern is diffuse or resembles female AGA, or, when there are changes suggestive of cicatricial alopecia (1,19). In females, a biopsy may be helpful when trying to exclude cicatricial alopecia, diffuse alopecia areata, and telogen effluvium (19).

The diagnostic specimens of choice are paired 4 mm punch biopsies from both involved (e.g., vertex or frontal) and uninvolved (usually occipital) regions of the scalp. A comparison of follicular size and number in the two specimens will allow for a definitive diagnosis (Fig. 9.4). In sufficiently advanced disease, a single biopsy from involved skin will also demonstrate diagnostic features (41). AGA was once considered a histological diagnosis of exclusion. The diagnostic "breakthrough" was the study of transverse (horizontal) sections of scalp biopsies, a technique popularized through the efforts of Headington

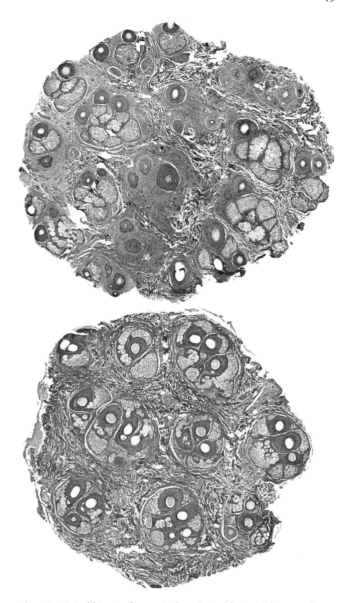

Figure 9.4 Paired biopsies from a single patient with AGA. The upper image reveals a normal number of follicles with variability in follicular size, scant patchy inflammation, and a slight catagen/telogen shift compared with the lower image from the unaffected occipital scalp.

and others (42). Since the microscopic diagnosis of AGA depends more on *quantitative* than *qualitative* features, the ability to identify all follicles within a biopsy specimen is required to establish the diagnosis. The Headington technique is ideally suited to this evaluation as it allows the assessment of all follicles at several levels throughout the scalp (42).

AGA, whether in males or females, is characterized by a gradual reduction in the duration of the anagen (growth) phase, coupled with follicular miniaturization (Fig. 9.5) over successive cycles (19,43). As follicular growth cycles are asynchronous, and follicles are not affected equally by AGA, miniaturized follicles will be randomly scattered at first. A biopsy will reveal a mix of hairs with various bulb depths and shaft diameters (Figs. 9.6–9.9). Ordinarily, the bulbs of full size (terminal) hairs reside in the subcutaneous fat (Figs. 9.10–9.14). Terminal follicles produce a hair shaft greater than 0.06 mm in diameter and thicker than the follicle's inner root sheath (IRS) (19). With progressive shortening of the duration of anagen, affected follicles spend proportionately more time in the catagen/telogen

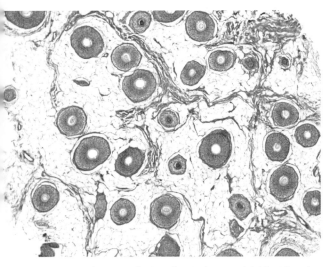

Figure 9.5 Horizontal section of AGA taken in the superficial fat. There is a marked variability in follicular size.

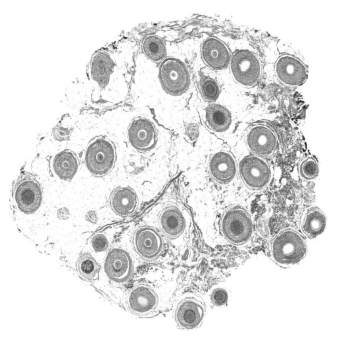

Figure 9.7 Horizontal section of the same case imaged in Fig. 9.6 taken at the superficial subcutaneous fat. Twenty-eight follicles as well as 8 stelae were identified. This suggests there were 36 terminal follicles overall, with 13 vellus follicles captured only in the superficial dermis. The 8 stelae can be tracked superficially to the base of miniaturized hairs whose bulbs reside in the dermis.

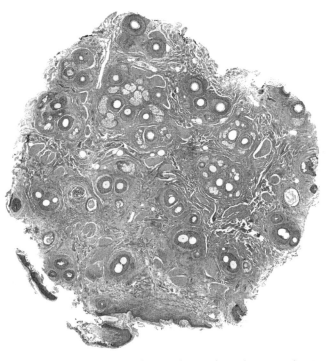

Figure 9.6 Horizontal section of AGA taken in the mid-to-upper dermis. There are normal number of follicles (approximately 49 visible in this image) with diminished sebaceous lobule size and solar elastosis.

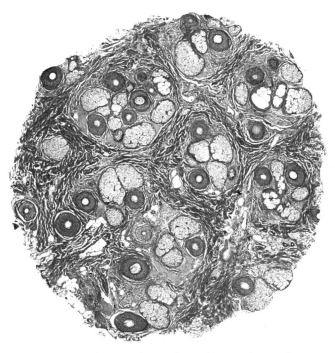

Figure 9.8 Horizontal section of AGA taken in the upper dermis. There are a normal number of follicles (approximately 27 visible in this image) with normal sebaceous lobules and no inflammation.

phase (2). Subsequent anagen phases fail to achieve the bulb depth of the preceding generation. In addition, the mesenchymal papilla, thought to influence the size of the follicular bulb and ultimately the diameter of the shaft itself, becomes smaller with successive growth cycles (2,8). Besides the narrowing of the shaft diameter (Fig. 9.15) and the diminished time spent lengthening, the hair shafts become progressively less pigmented, appearing nearly invisible at the scalp surface; some never emerge from the follicular ostium before returning to catagen phase (8,44).

Histologically, follicular miniaturization can be identified by follicular bulbs present in the mid-to-deep dermis, hair shafts thinner than their IRS, and shafts narrower than 0.06 mm. As terminal hairs cycle into catagen phase, the lower third of the

hair follicle (deep to the bulge zone) (45,46) involutes and the follicular papilla follows the involuting epithelium into the mid-dermis trailed by a ribbon of fibrovascular tissue known as a streamer or stela (Fig. 9.16). These stelae are easily identified in horizontal sections, marking the site of a terminal follicle that has cycled into catagen/telogen phase or of a miniaturized follicle (45). Identifying stelae does not necessarily indicate that miniaturization has taken place; however, the

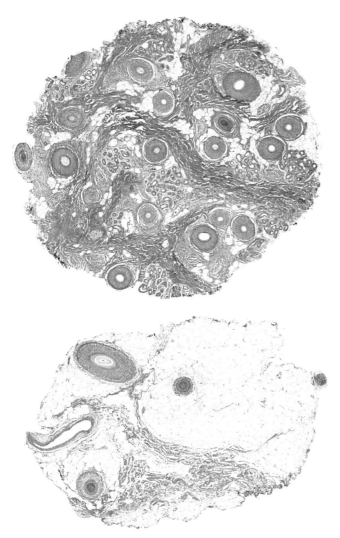

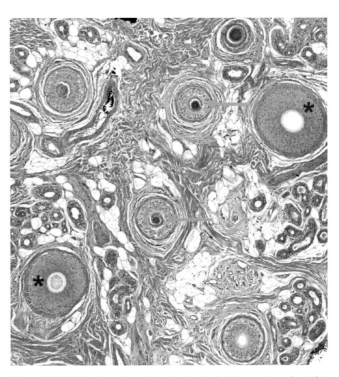

Figure 9.10 AGA horizontally sectioned at the level of the eccrine coils. At this level, any narrow caliber hairs (green arrows) must be miniaturized, as the bulbs of true vellus follicles do not reach this depth. Two normal-sized terminal follicles are marked with blue asterisks for comparison. Also present are two stelae that belong to other miniaturized follicles residing more superficially in the dermis.

Figure 9.9 Horizontal sections of the same specimen imaged in Fig. 9.8 taken at the mid-to-deep dermis (upper image) and subcutaneous fat (lower image). Seventeen follicles and 10 stelae were identified. Very few terminal bulbs actually reside in the subcutis.

discovery of many such stelae in the same specimen does indicate that a large proportion of follicles have shifted into the catagen/telogen phase, a finding commonly encountered in alopecias characterized by follicular miniaturization. Using successive horizontal sections it is possible to trace individual stelae from the subcutis superficially to the base of either a terminal catagen/telogen follicle or a miniaturized anagen follicle, thus establishing whether miniaturization is indeed present (Figs. 9.17–9.20) (30,41,45). Hair shafts less than the 0.06 mm diameter of terminal hairs, but greater than the 0.03 mm diameter of vellus hairs are termed "indeterminate" hairs (see chap. 3 for more information).

When one examines a specimen from a normal scalp sectioned transversely through the lower dermis, one gets the global impression that almost all hairs are terminal hairs of similar diameter. The normal ratio of terminal:vellus hairs (T:V ratio) should be at least 2:1, and authors who include indeterminate hairs in the terminal count will of course record higher ratios, such as 4:1 or greater. Specimens diagnostic of AGA show a reduction in this ratio. One study found a mean T:V of 2.3:1 in patients with AGA (compared with normal controls with a T:V ratio of 7:1) (46). Others have measured

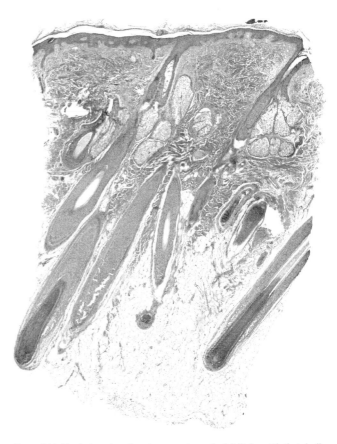

Figure 9.11 Vertical section showing several terminal follicles with their bulbs in the subcutis.

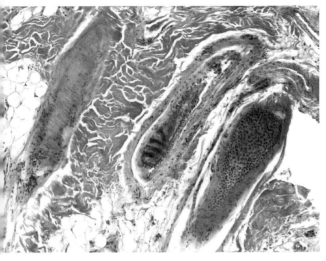

Figure 9.12 Higher magnification of Fig. 9.11 showing a miniaturized follicle with its bulb in the dermis. The findings are consistent with early AGA.

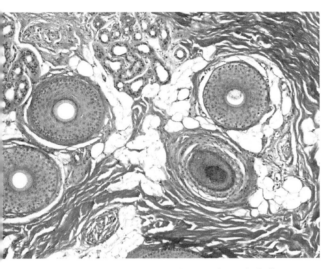

Figure 9.13 Horizontal section of AGA with two stelae and a bulb present at the level of eccrine coils. The presence of a follicular bulb at this level indicates the presence of miniaturization.

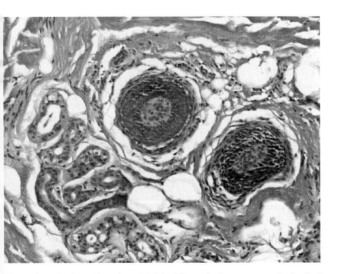

Figure 9.14 Horizontal section of AGA with two bulbs present at the level of an eccrine coil. The presence of follicular bulbs at this level indicates there is miniaturization.

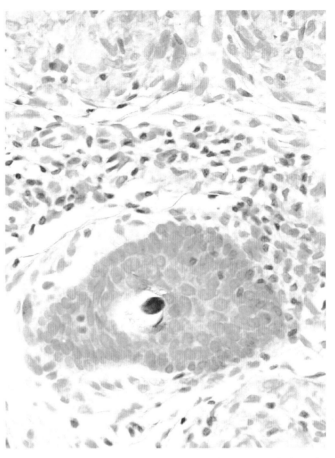

Figure 9.15 Hair shafts stain with the acid fast Ziehl–Neelsen method, a technique available in most histopathology laboratories. This technique may help identify markedly narrowed hair shafts.

the normal T:V ratio as being between 6:1 and 8:1 (47), with severe AGA measuring less than 4:1 (43). In advanced cases, the number of vellus and indeterminate hairs will actually *surpass* the number of terminal hairs. Early in the course of AGA, the *number* of follicles present remains normal (41). In very longstanding AGA, however, there is an actual decrease in follicular density as well as follicular size (19). AGA therefore shows a *biphasic* pattern of hair loss and may eventually resemble cicatricial alopecia.

Unlike most end-stage alopecias, sebaceous lobules are spared until very late in the course of AGA, appearing relatively more prominent than the miniaturized follicles to which they are attached (Figs. 9.21 and 9.22). Many observers have indicated sebaceous lobules are enlarged in AGA (30,46), while still others have suggested they are unchanged or even reduced in number (48). In late AGA the entire folliculosebaceous unit diminishes to the point that the resultant hair shaft is clinically not apparent either due to its small caliber and lack of pigmentation or due to its failure to emerge from the follicular ostium. At this stage the sebaceous lobules and follicles are markedly smaller than in a normal scalp, and the spacing between individual follicular units is quite marked (Figs. 9.23 and 9.24). In fair-skinned individuals, longstanding AGA often shows solar elastosis in the interfollicular areas due to ineffectual sun protection by the widely spaced, hypopigmented, and thinned shafts (Fig. 9.25).

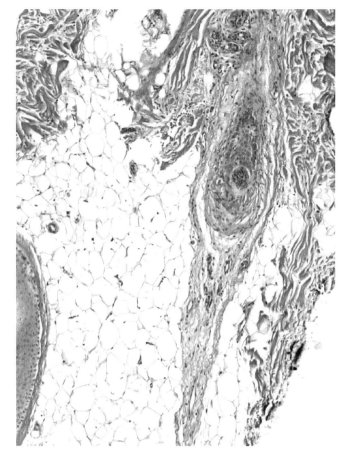

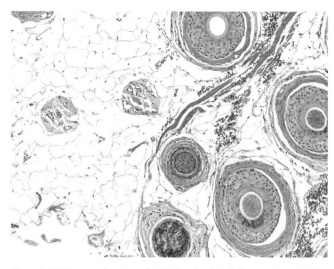

Figure 9.18 Horizontal section of AGA showing hair follicular size variability and two adjacent stelae. Note: the stelae contain grey staining elastic material and small caliber blood vessels.

Figure 9.16 This vertically sectioned biopsy of AGA shows a follicular stela (streamer) that tracks upward to the bulb of a miniaturized hair follicle located at the dermal-subcutaneous junction.

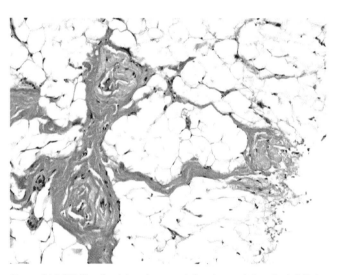

Figure 9.19 "Old" stelae lying dormant below long-miniaturized follicles tend to be amphophilic and relatively avascular, compared with "young" stelae (Fig. 9.20).

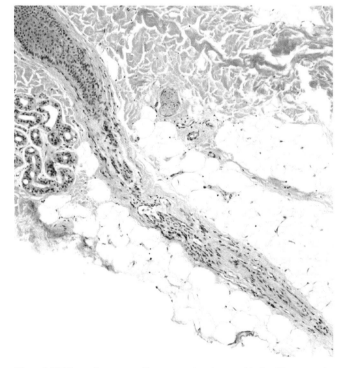

Figure 9.17 The stela acts as a fibroconnective tissue guide (and becomes the new fibrous root sheath) for the follicle once it re-enters the anagen phase.

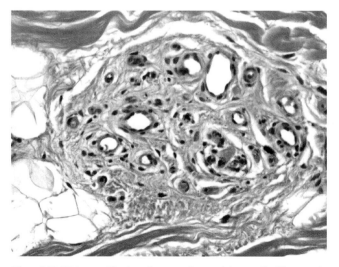

Figure 9.20 High magnification of a new stela containing small caliber vessels.

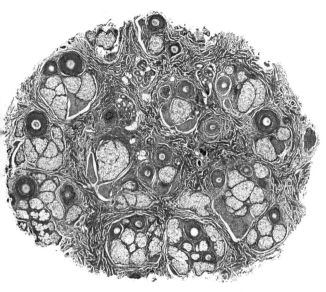

Figure 9.21 Scanning image of AGA sectioned at the sebaceous lobules demonstrating preserved full size sebaceous lobules, and two catagen-shifted follicles at the left edge. The eccrine coils present in the upper half of the image indicate the section was probably cut on a slight bias.

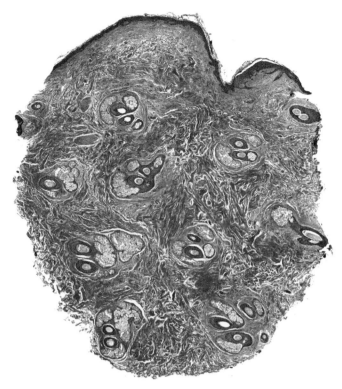

Figure 9.23 Scanning image of AGA at the level of the sebaceous glands. The folliculosebaceous structures are diminished overall, leaving large uniform gaps of dermis between them. No significant inflammation is apparent.

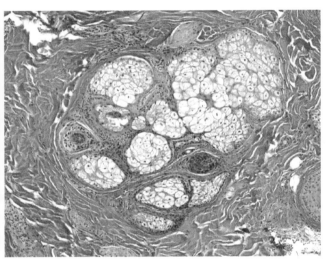

Figure 9.22 A folliculosebaceous unit in a patient with AGA showing prominent sebaceous lobules with small follicular epithelia.

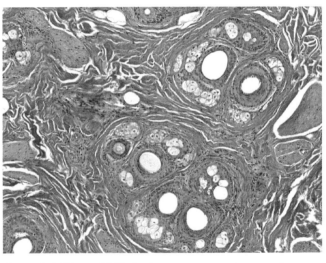

Figure 9.24 Well-spaced folliculosebaceous structures demonstrating somewhat atrophic sebaceous lobules in AGA.

Another measure of the severity of AGA is the anagen:telogen ratio. As hairs miniaturize, the average anagen phase becomes shorter. Therefore, the balding scalp shows an increase in the telogen count (the percentage of terminal hairs in the telogen phase), since miniaturized hairs spend a greater proportion of each hair cycle in the telogen phase (30,41). The telogen count can be based on the trichogram, in which only terminal hairs are sampled, or on a scalp biopsy, in which only terminal hairs are included in the calculation (41). A normal telogen count is approximately 5%–10% and values of 15%–20% are commonly encountered in AGA (19). In well-established AGA, the majority of telogen follicles will be miniaturized follicles.

Inflammation, seen histologically, has been reported in cases of AGA, however, it is not a consistent feature and has not been clearly associated with its pathogenesis. Many biopsy specimens of AGA show mild, perifollicular, lymphohistiocytic, upper dermal inflammation, sometimes associated with mild perifollicular

fibrosis (Fig. 9.25) (26,30,34,46,48–50). These changes are not only subtle and nonspecific, but also can be found in many normal scalp specimens (41). Mild, peri-infundibular chronic inflammation is especially common in African-American women and can be regarded as normal. Peribulbar or destructive inflammation is absent in common balding.

Two additional features are noteworthy. In 1972, Hori *et al.* found a reduction in the thickness of the epidermis, dermis, and subcutaneous tissue in advanced AGA ranging from 24% to 44% compared with normal skin (51). A subsequent study identified reductions in dermal thickness thought to be secondary to the loss of hair follicular volume *versus* the loss

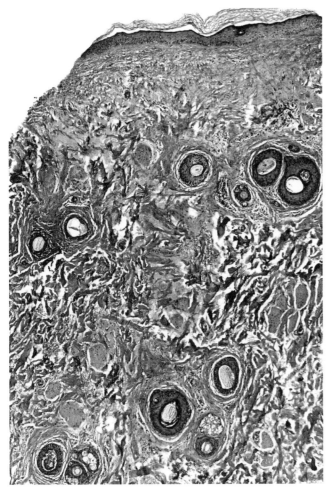

Figure 9.25 Diminished folliculosebaceous structures and solar elastosis are features of longstanding AGA.

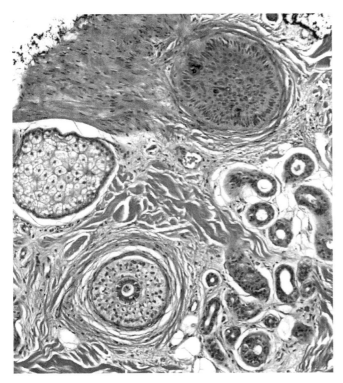

Figure 9.26 This image of AGA shows eccrine coils adjacent to sebaceous lobules, a finding suggestive of some degree of dermal atrophy. In addition, there is a small follicle adjacent to an eccrine coil, supporting miniaturization. Lastly, there is a follicle that has shifted to catagen phase (*top*).

of the dermal connective tissue itself (Fig. 9.26) (48). Finally, in 1978 Pinkus identified remnants of successively arranged Arao–Perkins bodies in fibrous streamers using elastic staining on vertically sectioned specimens (52). Experience has shown that obtaining a section with this serendipitous alignment is likely very challenging indeed, and although interesting, it is not a practical matter given the many easily accessible features of AGA outlined above.

Androgenetic Alopecia in Summary

Clinical correlation: symmetric thinning, predominantly affecting crown, vertex, and frontal regions, with relative sparing of the occiput; no evidence of scarring. "Christmas tree pattern" of a widened frontal part is a useful finding in female patients. Family history of balding usually elicited.

Histological findings:
❖ Normal total number of follicles [about 35 (Caucasian) or 20 (African-American) per 4 mm punch biopsy] when counted at the superficial dermis
❖ Reduced number of hairs (mixture of terminal and indeterminate) when counted at the dermal/fat junction (i.e., miniaturization), a T:V ratio of 2:1 or less is typical of AGA
❖ Presence of fibrous "streamers" below miniaturized hairs
❖ Slightly increased telogen count when compared with "unaffected" scalp (values of 15%–20% are typical)
❖ Sebaceous lobules preserved but may be reduced in size
❖ No significant inflammation
• Solar elastosis in well-established cases
• Variable dermal atrophy

Histological differential diagnosis:
• **Chronic telogen effluvium**: shares the preservation of folliculosebaceous structures, increased telogen count, mild nonspecific inflammation, and presence of stele, but lacks miniaturization
• **Alopecia areata**: shares the preservation of folliculosebaceous structures and miniaturization with stele but shows a much more marked catagen/telogen shift (50%–100%) with occasional "nanogen" hairs and, in early-active disease, peribulbar lymphocytic inflammation
• **Fibrosing alopecia in a pattern distribution**: shares the clinical pattern and all of the histologic features of AGA, but also shows focal interface dermatitis in a lichenoid pattern with loss of folliculosebaceous structures (follicular scars)

⚠ **Pitfalls**
Early changes of AGA may be unmasked by sudden new onset telogen effluvium. Paired biopsies from both involved (e.g., frontal or crown) and normal-appearing (e.g., occipital) scalp may be required to evaluate for the presence of one (or both) of the two diseases.

REFERENCES

1. Gonzalez ME, Cantatore-Francis J, Orlow SJ. Androgenetic alopecia in the paediatric population: a retrospective review of 57 patients. Br J Dermatol 2010; 163: 378–85.
2. Jahoda CA. Cellular and developmental aspects of androgenetic alopecia. Exp Dermatol 1998; 7: 235–48.
3. Ludwig E. Androgenetic alopecia. Arch Dermatol 1977; 113: 109.
4. Olsen EA, Hordinsky M, Roberts JL, Whiting DA. Female pattern hair loss. J Am Acad Dermatol 2002; 47: 795.
5. Norwood OT, Lehr B. Female androgenetic alopecia: a separate entity. Dermatol Surg 2000; 26: 679–82.
6. Price VH. Androgenetic alopecia in women. J Investig Dermatol Symp Proc 2003; 8: 24–7.
7. Kim BJ, Kim JY, Eun HC, et al. Androgenetic alopecia in adolescents: a report of 43 cases. J Dermatol 2006; 33: 696–9.
8. Whiting DA. Male pattern hair loss: current understanding. Int J Dermatol 1998; 37: 561–6.
9. Bedocs LA, Bruckner AL. Adolescent hair loss. Curr Opin Pediatr 2008; 20: 431–5.
10. Drake LA, Dinehart SM, Farmer ER, et al. Guidelines of care for androgenetic alopecia. American Academy of Dermatology. J Am Acad Dermatol 1996; 35: 465–9.
11. Sullivan JR, Kossard S. Acquired scalp alopecia. Part II: A review. Australas J Dermatol 1999; 40: 61–70; quiz 71–62.
12. Hamilton J. Male hormone stimulation is prerequisite and an incident in common baldness. Am J Anat. 1942; 71: 451–80.
13. Imperato-McGinley J, Guerrero L, Gautier T, Peterson RE. Steroid 5alpha-reductase deficiency in man: an inherited form of male pseudohermaphroditism. Science 1974; 186: 1213–5.
14. Schweikert HU, Milewich L, Wilson JD. Aromatization of androstenedione by isolated human hairs. J Clin Endocrinol Metab 1975; 40: 413–7.
15. Sawaya ME, Price VH. Different levels of 5alpha-reductase type I and II, aromatase, and androgen receptor in hair follicles of women and men with androgenetic alopecia. J Invest Dermatol 1997; 109: 296–300.
16. Chartier MB, Hoss DM, Grant-Kels JM. Approach to the adult female patient with diffuse nonscarring alopecia. J Am Acad Dermatol 2002; 47: 809–18; quiz 818–20.
17. Kuster W, Happle R. The inheritance of common baldness: two B or not two B? J Am Acad Dermatol 1984; 11: 921–6.
18. Chumlea WC, Rhodes T, Girman CJ, et al. Family history and risk of hair loss. Dermatology. 2004; 209: 33–9.
19. Olsen EA, Messenger AG, Shapiro J, et al. Evaluation and treatment of male and female pattern hair loss. J Am Acad Dermatol 2005; 52: 301–11.
20. Nyholt DR, Gillespie NA, Heath AC, Martin NG. Genetic basis of male pattern baldness. J Invest Dermatol 2003; 121: 1561–4.
21. Lee AT, Zane LT. Dermatologic manifestations of polycystic ovary syndrome. Am J Clin Dermatol 2007; 8: 201–19.
22. Kim Y, Marjoniemi VM, Diamond T, et al. Androgenetic alopecia in a postmenopausal woman as a result of ovarian hyperthecosis. Australas J Dermatol 2003; 44: 62–6.
23. Tosi A, Misciali C, Piraccini BM, Peluso AM, Bardazzi F. Drug-induced hair loss and hair growth. Incidence, management and avoidance. Drug Saf 1994; 10: 310–7.
24. Sinclair R. Male pattern androgenetic alopecia. BMJ 1998; 317: 865–9.
25. Millikan LE. Androgenetic alopecia: the role of inflammation and Demodex. Int J Dermatol 2001; 40: 475–6.
26. Aslani FS, Dastgheib L, Banihashemi BM. Hair counts in scalp biopsy of males and females with androgenetic alopecia compared with normal subjects. J Cutan Pathol 2009; 36: 734–9.
27. Price VH, Roberts JL, Hordinsky M, et al. Lack of efficacy of finasteride in postmenopausal women with androgenetic alopecia. J Am Acad Dermatol 2000; 43: 768–76.
28. Norwood OT. Incidence of female androgenetic alopecia (female pattern alopecia). Dermatol Surg 2001; 27: 53–4.
29. Sinclair RD. Management of male pattern hair loss. Cutis 2001; 68: 35–40.
30. Sullivan JR, Kossard S. Acquired scalp alopecia. Part I: A review. Australas J Dermatol 1998; 39: 207–19; quiz 220–201.
31. Lee DY, Lee JH, Yang JM, Lee ES. Sparse hairs below frontal hair line are early sign of androgenetic alopecia in men. J Eur Acad Dermatol Venereol 2009; 23: 721–2.
32. Birch MP, Lalla SC, Messenger AG. Female pattern hair loss. Clin Exp Dermatol 2002; 27: 383–8.
33. Ekmekci TR, Sakiz D, Koslu A. Occipital involvement in female pattern hair loss: histopathological evidences. J Eur Acad Dermatol Venereol 2010; 24: 299–301.
34. Whiting DA. Chronic telogen effluvium: increased scalp hair shedding in middle-aged women. J Am Acad Dermatol 1996; 35: 899–906.
35. Inui S, Nakajima T, Itami S. Scalp dermoscopy of androgenetic alopecia in Asian people. J Dermatol 2009; 36: 82–5.
36. Sewell LD, Elston DM, Dorion RP. "Anisotrichosis": a novel term to describe pattern alopecia. J Am Acad Dermatol 2007; 56: 856.
37. de Lacharriere O, Deloche C, Misciali C, et al. Hair diameter diversity: a clinical sign reflecting the follicle miniaturization. Arch Dermatol 2001; 137: 641–6.
38. Chamberlain AJ, Dawber RP. Methods of evaluating hair growth. Australas J Dermatol 2003; 44: 10–8.
39. Rathnayake D, Sinclair R. Male androgenetic alopecia. Expert Opin Pharmacother. 2010; 11: 1295–304.
40. Eun HC, Kwon OS, Yeon JH, et al. Efficacy, safety, and tolerability of dutasteride 0.5 mg once daily in male patients with male pattern hair loss: a randomized, double-blind, placebo-controlled, phase III study. J Am Acad Dermatol 2010; 63: 252–8.
41. Sperling LC, Lupton GP. Histopathology of non-scarring alopecia. J Cutan Pathol 1995; 22: 97–114.
42. Headington JT. Transverse microscopic anatomy of the human scalp. A basis for a morphometric approach to disorders of the hair follicle. Arch Dermatol 1984; 120: 449–56.
43. Sundberg JP, Beamer WG, Uno H, Van Neste D, King LE. Androgenetic alopecia: in vivo models. Exp Mol Pathol 1999; 67: 118–30.
44. Messenger AG, Sinclair R. Follicular miniaturization in female pattern hair loss: clinicopathological correlations. Br J Dermatol 2006; 155: 926–30.
45. Horenstein MG, Jacob JS. Follicular streamers (stelae) in scarring and non-scarring alopecia. J Cutan Pathol 2008; 35: 1115–20.
46. El-Domyati M, Attia S, Saleh F, Abdel-Wahab H. Androgenetic alopecia in males: a histopathological and ultrastructural study. J Cosmet Dermatol 2009; 8: 83–91.
47. Whiting DA. Diagnostic and predictive value of horizontal sections of scalp biopsy specimens in male pattern androgenetic alopecia. J Am Acad Dermatol 1993; 28: 755–63.
48. Lattanand A, Johnson WC. Male pattern alopecia a histopathologic and histochemical study. J Cutan Pathol 1975; 2: 58–70.
49. Deloche C, de Lacharriere O, Misciali C, et al. Histological features of peripilar signs associated with androgenetic alopecia. Arch Dermatol Res 2004; 295: 422–8.
50. Sueki H, Stoudemayer T, Kligman AM, Murphy GF. Quantitative and ultrastructural analysis of inflammatory infiltrates in male pattern alopecia. Acta Derm Venereol 1999; 79: 347–50.
51. Hori H, Moretti G, Rebora A, Crovato F. The thickness of human scalp: normal and bald. J Invest Dermatol 1972; 58: 396–9.
52. Pinkus H. Differential patterns of elastic fibers in scarring and non-scarring alopecias. J Cutan Pathol 1978; 5: 93–104.

10 Telogen effluvium

A telogen effluvium (TE) occurs when abnormally large numbers of anagen hairs from all areas of the scalp enter the telogen phase (1). This may be caused by some sort of endogenous stress to the follicles, such as a metabolic disturbance, nutritional deficiency, or serious systemic illness. Other cases of TE are "physiologic" and not indicative of disease. Some of the many possible causes are listed in Table 10.1. In response to the etiologic insult, many hairs prematurely enter the catagen phase. This is a committed step for follicles, and having entered catagen they must proceed through the telogen phase and ultimately exogen (shedding).

Headington proposed five functional subtypes of TE distinguishable by different perturbations of follicular cycling that ultimately result in increased shedding of telogen club hairs (10). These subtypes may account for the many different types of triggers and slight variations in presentation and symptom duration that can be experienced by patients with TE.

CLINICAL FINDINGS

TE is probably the most common form of hair loss associated with systemic disease, especially chronic and debilitating conditions (11). However, only the most dramatic cases of TE, resulting in a greater than 25% hair loss, are likely to come to clinical attention. An apparent reduction of hair density is often not appreciated until a substantial amount of hair has been lost—some authors claim that a 50% reduction in density is required for clinically obvious thinning (10,12). The majority of drugs that have been associated with alopecia (with the important exception of anticancer medicines, other toxins, and biologic immunomodulatory agents) cause hair loss through the mechanism of a telogen effluvium (13).

Physiological forms of TE include postpartum and neonatal hair loss. During pregnancy, numerous follicles are artificially maintained in the anagen state under the influence of gestational hormones. This is reflected in the lower telogen counts that occur in the second two trimesters of pregnancy (1,14). After parturition, numerous follicles synchronously enter the catagen/telogen phase, followed by synchronous shedding of hairs approximately three months later. An analogous drug-induced effluvium can be seen after discontinuation (and occasionally after the initiation) of estrogenic oral contraceptives due to synchronized shifting of follicles into or out of an artificially prolonged anagen stage (13).

TE of the newborn represents the nearly universal shedding of scalp hair during the first six months of life. This may occur rapidly, resulting in obvious alopecia, or may proceed slowly and imperceptibly. In either case, large numbers of anagen hairs enter telogen within a period of months. It is presumed that changes in the hormonal milieu precipitated by childbirth contribute at least partially to the effluvium in the infant. The telogen counts can be elevated beyond what is typically seen in adult TE, with observations in the 70th percentile(1); this is presumed to be due to the synchronization of the majority of the follicles in the first pelage of the neonate (1).

Many adult women suffer from an ongoing TE with no definable precipitating event (15). Effluvium lasting more than 6 months has been termed "chronic telogen effluvium" and is a diagnosis of exclusion (15). Many or most of these women experience an insidious onset of disease. The course is frequently self-limited, although the condition may last for years prior to

Table 10.1 Causes of Telogen Effluvium

Physiological (not pathological)
Physiological effluvium of the newborn
Postpartum telogen effluvium

Injury or stress (pathologic)
Postfebrile (extremely high fevers, e.g., malaria)
Severe infection
Severe chronic illness
Severe, prolonged psychological stress
Postsurgical (implies major surgical procedure)
Hypothyroidism, hyperthyroidism, and other endocrinopathies
Crash or liquid protein diets; starvation

Drugs
ACE-inhibitors (e.g., captopril, enalapril, ramipril) (2)
allopurinol (2)
amphetamines (2)
androgens (2)
Anticoagulants (especially heparin) (1)
Antithyroid (propylthiouracil, methimazole)
Anticonvulsants (e.g., phenytoin, valproic acid)
Antifungals (e.g., terbinafine, fluconazole, itraconazole, clotrimazole) (2)
Antihistamines (e.g., cimetidine, ranitidine)
Antiretrovirals (e.g., indinavir, acyclovir) (3,4)
Beta-blockers (e.g., metoprolol, propranolol) (2)
Dopamine agonists (e.g., pramipexole, bromocriptine, pergolide) (5)
Ethambutol (2)
Dopamine precursor (levodopa) (5)
Fibrates (clofibrate, fenofibrate) (2)
Heavy metals
Interferons (6)
Leflunomide (2)
Lithium (especially if induces hypothyroidism) (2)
Minoxidil (either initiation or discontinuation of) (2,7)
Nicotinic acid (2)
Nonsteroidal anti-inflammatories (e.g., naproxen, ibuprofen) (2)
Oral contraceptives (either initiation or discontinuation of) (8)
Retinoids, vitamin A and its derivatives (acitretin, etretinate, isotretinoin) (2,9)
Salicylates (2)
Serotonin re-uptake inhibitors (e.g., fluoxetine) (2)
Spironolactone (2)
Tricyclic antidepressents (e.g., amytriptiline, doxepin) (2)

spontaneous resolution. This form of TE is speculated to result in part from a shortened duration of the anagen phase (10).

The early stage of androgenetic alopecia is akin to a *localized* form of chronic TE (10). The affected hairs of the balding (typically vertex and frontal) scalp experience a marked reduction in the length of anagen. A much higher proportion of hairs are thus entering telogen at any given time. Hair shedding is only obvious during the early stages of the balding process, when large, terminal hairs are being shed. As androgenetic alopecia becomes more chronic, the hairs miniaturize and the turnover and shedding of vellus telogen hairs is not apparent.

Patients with acute forms of TE notice hair loss about three or four months after the precipitating event. This corresponds to the time it takes for a hair to move through catagen and the early stages of telogen. Scalp hair density may appear normal to outside observers, despite the patient's complaint of profuse hair loss. If alopecia is clinically obvious, the loss appears diffuse and affects all parts of the scalp equally (Figs. 10.1 and 10.2). A gentle hair pull yields several hairs with the depigmented, cornified, clubbed morphology of telogen hair roots (Fig. 10.3). Dystrophic anagen hairs are not expected in a diagnosis of TE; if they are found, this may point to a diagnosis of alopecia areata incognita (16). A forcible hair pluck produces a mixture of normal anagen (dysmorphic due to plucking but not dystrophic) and telogen hairs, as well as an occasional catagen hair (Fig. 10.4).

In TE the percentage of telogen hairs will be increased to more than 20%, a criterion without which this diagnosis cannot be established with certainty. Counts between 15% and 20% can be regarded as "suspicious." In the typical case of TE,

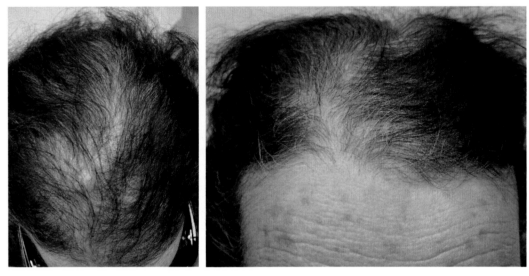

Figure 10.1 This patient with chronic *Mycobacterium avium intracellulare* lung infection treated with combination drug therapy including ethambutol, complained of diffuse thinning of the hair throughout her scalp.

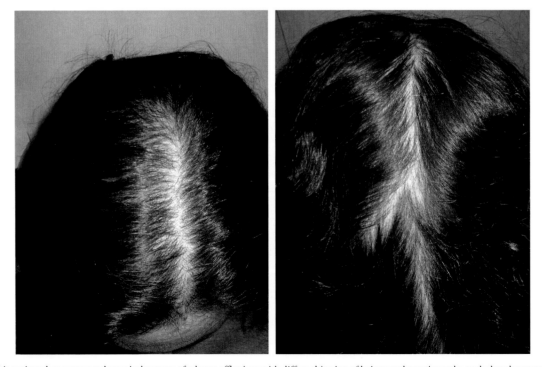

Figure 10.2 This patient demonstrates the typical pattern of telogen effluvium with diffuse thinning of hair over the entire scalp, such that the part width is equally widened over the frontal scalp and crown (*left panel*) and the posterior vertex and occiput (*right panel*).

the telogen count does not exceed 50%. However, exceptions to this rule can occur, and a unique case of effluvium following heparin administration with a telogen count of 80% has been documented (1). Figures exceeding 80% are inconsistent with a simple case of TE. The vast majority of cases we have seen have counts less than 50%.

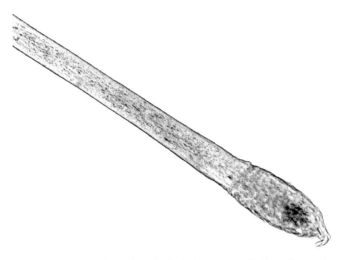

Figure 10.3 An example of a forcibly plucked or gently pulled late telogen hair. The club is depigmented and completely cornified.

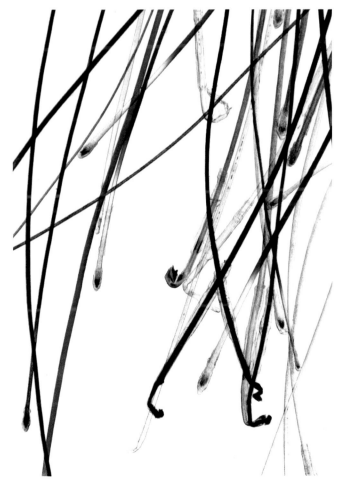

Figure 10.4 Portion of a forcible hair pluck (trichogram) obtained from the scalp of a young woman with telogen effluvium. There is a mixture of normal-appearing anagen and telogen bulbs, but the telogen bulbs are over-represented (nine telogen bulbs are visible in this image). When all hairs were counted, the telogen count was 35%.

Treatment is aimed at identifying the cause of the TE and ameliorating the condition when possible. A thorough history addressing the potential triggers of various physiologic conditions, symptoms, disease states, and medications in the preceding three months is imperative. This is followed by appropriate physical exam and laboratory testing as guided by the history. When one or more of the medications closely associated with TE are being taken by the patient, a dialog with the primary prescribing physician and a search for alternative agents is a worthwhile endeavor. Vitamin A supplements should be limited, hormone therapies stabilized and diets should be balanced (17). The relationship of iron deficiency to alopecia, and TE in particular, has been a topic of ongoing investigation (18). Recent studies support that iron deficiency, although common in women in general, is not more common in patients with chronic TE as compared with patients with female pattern hair loss or control patients (19). There are no solid data to support the contention that iron supplementation in iron-deficient patients improves hair regrowth. Nevertheless, many clinicians provide iron supplementation with a goal of achieving a serum ferritin greater than $40\,\mu g/L$ in otherwise healthy individuals. Topical minoxidil may hasten regrowth, but the medication can itself lead to a temporary effluvium upon initiation of use, due to conversion of telogen follicles into exogen in preparation for new anagen hair growth (13). Furthermore, discontinuation of minoxidil can lead to a synchronized transition of follicles (previously maintained in anagen by the drug) into telogen, with subsequent shedding after 2–3 months (13). Reassurance and stress management are important aspects of counseling patients with TE (20).

HISTOLOGICAL FINDINGS

Just as in androgenetic alopecia, the histological diagnosis of TE depends more on *quantitative* than *qualitative* features (21). The only abnormality in a "pure" case of TE is an increase in the percentage of terminal telogen follicles (Fig. 10.5). Therefore, the total number of hairs in the specimen will be normal, but there will appear to be a reduced number of terminal hairs when counted at the level of the subcutis or the deep reticular

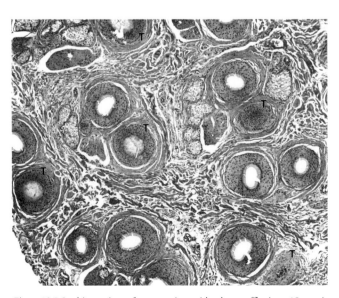

Figure 10.5 In this specimen from a patient with telogen effluvium, 15 terminal follicles can be identified; of these, five are in the catagen/telogen phase (labeled "T"). This is a catagen/telogen percentage of approximately 33%, within the typical range seen in telogen effluvium.

dermis. Fibrous "streamers" (stelae) replace the "missing" terminal hairs at this level (Figs. 10.6–10.8). These streamers lie deep to the bulbs of the terminal telogen hairs, which are found in the mid-dermis. The telogen hairs are increased in number, and the telogen count (number of terminal telogen hairs divided by the total number of terminal hairs) will be greater than 20% (Figs. 10.6–10.8).

It is important to realize, however, that a telogen count lower than 20% does *not* exclude the diagnosis of TE. If a patient's normal telogen count happens to be 5%, a telogen count of 15% would be clearly abnormal for that patient. Unfortunately, we do not know the "baseline" telogen counts for specific individuals, so numbers less than 20% must be regarded as equivocal. In cases of chronic, low-grade TE, values are

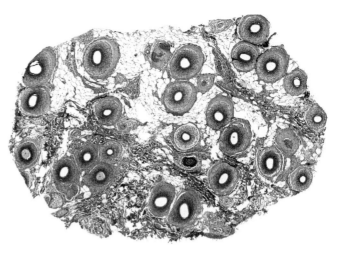

Figure 10.8 This case of telogen effluvium, also sectioned at the dermal/subcutaneous junction, is slightly subtler. In this section there are 25 anagen follicles, three catagen/telogen follicles, and four stelae (underlying telogen follicles). The catagen/telogen percentage is 22%.

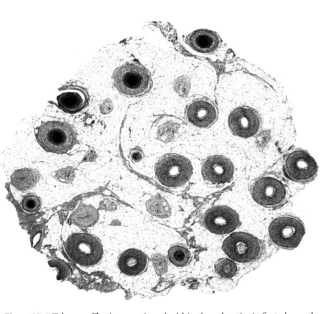

Figure 10.6 Telogen effluvium sectioned within the subcutis. At first glance the total follicular count might seem decreased for this Caucasian patient, however, when the catagen/telogen follicles (2) and numerous streamers (11) are counted along with the anagen follicles (19), the total follicular count is normal (32 total follicles). The catagen/telogen percentage is approximately 40%.

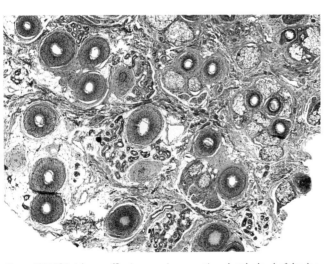

Figure 10.7 This telogen effluvium specimen, sectioned at the level of the dermal/subcutaneous junction, also demonstrates a reduced number of terminal anagen hairs. The terminal anagen hairs present are all roughly similar in diameter. Catagen/telogen hairs are seen, as well as several stelae (underlying additional catagen/telogen hairs). The total follicular number is normal but the percentage of telogen hairs is elevated to 36%.

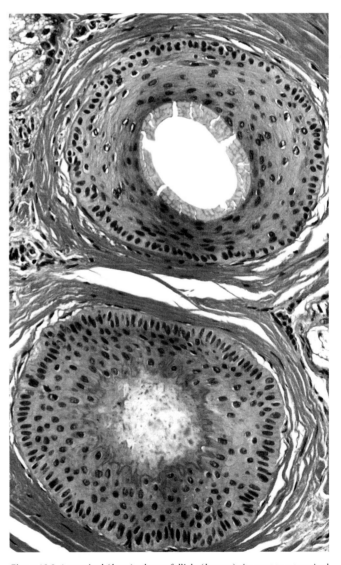

Figure 10.9 A terminal (*large*) telogen follicle (*bottom*) sits next to a terminal anagen follicle (*top*) in a high power view of a biopsy from a patient with telogen effluvium. The sizes of the two follicles are comparable.

often lower than typically seen in acute effluvium, in the range of 15%–20%; Whiting cites an even lower range of 10%–20%, with an average of 11% (15).

The size of hairs is not affected in TE. Abnormally high numbers of terminal anagen hairs are converted into terminal telogen hairs which regress normally leaving streamers behind, but miniaturization does not occur (Figs. 10.9 and 10.10). Therefore, the terminal:vellus hair ratio is normal (greater than 2:1) (Figs. 10.11 and 10.12).

In a simple case of TE, all parts of the scalp are affected equally, resulting in truly diffuse hair loss. In fact, all body hair is affected by the disease. This is clinically demonstrable by thinned eyebrows, pubic hair, and axillary hair. If paired biopsy specimens (frontal and occipital scalp) are obtained, the histological findings will be very similar at both sites; this is in contrast to androgenetic alopecia, which preferentially affects the frontal and/or vertex scalp while the occipital scalp remains normal.

TE is a non-inflammatory form of hair loss, and accordingly, no significant inflammatory infiltrate is found. In particular, peribulbar inflammation and inflammation affecting the lower two-thirds of the follicles is *absent* (Fig. 10.13). If inflammation (or miniaturization) is found, the patient may, in fact, have the diffuse form of alopecia areata known as alopecia areata incognita (see chap. 15 for more information), a potential diagnostic pitfall, as the clinical presentations can be remarkably similar.

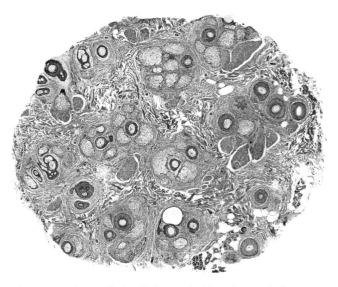

Figure 10.11 Telogen effluvium is characterized by an increase in the percentage of catagen/telogen hairs without a decrease in the overall size of hairs. The terminal: vellus hair ratio in this section taken at the level of the sebaceous glands where vellus hairs are evident, is much greater than 2:1.

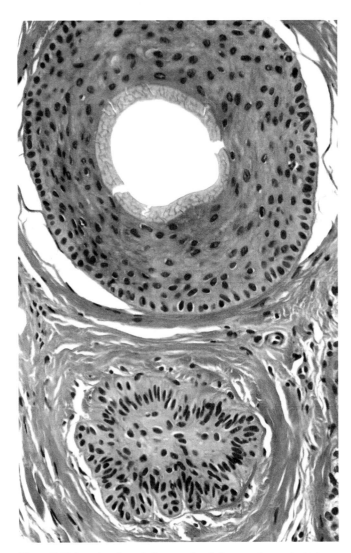

Figure 10.10 A section through the secondary hair germ of a terminal telogen hair (inferior) sits next to a terminal anagen follicle (superior) in a high power view of a biopsy from a patient with telogen effluvium. The condensed structure of the secondary hair germ is smaller than the terminal anagen follicle, but this does not represent miniaturization.

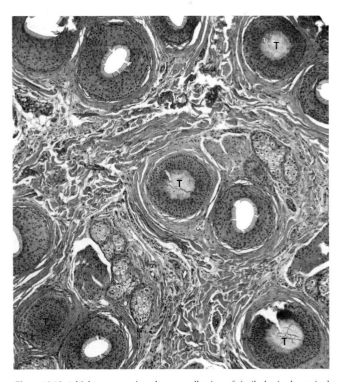

Figure 10.12 A higher power view shows a collection of similarly sized terminal telogen hairs (T) and terminal anagen hairs without evidence of miniaturization.

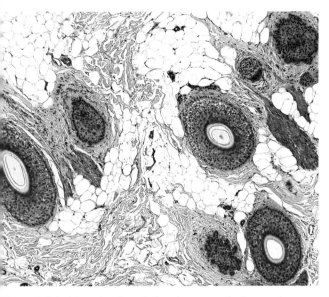

Figure 10.13 In this section through the subcutaneous fat there are three ana-gen follicles, three catagen/telogen follicles, and a single bulb; there is no inflammation to account for the shift, concordant with a diagnosis of telogen effluvium.

Telogen Effluvium in Summary

Clinical correlation: a patient reports diffuse hair loss/ increased shedding of hair into the brush or comb, on the pillow, or in the shower drain. A history of a precipitating event (approximately 3 months prior to onset of hair loss) is often obtainable, such as childbirth, major surgery or severe illness, use of certain medications, etc. Many cases of chronic TE do not have an identifiable cause.

Histological findings:

❖ Normal *total* number of follicles
❖ Increased *percentage* of terminal catagen/telogen hairs (rarely exceeds 50%)
❖ Normal size of follicles (miniaturization is not a feature) and, therefore, a normal terminal: vellus hair ratio
❖ Presence of fibrous "streamers" indicating conversion to telogen hairs
❖ Absence of significant inflammation
• In chronic TE the catagen/telogen rate can be quite vari-able because of a waxing and waning course

Histological Differential diagnosis:

• **Acute traction alopecia:** shares with TE normal follicu-lar size and count with an increased catagen/telogen shift. Trichomalacia and pigment casts (not features of TE) may occasionally be found. The clinical history is especially important
• **Trichotillomania:** also demonstrates normal follicular size and counts, and frequently shows an increased cata-gen/telogen percentage. Incomplete, disrupted follicular anatomy is diagnostic but not always present
• **Androgenetic alopecia:** can show a slight shift to the catagen/telogen phase but miniaturization of follicles is also present

• **Postoperative (pressure-induced) alopecia:** shows a mas-sive conversion into the catagen/telogen phase, far sur-passing the typical 20–50% range of TE. Trichomalacia, vascular thrombosis and fat necrosis can be seen in this entity but not in TE. The clinical history is also distinctive
• **Alopecia areata:** demonstrates a higher catagen/telogen shift (typically well above 50%) than TE; miniaturiza-tion is a prominent feature in alopecia areata (especially with chronic disease)
• **Psoriatic alopecia and TNF-alpha-inhibitor associated psoriasiform alopecia:** also show very elevated catagen/ telogen percentages (typically > 50%), however they have additional findings (most notably inflammation) that help to distinguish them from TE

⚠ **Pitfalls**

• The diffuse variant of alopecia areata (alopecia areata incognita) is a deceptive clinical mimic of TE; careful evaluation of the histopathology is required.
• New onset TE not uncommonly unmasks the early stages of androgenetic alopecia. Paired biopsies from both involved (e.g., frontal or crown) and normal-appearing (e.g., occipital) scalp may be required to eval-uate for the presence of one (or both) of the two diseases.

Abbreviation: TE, telogen effluvium.

REFERENCES

1. Kligman A. Pathologic dynamics of human hair loss: I, Telogen effluvium. Arch Dermatol 1961; 83: 175–98.
2. Piraccini BM, Iorizzo M, Rech G, Tosti A. Drug-induced hair disorders. Curr Drug Saf 2006; 1: 301–5.
3. Calista D, Boschini A. Cutaneous side effects induced by indinavir. Eur J Dermatol 2000; 10: 292–6.
4. Ward HA, Russo GG, Shrum J. Cutaneous manifestations of antiretroviral therapy. J Am Acad Dermatol 2002; 46: 284–93.
5. Katz KA, Cotsarelis G, Gupta R, Seykora JT. Telogen effluvium associated with the dopamine agonist pramipexole in a 55-year-old woman with Parkinson's disease. J Am Acad Dermatol 2006; 55: S103–4.
6. Tosti A, Misciali C, Bardazzi F, Fanti PA, Varotti C. Telogen effluvium due to recombinant interferon alpha-2b. Dermatology 1992; 184: 124–5.
7. Bamford JT. A falling out following minoxidil: telogen effluvium. J Am Acad Dermatol 1987; 16: 144–6.
8. Hair loss and contraceptives. Br Med J 1973; 2: 499–500.
9. Berth-Jones J, Shuttleworth D, Hutchinson P. A study of etretinate alope-cia. Br J Dermatol 1990; 122: 751–5.
10. Headington JT. Telogen effluvium. New concepts and review. Arch Der-matol 1993; 129: 356–63.
11. Sperling LC. Hair and systemic disease. Dermatol Clin 2001; 19: 711–26, ix.
12. Gordon KA, Tosti A. Alopecia: evaluation and treatment. Clin Cosmet Investig Dermatol 2011; 4: 101–6.
13. Tosti A, Pazzaglia M. Drug reactions affecting hair: diagnosis. Dermatol Clin 2007; 25: 223–31, vii.
14. Lynfield YL. Effect of pregnancy on the human hair cycle. J Invest Derma-tol 1960; 35: 323–7.
15. Whiting DA. Chronic telogen effluvium: increased scalp hair shedding in middle-aged women. J Am Acad Dermatol 1996; 35: 899–906.
16. Quercetani R, Rebora AE, Fedi MC, et al. Patients with profuse hair shed-ding may reveal anagen hair dystrophy: a diagnostic clue of alopecia areata incognita. J Eur Acad Dermatol Venereol 2011; 25: 808–10.
17. Ross EK, Shapiro J. Management of hair loss. Dermatol Clin 2005; 23: 227–43.

18. Kantor J, Kessler LJ, Brooks DG, Cotsarelis G. Decreased serum ferritin is associated with alopecia in women. J Invest Dermatol 2003; 121: 985–8.

19. Olsen EA, Reed KB, Cacchio PB, Caudill L. Iron deficiency in female pattern hair loss, chronic telogen effluvium, and control groups. J Am Acad Dermatol 2010; 63: 991–9.

20. Hadshiew IM, Foitzik K, Arck PC, Paus R. Burden of hair loss: stress and the underestimated psychosocial impact of telogen effluvium and androgenetic alopecia. J Invest Dermatol 2004; 123: 455–7.

21. Sperling LC, Lupton GP. Histopathology of non-scarring alopecia. J Cutan Pathol 1995; 22: 97–114.

11 Trichotillomania

The term "trichotillomania" was coined in 1889 by Hallopeau to describe the "morbid impulse to pull one's own hair" (1). The Diagnostic and Statistical Manual of Mental Disorders (DSM-IV) describes trichotillomania (TT) as an impulse control disorder (2,3). While there is no consensus regarding prevalence, it is estimated that 8 million Americans are affected (1,4). TT is seven times more frequent in children than adults (1). The mean age of onset for males is 8 years, while in females it is 12 (3). With increasing age, females represent a larger proportion of affected patients; those older than 40 years are five times more likely to be women (5). Patients frequently engage in rituals for hair removal that might include removal of individual strands, hair chewing, licking, or swallowing. In later adolescence and adult years the behavior is often classified as obsessive-compulsive (1). In many patients, no underlying mental or emotional issue can be identified, although careful questioning may reveal a history of significant stress or turmoil at school, home, or work.

CLINICAL FINDINGS

TT patients will often present with a history of hair or eyelashes "falling out" without explanation (3). They may describe hair that does not grow (6). While the diagnosis of TT is usually made by clinical examination, often both child and parents deny the possibility of pulling or plucking as a cause of hair loss (1,3,4). Typically patients will present with a sharply demarcated, unusually shaped (geographic, linear, curved, or circular) area of alopecia comprising hairs that are short or broken off at varying lengths (Figs. 11.1–11.3) (4,7,8).

A round patch of incomplete alopecia on the central crown or vertex, surrounded by a rim of unaffected hair, is characteristic of TT. This pattern is known as the "Friar Tuck Sign" or the "tonsure" pattern (Fig. 11.3A) (4,9). In the most severe cases, almost all hairs within reach may be broken off (7). Any part of the body may be affected, although central scalp, eyebrows, and eyelashes represent the most commonly involved areas in decreasing frequency (2,3). Underlying skin is free of scaling and erythema, although signs of excoriation may be observed, and the patient may complain of pruritus (2,4). In instances where trichophagia is a component of the disorder, a trichobezoar may form. In such cases, clinical examination may reveal a freely movable mass in the left upper quadrant or mid-epigastrium (2,4).

The clinical differential of TT includes tinea capitis, alopecia areata, traction alopecia, disorders of hair fragility, such as trichorrhexis nodosa, and syphilitic alopecia. Tinea capitis has one or more patches of broken hairs, but these usually are fractured at their bases; the scalp may or may not be inflamed. Alopecia areata typically manifests as a smooth, well-demarcated patch of alopecia, frequently with very short, easily extractable "exclamation point" hairs. These exclamation point hairs demonstrate a frayed, broken shaft that is narrowed proximally, terminating in a resting club (10). The short hairs in TT are not

easily extractable nor should they have a frayed distal end. Traction alopecia shows noninflamed, often linear areas of alopecia adjacent to areas of tight braiding or ponytails. Disorders of hair fragility also contain hairs broken off at varying lengths and can be localized to regional areas of the scalp, especially those under greater frictional or chemical stress (Fig. 36.1). Trichorrhexis nodosa and many other shaft disorders can be evaluated by light microscopy. Syphilitic alopecia is classically described as "moth eaten" in appearance and can be evaluated by serologic (e.g., rapid plasma reagin) testing (4).

Treatment of TT depends on the clinical scenario. In many children the behavior is regarded as a tic, similar to nail

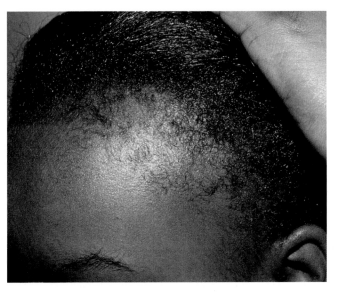

Figure 11.1 Trichotillomania. There is an unusually shaped, unilateral patch of alopecia showing hairs of varying lengths. The pattern of hair loss seen in this patient resembles end-stage traction alopecia, but her hair loss was sudden in onset, and the biopsy was confirmatory.

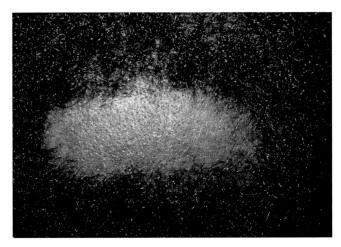

Figure 11.2 Trichotillomania. This patch of alopecia has an unusual, sharply defined, geometric shape.

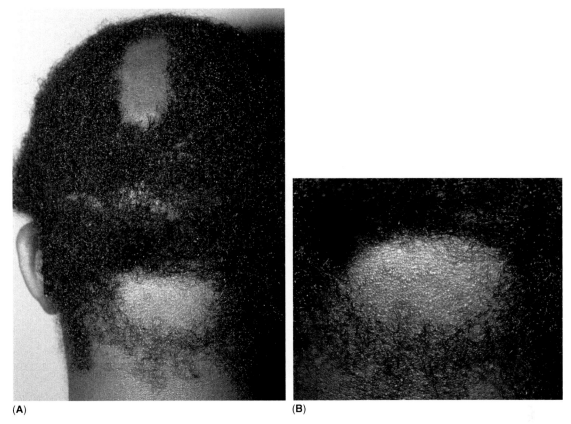

(A) **(B)**

Figures 11.3 Trichotillomania. (**A** and **B**) There is a well-demarcated area of alopecia on the vertex surrounded by normal hair, the "Friar Tuck" sign. The lower occipital lesion bears a close resemblance to alopecia areata, but the biopsy was confirmatory.

biting, and requires no specific attention (7). In others, bringing the child's attention to the behavior and reassurance is enough to stop it (7). In some cases the child's attention can be diverted (1). If symptoms persist for over three months, consultation with a child psychiatrist should be sought (1). The most common treatment is a combination of drug and behavioral therapy (3).

HISTOLOGICAL FINDINGS
Because patients frequently deny hair plucking, a biopsy specimen can be crucial for establishing a convincing diagnosis (for the doctor *and* patient/parent). The most fruitful biopsies of TT are obtained within eight weeks of onset (5). The most distinctive and diagnostic histological feature of trichotillomania is incomplete, distorted follicular anatomy (Figs. 11.4–11.6) (11). This is a direct result of forcible hair shaft extraction. Traumatically disrupted follicles were identified in 21% of TT cases in one large study using vertical sections, and were considered a specific finding (5). Utilizing horizontal sectioning, this finding may be seen in 50% of cases (Figs. 11.7–11.14) (11). In addition, completely normal hairs may be intermixed among follicles showing evidence of traumatic avulsion (Fig. 11.9). Vellus hairs, by virtue of their smaller size, are not typically plucked (12).

Ordinarily, the inner root sheath surrounds either a hair shaft or the oval space occupied by the shaft before processing (as in Fig. 11.9, *upper right*). A collapsed inner root sheath indicates prior extraction of the hair shaft and is the most common histological defect encountered in trichotillomania.

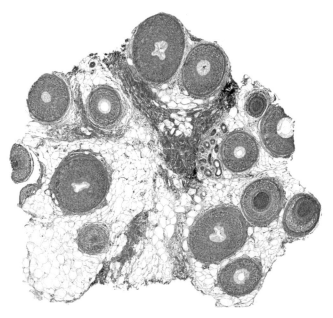

Figure 11.4 Trichotillomania. Low magnification reveals a noninflammatory alopecia with several follicles manifesting distortion and collapse of the inner root sheath where hair shafts have been forcefully removed.

Partially extracted and distorted residual root sheath material may be identified within the follicular lumen, along with fragments of pigmented hair matrix or superficially displaced cortical cells (8). These "pigment casts" are identified in as many as 70% of cases of TT, and more than one can be seen in up to one-third of cases (Fig. 11.13) (5,12). When both the

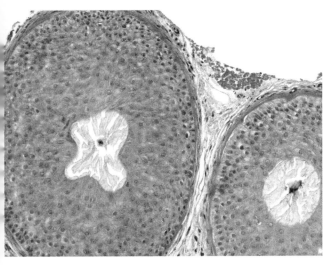

Figure 11.5 Trichotillomania. High magnification of the same specimen shown in Fig. 11.4 reveals follicles with missing shafts and distorted and collapsed inner root sheaths.

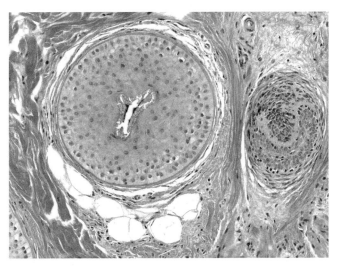

Figure 11.7 Trichotillomania. There is a follicle with a collapsed inner root sheath adjacent to a catagen/telogen follicular bulb (*right side*).

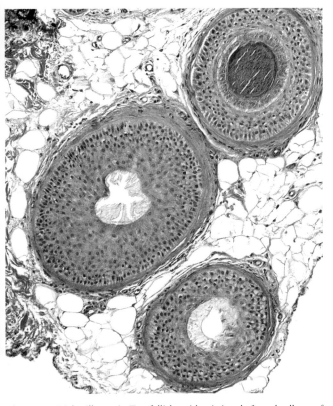

Figure 11.6 Trichotillomania. Two follicles with missing shafts and collapse of the inner root sheath; adjacent (*upper right*) is a single unaffected follicle.

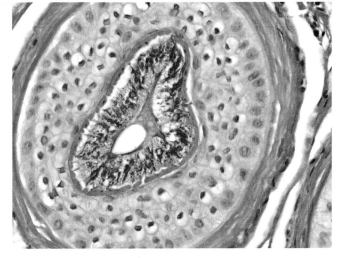

Figure 11.8 Trichotillomania. Distorted (collapsed) inner root sheath manifesting the trichohyaline granules characteristic of the suprabulbar (stem) portion of the hair follicle.

shaft and inner root sheath are extracted, the outer root sheath collapses upon itself (Fig. 11.14). Although absence of hair shafts is a common finding in TT, absent hair shafts *without distortion of the inner root sheath* are routine artifacts of histologic processing, and should not be confused with the findings described above (5).

In up to 20% of cases, hair bulbs are traumatically distorted or extracted, a feature considered diagnostic of TT (5,12). Infrequently, all or most of the follicular epithelium is removed, and the fibrous root sheath, along with any retained epithelial

fragments and extravasated red blood cells form a vertical column (8). Hemorrhage within the fibrous connective tissue sheath may also be seen (Fig. 11.15).

Traumatically disrupted hair follicular germinative epithelium may produce an abnormally formed, distorted hair shaft of diminished caliber and with irregular pigmentation (8). This feature, known as *trichomalacia*, has been noted in up to 40% of TT patients (Figs. 11.16–11.18), but may occasionally be seen in alopecia areata (8,12).

A rare but specific feature of TT consists of longitudinally fractured shafts containing hemorrhage within the cleft, forming the so-called "hamburger sign" when the shaft is sectioned crosswise (Fig. 11.19) (13). Traumatic rifts within hair matrix were noted in 50% of TT cases in one study (12). Melanin spillage into the adjacent fibrous connective tissue sheath, seen in about one quarter of cases, has been advocated as a specific feature of trichotillomania, but this finding also occurs in alopecia areata (5,12).

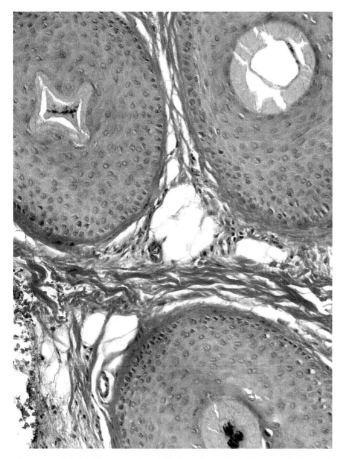

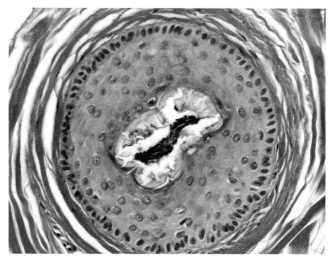

Figure 11.11 Trichotillomania. There is inner root sheath disruption with an ectopic fragment of superficially translocated pigmented and nucleated cortical cells.

Figure 11.9 Trichotillomania. Two follicles with variably distorted (collapsed) inner root sheaths and some retained intrafollicular pigment. Adjacent (*upper right*) is an unaffected folllicle; its shaft was lost during processing.

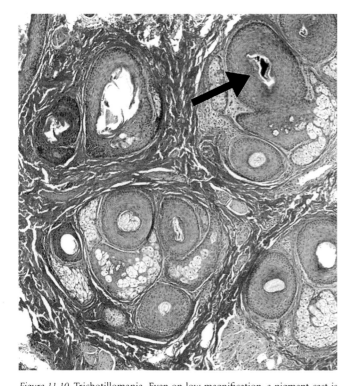

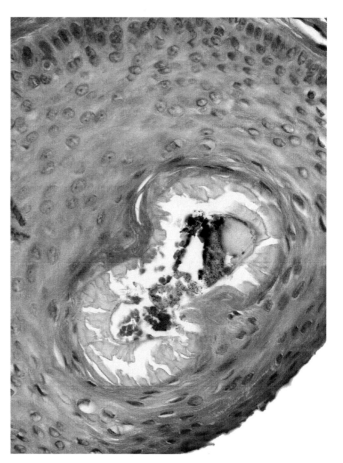

Figure 11.12 Trichotillomania. There is trichomalacia, inner root sheath disruption, and intrafollicular hemorrhage.

Figure 11.10 Trichotillomania. Even on low magnification, a pigment cast is identifiable within a follicle (*arrow*).

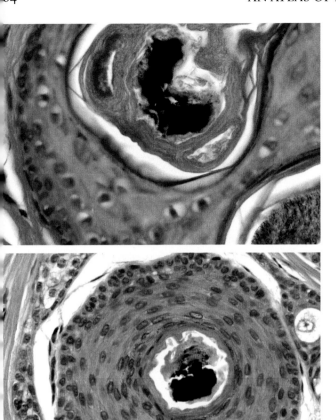

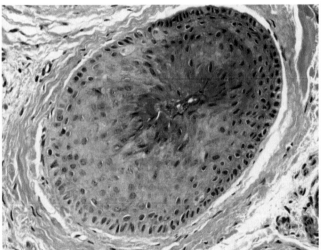

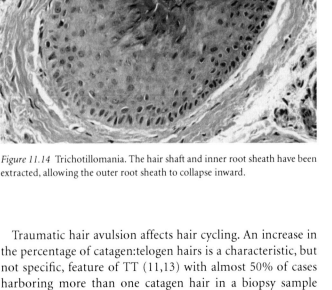

Figure 11.13 Trichotillomania. Pigment casts.

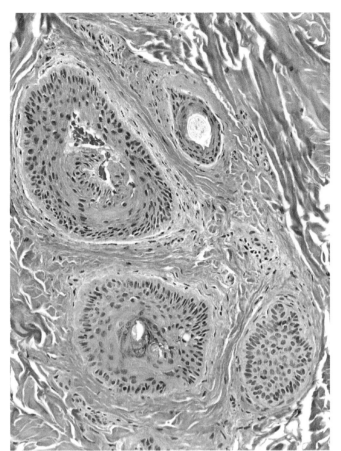

Figure 11.15 Trichotillomania. Intrafollicular hemorrhage.

Figure 11.14 Trichotillomania. The hair shaft and inner root sheath have been extracted, allowing the outer root sheath to collapse inward.

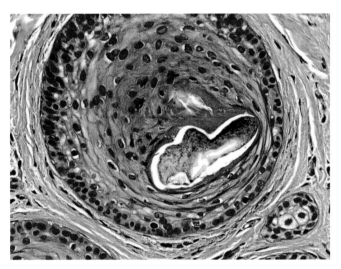

Figure 11.16 Trichotillomania. A deformed, irregular pigmented shaft characteristic of trichomalacia.

Traumatic hair avulsion affects hair cycling. An increase in the percentage of catagen:telogen hairs is a characteristic, but not specific, feature of TT (11,13) with almost 50% of cases harboring more than one catagen hair in a biopsy sample (Fig. 11.20) (5). As the catagen phase only lasts a couple of weeks, the increased numbers of catagen follicles soon cycle into the much longer telogen phase. Therefore, finding numerous telogen hairs has the same diagnostic significance. Traumatic changes may also be seen in sebaceous lobules, with one study describing distorted sebaceous lobules in up to 30% of cases (12) (Fig. 11.21).

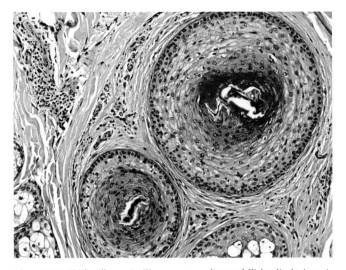

Figure 11.17 Trichotillomania. There are two adjacent follicles displaying trichomalacia and intrafollicular pigment casts.

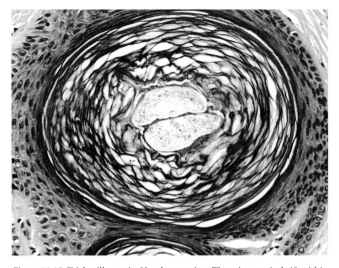

Figure 11.19 Trichotillomania. Hamburger sign. There is a vertical rift within the shaft and hemorrhage within the space.

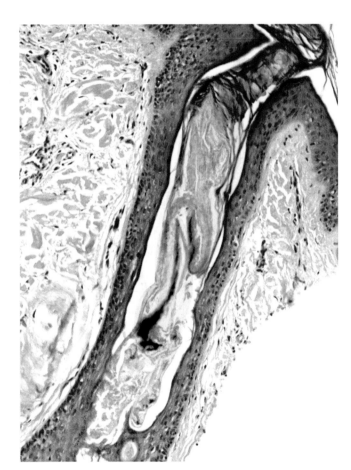

Figure 11.18 Trichotillomania. Vertical section showing both pigment cast formation and trichomalacia.

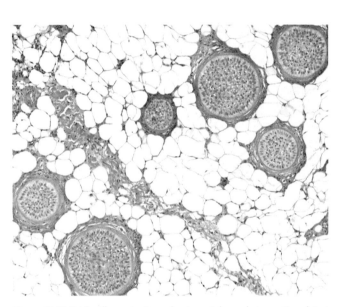

Figure 11.20 Trichotillomania. Several catagen/telogen hairs sectioned just below the forming club.

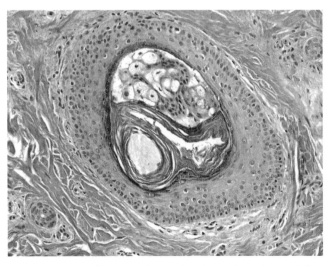

Figure 11.21 Trichotillomania. Sebocytes have been relocated to the infundibulum by forcible extraction.

Trichotillomania in Summary

Clinical correlation: Typically a child or young adult with a sharply demarcated, unusually shaped (geographic, linear, curved, or circular) area of alopecia containing hairs that are short or broken off at varying lengths. A round patch of incomplete alopecia surrounded by a rim of unaffected hair may be seen (Friar Tuck sign, tonsure pattern).

Histological findings:
❖ Distorted follicular anatomy
❖ Absence of peribulbar lymphocytic infiltrates
• Pigment casts
• Trichomalacia
• Melanin pigment in collapsed fibrous root sheaths
• Fractured hair shafts
• Peri- and intrafollicular hemorrhage
• Variably increased catagen/telogen count

Histological differential diagnosis:
• **Acute traction alopecia**: shows features akin to a "mild" trichotillomania with normal follicular size, normal follicular counts, increased catagen/telogen counts, and incomplete follicular anatomy. Occasional trichomalacia and pigment casts may be found, but only rare follicular/shaft distortion and miniaturization
• **Alopecia areata**: shares with TT a variable catagen/telogen shift (although the shift is typically much greater in alopecia areata) and occasional pigment casts; TT differs by mild peribulbar inflammation and lack of traumatic follicular/shaft distortion, and miniaturization
• **Postoperative alopecia**: shares with TT a variable catagen/telogen shift (although the shift is typically much greater in postoperative alopecia) and occasional pigment casts; TT differs by the history of a prior operative procedure/prolonged period of pressure, and by the absence of follicular distortion
• **Telogen effluvium**: shares with TT a catagen/telogen shift, normal follicular counts and size, and an absence of significant inflammation. Distorted, incomplete follicular anatomy is absent in TE

⚠ Pitfalls
Absent hair shafts without distortion of the inner root sheath are a common finding in routine histological processing and should not be confused with the findings described above.

REFERENCES

1. Schneider D, Janniger CK. Trichotillomania. Cutis. 1994; 53: 289–90, 294.
2. Walsh KH, McDougle CJ. Trichotillomania. Presentation, etiology, diagnosis and therapy. Am J Clin Dermatol. 2001; 2: 327–33.
3. Mawn LA, Jordan DR. Trichotillomania. Ophthalmology. 1997; 104: 2175–8.
4. Dimino-Emme L, Camisa C. Trichotillomania associated with the "Friar Tuck sign" and nail-biting. Cutis 1991; 47: 107–10.
5. Muller SA. Trichotillomania: a histopathologic study in sixty-six patients. J Am Acad Dermatol. 1990; 23: 56–62.
6. Steck WD. The clinical evaluation of pathologic hair loss with a diagnostic sign in trichotillomania. Cutis. 1979; 24: 293–5, 298–301.
7. Price VH. Disorders of the hair in children. Pediatr Clin North Am. 1978; 25: 305–20.
8. Mehregan AH. Histopathology of alopecias. Cutis. 1978; 21: 249–53.
9. Muller SA. Trichotillomania. Dermatol Clin. 1987; 5: 595–601.
10. Ihm CW, Han JH. Diagnostic value of exclamation mark hairs. Dermatology. 1993; 186: 99–102.
11. Sperling LC, Lupton GP. Histopathology of non-scarring alopecia. J Cutan Pathol. 1995; 22: 97–114.
12. Lachapelle JM, Pierard GE. Traumatic alopecia in trichotillomania: a pathogenic interpretation of histologic lesions in the pilosebaceous unit. J Cutan Pathol. 1977; 4: 51–67.
13. Royer MC, Sperling LC. Splitting hairs: the 'hamburger sign' in trichotillomania. J Cutan Pathol. 2006; 33 Suppl. 2: 63–64.

12 Traction alopecia

Like trichotillomania, traction alopecia is a form of mechanical, traumatic alopecia. However, trauma to the hair is usually mild and chronic. Although vigorous scratching or combing may cause traction alopecia, most cases are caused by hairstyles involving tight braiding or banding of the hair (1).

CLINICAL FINDINGS

The condition is most common among African-American girls whose hairstyles involve frequent braiding (2,3). However, the identical pattern of hair loss can be seen in persons of all races (4–6). Some girls develop the condition after wearing tight "ponytail" type hairstyles, such as has been popular among female cheerleaders. It has also been related to the tight buns worn by ballet dancers. The hair loss tends to be a peripheral or marginal form of alopecia, that is, involving the frontal, temporal, parietal, and occasionally occipital margins of the scalp (Fig. 12.1). In girls who wear tight braids, perifollicular erythema and pustule formation may be seen. Whether this inflammation is caused by traction or by cosmetics used in conjunction with hairstyling is unknown.

Traction alopecia is a biphasic form of hair loss. Initially the hair loss is temporary, hair regrowth occurs, and the condition is similar to a noncicatricial form of alopecia. However, if excessive traction is maintained for years, the hair loss may eventually become permanent (end stage or "burnt out"; Figs. 12.2–12.5).

There may be a lag period of a decade or more between the period of traction and the onset of permanent hair loss. Consequently, many African-American women present in their 30s and 40s with a several-year history of persistent, bitemporal or frontal hair loss. These women may deny having worn tight braids since childhood, although often other forms of traumatic styling (e.g., curlers) have been used (Fig. 12.3). However, the lack of a history of severe traction or harsh styling practices in half the patients casts doubt on whether or not traction is the only causative factor (7). Recent evidence suggests that an immune-mediated mechanism, akin to that proposed for lichen planopilaris, is unlikely in the pathogenesis of traction alopecia (8).

HISTOLOGICAL FINDINGS

The histological findings in acute, reversible traction alopecia and permanent, long-standing, "burnt out" traction alopecia are entirely different (9). The acute form, most commonly seen in African-American girls or after a short-lived, traumatic hairstyle (such as a hair weave or "corn rows"), resembles a mild form of trichotillomania. Occasionally, distorted or incomplete follicular anatomy is seen. More often, there is an increase in catagen/telogen hairs (10), pigment casts and subtle trichomalacia. Follicular numbers are normal.

In end-stage disease, most commonly found in adult African-American women, the total number of hairs is markedly reduced (Fig. 12.6). This is accounted for by the loss of terminal hairs, because vellus hairs are still present in normal numbers (Fig. 12.7). Sometimes the missing follicles appear to have disappeared without a trace because the dermal collagen appears normal, but often some "old" stelae can be found when deeper levels are examined (Figs. 12.8 and 12.9). In many cases, distinct columns of connective tissue replace some follicles, leaving obvious "blank spaces" (Fig. 12.10).

The sebaceous glands associated with the remaining hairs are still intact, and often persist in follicular units that seem to

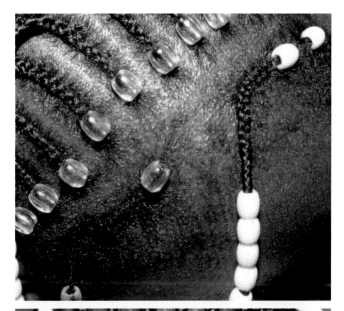

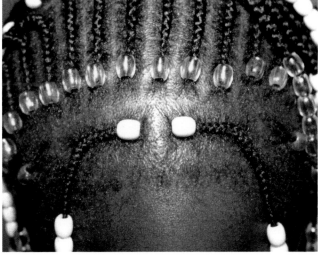

Figure 12.1 Young girl with marginal traction alopecia. With cessation of braiding, regrowth occurred.

have lost *all* their follicles (Fig. 12.11). The presence of sebaceous glands and relative normality of the dermal architecture, despite marked hair loss, is highly characteristic of end-stage traction alopecia. Usually, no significant perifollicular inflammation is present in either early or late disease. However, occasionally within an otherwise typical example of end-stage traction alopecia, a single follicle will be found in some phase of destruction. More often, one or two follicular units will be devoid of sebaceous glands (Fig. 12.12). It is unclear whether this represents a variant of end-stage traction or indicates the coincidental presence of a second form of alopecia (cicatricial). Further study will be required to clarify this.

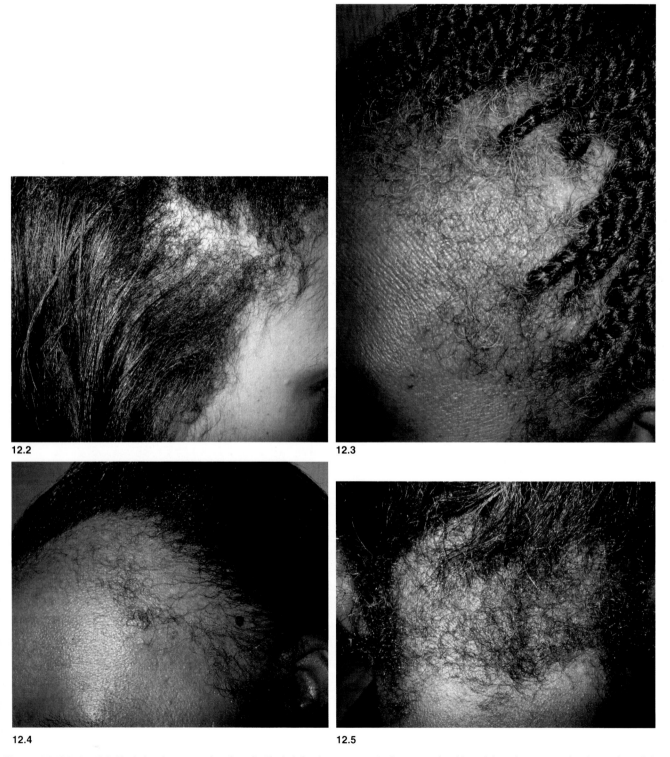

12.2

12.3

12.4

12.5

Figures 12.2,12.3,12.4,12.5 Typical end-stage traction alopecia. The hair loss is most severe in the temporal and lateral frontal regions, and is almost always bilateral. The occiput can also be involved (as in Fig. 12.5).

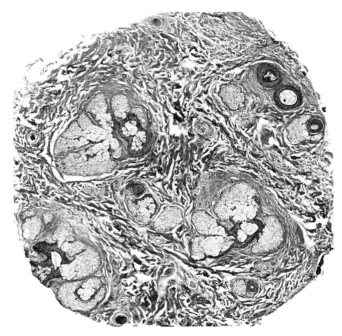

Figure 12.6 End-stage traction alopecia. A reduction in the expected number of follicles is obvious.

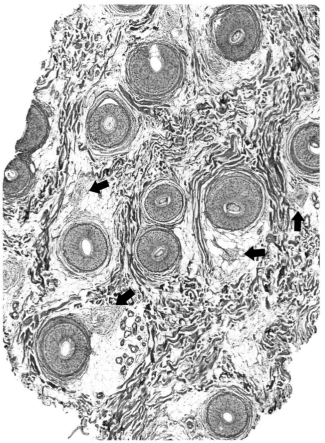

12.8

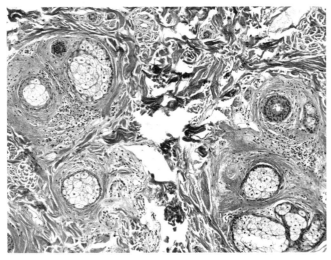

Figure 12.7 Vellus hairs tend to be retained in end-stage traction alopecia.

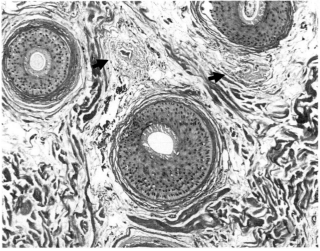

12.9

Figures 12.8 and 12.9 "Old" stelae in specimens from patients with end-stage traction alopecia. When sectioned transversely, these stelae appear as roughly oval amphophilic condensations of connective tissue (*arrows*) containing a few small vascular spaces.

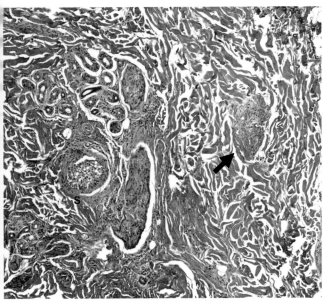

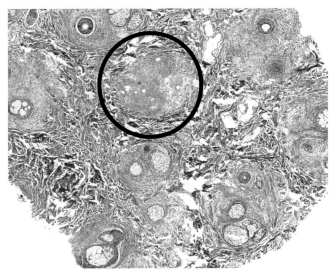

Figure 12.12 Most follicular units in this example of end-stage traction alopecia have retention of sebaceous glands, except for a single unit (*circled*).

Figure 12.10 A column of connective tissue marking the site of a former follicle (*arrow*) is quite obvious in this case of traction alopecia. In some cases, each column may represent the former site of an entire follicular unit. *Abbreviation*: S, sebaceous gland.

Traction Alopecia in Summary

Clinical correlation:

Early or acute disease: The patient is often an African-American child whose hair is tightly braided with alopecia of the scalp margin or around braids.

End-stage disease: The patient is usually an African-American woman with symmetrical thinning of the temples and/or frontal regions.

Histological findings:
Early or acute disease:

❖ Normal size of follicles

❖ Total number of hairs (both terminal and vellus) is normal

❖ Increased number of terminal catagen and/or telogen hairs (the most prominent finding)

❖ No significant inflammation (peribulbar inflammation *absent*)

• Fibrous "streamers" may be present if telogen hairs are increased in number

• Occasional trichomalacia and pigment casts with incomplete, disrupted follicular anatomy rarely found

End-stage or "burnt out" disease:

❖ Marked decrease in total number of follicles and terminal follicles with retention of vellus hairs

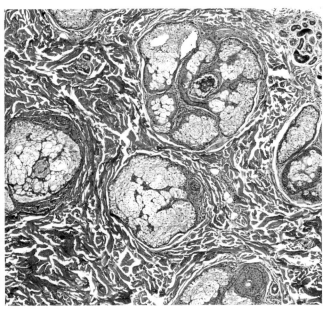

Figure 12.11 Several follicular units in this field have no hair follicles despite intact and non-inflamed sebaceous glands.

* ❖ Many or most follicular units still have associated sebaceous glands
* ❖ No significant inflammation (peribulbar inflammation
  absent)
* Dermal collagen appears relatively normal except for
  occasional fibrous tracts at sites of former follicles

Histological differential diagnosis:

* **Temporal triangular alopecia:** shares many features with
  end-stage traction alopecia. No fibrous tracts or stelae
  should be found in temporal triangular alopecia. Clinical information should help to differentiate
* **Androgenetic alopecia:** shows true miniaturization with
  the presence of stelae and a slightly increased catagen/
  telogen count

⚠ **Pitfalls**

Decreased T:V ratio (due to selective loss of terminal hairs)
should not be misinterpreted as evidence of miniaturization.

REFERENCES

1. Aaronson CM. Etiologic factors in traction alopecia. South Med J. 1969;
   62: 185–6.
2. Scott DA. Disorders of the hair and scalp in blacks. Dermatol Clin. 1988;
   6: 387–95.
3. Rudolph RI, Klein AW, Decherd JW. Corn-row alopecia. Arch Dermatol.
   1973; 108: 134.
4. Renna FS, Freedberg IM. Traction alopecia in nurses. Arch Dermatol.
   1973; 108: 694–5.
5. Trueb RM. "Chignon alopecia": a distinctive type of nonmarginal traction
   alopecia. Cutis; Cutaneous Medicine for the Practitioner. 1995; 55: 178–9.
6. Hwang SM, Lee WS, Choi EH, Lee SH, Ahn SK. Nurse's cap alopecia. Int J
   Dermatol. 1999; 38: 187–91.
7. Goldberg LJ. Cicatricial marginal alopecia: is it all traction? Br J Dermatol.
   2009; 160: 62–8.
8. Hutchens KA, Balfour EM, Smoller BR. Comparison between Langerhans
   cell concentration in lichen planopilaris and traction alopecia with possible immunologic implications. Am J Dermatopathol. 2011; 33: 277–80.
9. Sperling LC, Lupton GP. Histopathology of non-scarring alopecia.
   J Cutan Pathol. 1995; 22: 97–114.
10. Steck WD. Telogen effluvium: a clinically useful concept, with traction
    alopecia as an example. Cutis. 1978; 21: 543–48.

13 Postoperative (pressure-induced) alopecia

This form of hair loss is seen most commonly in patients who have undergone lengthy surgical procedures and had one portion of their scalp (usually the occiput) in prolonged contact with the operating table (1–5). The notion that this condition is caused solely by pressure between the skull and operating table has been challenged (6,7), and other factors, such as coma (8) or prolonged immobility (9) may be involved in certain cases. Postoperative alopecia can occur at any age and is often associated with gynecologic and open-heart procedures requiring tracheal intubation. Less commonly, the condition is found in patients who sustain blunt trauma to the scalp.

CLINICAL FINDINGS

Postoperative alopecia typically presents as a solitary, roughly oval patch on the upper occiput (Figs. 13.1 and 13.2). Early in the course of the condition (the first 2–3 postoperative days), erythema and induration are found in the central portion of the lesion. Nearly total hair loss with fairly sharp demarcation from the surrounding scalp is found just 2–3 weeks after the initial trauma (9). Complete hair regrowth may occur, although several cases of permanent (i.e., cicatricial) hair loss have been reported (9), including some cases seen by the authors of this text. Presumably the severity of local anoxia determines the extent of injury to the follicles and the ultimate prognosis. Alopecia develops up to 28 days following the surgical procedure. Treatment during the initial weeks of the disease is neither necessary nor possible. Partial or complete regrowth of hair is expected, and it would be prudent to wait at least 12 months before any corrective procedure is attempted for residual alopecia.

HISTOLOGICAL FINDINGS

The histological findings in postoperative alopecia change as the lesion evolves. Early in the course of the disease, before hair loss is complete, vascular thrombosis, inflammation, and adnexal necrosis may be seen in the dermis. In the typical case of postoperative alopecia, nearly all terminal follicles will be in the catagen or telogen phases (Fig. 13.3). This synchronized conversion of most or all terminal hairs to the catagen/telogen phase is highly characteristic of postoperative alopecia. Trichomalacia may be present but not the distorted or incomplete follicular anatomy sometimes found in trichotillomania (Fig. 13.4). Apoptotic bodies are often seen within the follicular epithelium (10) (Fig. 13.4). Pigment casts are also commonly found (Fig. 13.5). Melanin pigment is usually found in the collapsed root sheaths deep to catagen/telogen follicles.

Variable degrees of dermal fibrosis and chronic inflammation are present in the papillary and upper reticular dermis. Focal vascular and tissue necrosis may be present along with an associated chronic inflammatory infiltrate. Fat necrosis is often found, associated with an infiltrate of foamy macrophages and mononuclear cells (Fig. 13.6). Inflammation is mild relative to the degree of apparent tissue damage. The inflammation does not seem to be centered on hair follicles, but is usually associated with foci of vascular and tissue necrosis. Postoperative alopecia has several histologic features that are shared with trichotillomania. However, it can be distinguished from trichotillomania by the absence of follicular distortion or by the presence of deep, dermal/adipose degenerative changes.

During the early stages of the disease, the total number of follicles remains normal. However, permanent hair loss can occur, especially in the central portion of the lesion. A biopsy of any long-standing, residual bald spot will resemble an end-stage cicatricial alopecia. The most distinctive histological features of the condition are found during the first several postoperative weeks.

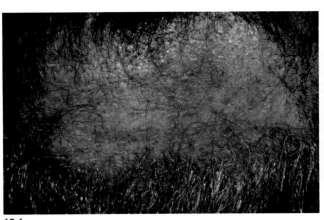
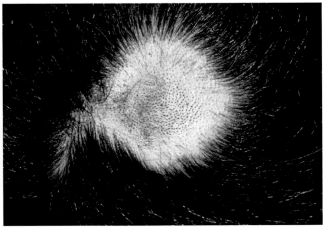

13.1　　**13.2**

Figures 13.1 and 13.2 Postoperative alopecia. In both cases, a large, nearly hairless, occipital patch was noted two weeks after a prolonged surgical procedure. In Figure 13.2, the patient's hair dye accentuates the shaftless, keratin-filled follicular ostia in the central portion of the lesion.

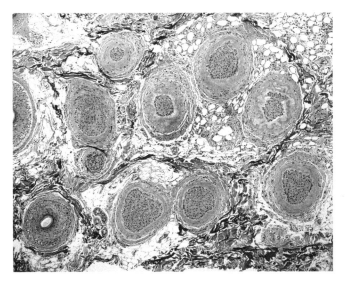

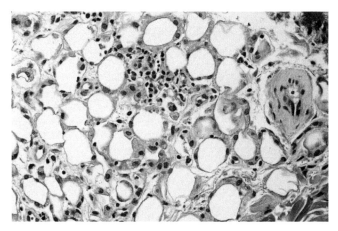

Figure 13.6 Foamy macrophages and other chronic inflammatory cells infiltrate a zone of fat necrosis.

Figure 13.3 Early lesion of postoperative alopecia. In the first few postoperative weeks, most if not all follicles will be in the catagen/telogen phase.

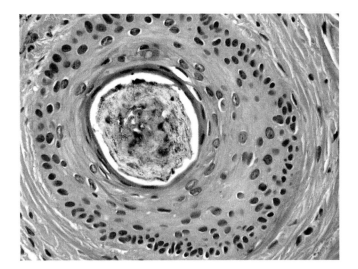

Figure 13.4 Trichomalacia is commonly seen in postoperative alopecia, but the abnormal shaft is centrally placed and ovoid, not the distorted and incomplete shape seen in trichotillomania. Keratinocyte apoptosis is seen.

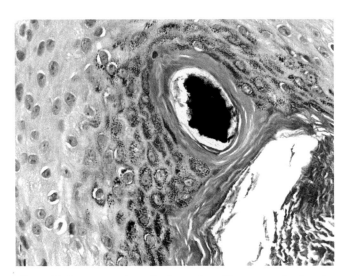

Figure 13.5 Pigment cast formation in a patient with postoperative alopecia.

Postoperative (Pressure-induced) Alopecia in Summary

Clinical correlation: A patch of occipital hair loss occurring within a few weeks of a prolonged surgical procedure requiring general anesthesia. Hair regrowth may or may not occur, and the amount of regrowth (if present) is highly variable.

Histological findings:
❖ Normal or nearly normal total number of follicles (in "early" disease)
❖ Almost all hairs in the catagen or telogen phase
❖ Trichomalacia
❖ Melanin pigment in collapsed fibrous root sheaths
• Vascular thrombosis or necrosis with a relatively mild perivascular and perifollicular inflammatory infiltrate
• Fat necrosis with secondary infiltration by foamy macrophages and a few lymphoid cells
• In "late" disease, findings resemble an end-stage cicatricial alopecia

Histological differential diagnosis:
• **Trichotillomania**: differs from POA by the suggestive clinical history (and absence of a history of a prior operative procedure/prolonged period of pressure), and by the presence of follicular distortion
• **Alopecia areata**: shares with POA the high degree of catagen/telogen shift and occasional pigment casts; differs by the presence of miniaturization and mild peribulbar inflammation

⚠ **Pitfalls**
Biopsy must be performed within the first several weeks to capture diagnostic changes.

Abbreviation: POA, Postoperative Alopecia

REFERENCES

1. Matsushita K, Inoue N, Ooi K, Totsuka Y. Postoperative pressure-induced alopecia after segmental osteotomy at the upper and lower frontal edentulous areas for distraction osteogenesis. Oral Maxillofac Surg 2011; 15: 161–3.
2. Boyer JD, Vidmar DA. Postoperative alopecia: a case report and literature review. Cutis 1994; 54: 321–2.
3. Patel KD, Henschel EO. Postoperative alopecia. Anesth Analg 1980; 59: 311–3.
4. Wiles JC, Hansen RC. Postoperative (pressure) alopecia. J Am Acad Dermatol. 1985; 12: 195–8.
5. Abel RR, Lewis GM. Postoperative (pressure) alopecia. Arch Dermatol 1960; 81: 34–42.
6. Lee WS, Lee SW, Lee S, Lee JW. Postoperative alopecia in five patients after treatment of aneurysm rupture with a Guglielmi detachable coil: pressure alopecia, radiation induced, or both? J Dermatol 2004; 31: 848–51.
7. Khalaf H, Negmi H, Hassan G, Al-Sebayel M. Postoperative alopecia areata: is pressure-induced ischemia the only cause to blame? Transplant Proc 2004; 36: 2158–9.
8. Chow IJ, Balakrishnan C, Meininger MS. Alopecia of the unburned scalp. Burns 1996; 22: 250–1.
9. Kosanin RM, Riefkohl R, Barwick WJ. Postoperative alopecia in a woman after a lengthy plastic surgical procedure. Plast Reconstr Surg 1984; 73: 308–9.
10. Hanly AJ, Jorda M, Badiavas E, Valencia I, Elgart GW. Postoperative pressure-induced alopecia: report of a case and discussion of the role of apoptosis in non-scarring alopecia. J Cutan Pathol 1999; 26: 357–61.

14 Temporal triangular alopecia

Also known as congenital triangular alopecia (1–3), temporal triangular alopecia (TTA) may be present at birth or first noticed during the first decade of life (4,5). Whether or not the zone of alopecia can develop after birth has never been established with certainty. Lesions outside the temporal area (Fig. 14.1), and ones seemingly acquired in adulthood (Fig. 14.2), can rarely occur (6–8). Clinicians unfamiliar with TTA may confuse this condition with alopecia areata (9).

The condition has been reported in association with aplasia cutis congenita (10), Down syndrome (11), mental retardation and epilepsy (12), phakomatosis pigmentovascularis (13,14), and congenital heart disease (15,16). Several familial cases have been described (17), and it has been suggested that the disorder is inherited as a paradominant trait, with expression only when there is a postzygotic somatic mutation (13). Treatment of TTA is seldom required, but some patients are bothered by the bald spot. Topical minoxidil solution would seem like a rational approach, but this has never been tested for efficacy and would probably not be a permanent solution. Hair transplantation could be used to fill in these relatively small areas (18), and in some cases simply excising the lesion is sufficient for cosmetic improvement.

CLINICAL FINDINGS

The lancet-shaped lesions (Fig. 14.3) are a few centimeters in width, may be unilateral or bilateral (Fig. 14.4). The lesions oriented so that the tip of the "lancet" points superiorly and posteriorly. Sometimes a good imagination is required to appreciate this orientation. Lesions appear hairless, but very fine vellus hairs can be seen with magnification. Both we, and others, have seen cases with a centrally placed tuft of terminal hairs (Fig. 14.5) (19,20). Once present, the patches of alopecia persist for life.

HISTOLOGIC FINDINGS

Microscopically, there are *normal* numbers of follicles but almost all are vellus hairs. The small size of the hairs necessitates transverse sectioning for adequate assessment (Fig. 14.6). There are no stelae below these small hairs, and in this regard they resemble primary vellus hairs. Therefore, such follicles will only be found in sections through the mid- to upper dermis. Transverse sections (Figs. 14.7–14.10) reveal that the total number of hairs is normal or nearly normal, although a case with diminished numbers has been reported (20). All other features of the epidermis, dermis, and other adnexae, including sebaceous glands, are entirely normal, and inflammation is absent. The dominant histologic feature is a population of vellus-only hairs confined to a small, lancet-shaped area of the temporal region, resulting in the characteristic "bald" spot. Congenital cases presumably undergo the process of follicular miniaturization in utero (or terminal hair formation never occurs). If postnatal development of the condition truly exists, then terminal hairs must miniaturize, akin to the situation in androgenetic alopecia. However, fibrous "streamers" (stelae) as found in androgenetic alopecia, are not found in TTA (Figs. 14.7 and 14.8).

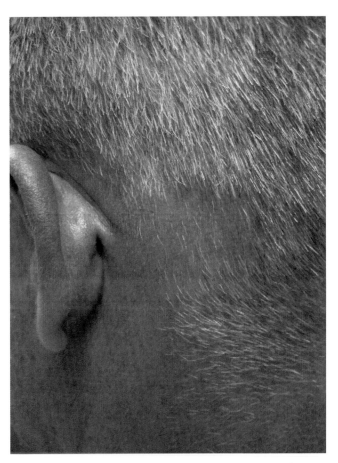

Figure 14.1 Lesion of temporal triangular alopecia in the occipital region. *Source*: Photograph courtesy of Dr. Rebecca Luria.

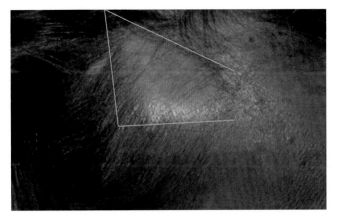

Figure 14.2 Temporal triangular alopecia acquired in adulthood. Blue lines demarcate the lesion, which merges with the patient's temporal recession from common balding, but this unilateral lesion could be distinguished both clinically and histologically.

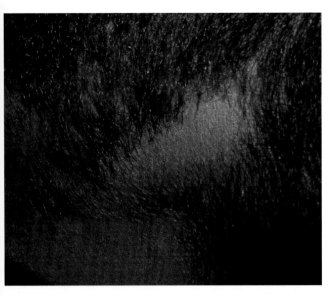

Figure 14.3 Temporal triangular alopecia. This unilateral lesion was first noted when the patient was an infant.

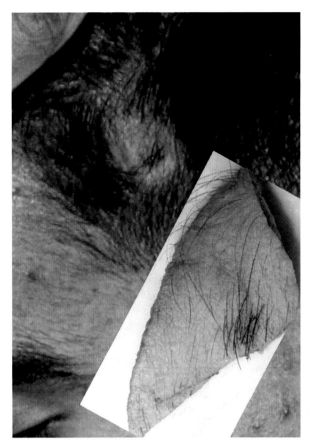

Figure 14.5 Temporal triangular alopecia with centrally placed tuft of terminal hairs. The inset shows an enlarged view of the excisional biopsy specimen.

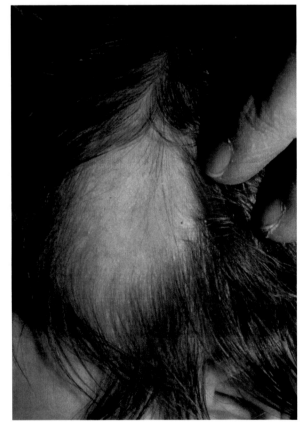

Figure 14.4 Temporal triangular alopecia. This is one of two bilateral lesions that were noted at birth.

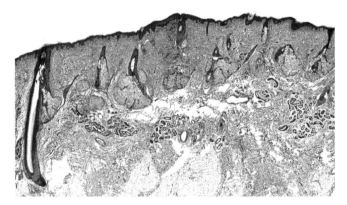

Figure 14.6 A vertical section from a patient with temporal triangular alopecia reveals several vellus follicles. It is almost impossible to quantify the total number and average size of follicles using vertical sections, but in this very generous section, a normal terminal hair at the border of lesion (*left side*) highlights the degree of miniaturization.

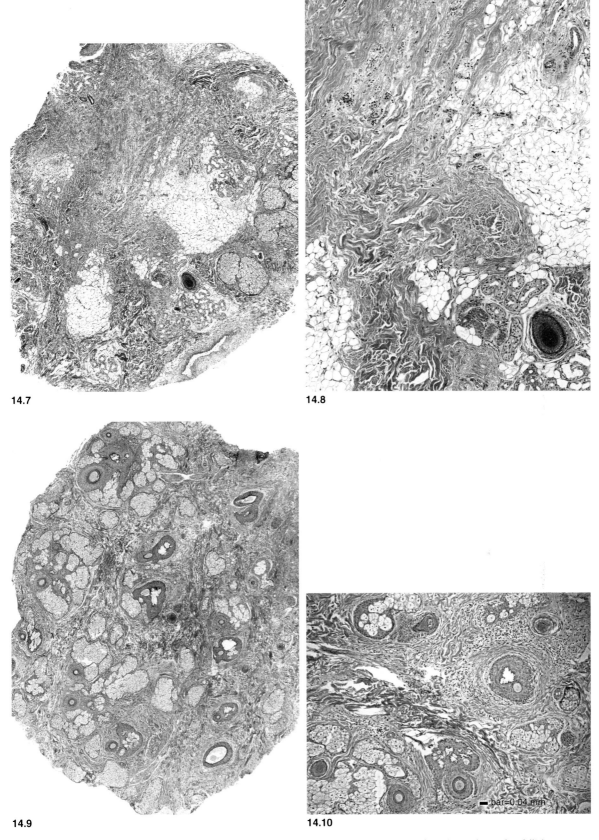

Figures 14.7,14.8,14.9,14.10 Temporal triangular alopecia. Sections through the deep dermis (Figs. 14.7 and 14.8) reveal very few follicles. However, sections through the upper dermis (Figures 14.9 and 14.10) demonstrate a normal number of follicles, almost all of which are very small. The small size of hairs in lesional skin from patients with temporal triangular alopecia is easily appreciated in Fig. 14.10, where the black bar represents 0.04 mm.

Temporal Triangular Alopecia in Summary

Clinical correlation: Lancet-shaped bald spot (may be bilateral) discovered on the temporal region of a newborn or young child; the remainder of the scalp is normal.

Histological findings:
❖ Normal or nearly normal *total* number of hairs
❖ Almost all hairs vellus hairs with few, if any, terminal hairs
❖ No significant inflammation or other epidermal or dermal abnormality
❖ No apparent fibrous "streamers" (stelae)
• Rare cases have shown a reduced number of hairs (20)

Histological differential diagnosis:
• **End-stage traction alopecia:** shares a marked reduction in terminal follicles, leaving vellus hairs with intact sebaceous lobules. The presence of stelae favors traction alopecia. Clinical information should help to differentiate.
• **Androgenetic alopecia:** shows miniaturization (with a mixture of large, medium, and small hair shafts) and underlying stelae.

⚠ **Pitfalls**

Vertical sections are insufficient to establish a definitive diagnosis. If only upper dermal levels of horizontal sections are examined, TTA may be mistaken for androgenetic alopecia.

REFERENCES

1. Kubba R, Rook A. Congenital triangular alopecia. Br J Dermatol 1976; 95: 657–9.
2. Bargman H. Congenital temporal triangular alopecia. Can Med Assoc 1984; 131: 1253–4.
3. Feuerman EJ. Congenital temporal triangular alopecia. Cutis 1981; 28: 196–7.
4. Yamazaki M, Irisawa R, Tsuboi R. Temporal triangular alopecia and a review of 52 past cases. J Dermatol 2010; 37: 360–2.
5. Trakimas C, Sperling LC, Skelton HG, 3rd, Smith KJ, Buker JL. Clinical and histologic findings in temporal triangular alopecia. J Am Acad Dermatol 1994; 31: 205–9.
6. Trakimas CA, Sperling LC. Temporal triangular alopecia acquired in adulthood. J Am Acad Dermatol 1999; 40: 842–4.
7. Akan IM, Yildirim S, Avci G, Akoz T, Karadayi N. Bilateral temporal triangular alopecia acquired in adulthood. Plast Reconstr Surg 2001; 107: 1616–7.
8. Tosti A. Congenital triangular alopecia. J Am Acad Dermatol 1987; 16: 991–3.
9. Laffitte E, Panizzon RG, Saurat JH. Delayed wound healing on the scalp following treatment of actinic keratoses: erosive pustular dermatosis of the scalp. Dermatol Surg 2004; 30: 1610.
10. Kenner JR, Sperling LC. Pathological case of the month. Temporal triangular alopecia and aplasia cutis congenita. Arch Pediatr Adolesc Med 1998; 152: 1241–2.
11. Bordel-Gomez MT. Congenital triangular alopecia associated with Down's syndrome. J Eur Acad Dermatol Venereol 2008; 22:1506–7.
12. Ruggieri M, Rizzo R, Pavone P, et al. Temporal triangular alopecia in association with mental retardation and epilepsy in a mother and daughter. Arch Dermatol 2000; 136: 426–7.
13. Happle R. Congenital triangular alopecia may be categorized as a paradominant trait. Eur J Dermatol 2003; 13: 346–7.
14. Kim HJ, Park KB, Yang JM, Park SH, Lee ES. Congenital triangular alopecia in phakomatosis pigmentovascularis: report of 3 cases. Acta Derm Venereol 2000; 80: 215–6.
15. Leon-Muinos E, Monteagudo B, Labandeira J, Cabanillas M. [Bilateral congenital triangular alopecia associated with congenital heart disease and renal and genital abnormalities]. Actas Dermosifiliogr 2008; 99: 578–9.
16. Park SW, Choi YD, Wang HY. Congenital triangular alopecia in association with congenital heart diseases, bone and teeth abnormalities, multiple lentigines and cafe-au-lait patches. Int J Dermatol 2004; 43: 366–7.
17. Patrizi A, Morrone P, Fiorentini C, Bianchi T. An additional familial case of temporal triangular alopecia. Pediatr Dermatol 2001; 18: 263–4.
18. Burkhart CG, Burkhart CN. Trichorrhexis nodosa revisited. Skinmed 2007; 6: 57–8.
19. Assouly P, Happle R. A hairy paradox: congenital triangular alopecia with a central hair tuft. Dermatology 2010; 221: 107–9.
20. Silva CY, Lenzy YM, Goldberg LJ. Temporal triangular alopecia with decreased follicular density. J Cutan Pathol 2010; 37: 597–9.

15 Alopecia areata

Alopecia areata (AA) is a common form of noncicatricial hair loss affecting males and females of all ages and ethnicities. Data from the First National Health and Nutrition Examination Survey in the early 1970s placed the prevalence at 0.1–0.2% (1). Another community-based study estimated a lifetime risk of 1.7%, with similar rates between the sexes and over all age groups (2). Children are frequently affected, as the majority (60%) of patients experience onset of disease before the age of 20 years (3). The disease can affect any part of the body (Fig. 15.1), but scalp hair loss is the most common complaint. The degree of involvement ranges from a small, circumscribed bald spot to total scalp hair loss (*alopecia totalis*), and even total body hair loss (*alopecia universalis*). Prognosis is variable between the types but frequently mirrors the severity of disease at the time of presentation (4). AA stems from a loss of the immune privilege of the follicle (5,6), opening the door for a lymphocyte-mediated autoimmune attack recognized histologically as the "swarm of bees" around hair bulbs (7). The various susceptibility loci identified by a genome-wide association study provide evidence that defects in both acquired and innate immunity, many of which are common to other autoimmune diseases, are involved in the pathogenesis of AA (8).

CLINICAL FINDINGS

Several patterns of partial hair loss are recognized, including circumscribed (isolated round-to-oval patches; Figs. 15.2 and 15.3), which can coalesce (Fig. 15.4), reticular or mosaic (innumerable small patches; Fig. 15.5), ophiasis (marginal involvement of the posterolateral scalp, Fig. 15.6), the very rare inverse ophiasis pattern or "sisapho" (a band of hair loss along the frontotemporal to parietal scalp) and diffuse AA.

Diffuse AA can present a diagnostic challenge. There are reported cases where the clinical presentation is an acute and diffuse alopecia involving the whole scalp. In this form, also known as AA incognita (9–11), the hair density is typically diffusely diminished throughout the scalp (Fig. 15.7), although it may be more pronounced in the androgen-dependent areas. Circumscribed bald patches are absent. The clinical picture has been described as mimicking a severe telogen effluvium (12). Histological confirmation is required to establish the diagnosis.

The reports of a rapidly progressive form of complete hair loss termed "acute diffuse and total alopecia" seen primarily in young Asian women may represent cases of AA incognita (13) or a similar variant with a unique natural history of rapid regrowth (14–17). Additional study of similar cases is necessary. If steadily and rapidly shedding hair proceeds to baldness without short-term recovery, the diagnosis of alopecia totalis

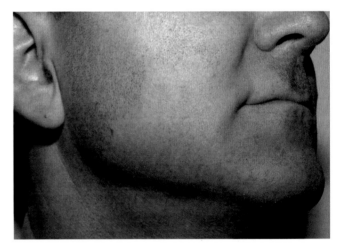

Figure 15.1 Alopecia areata affecting the beard area. This patient had no scalp hair loss.

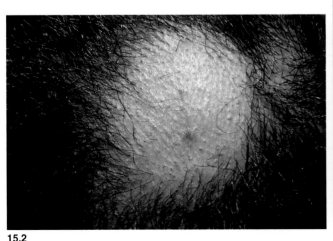

15.2

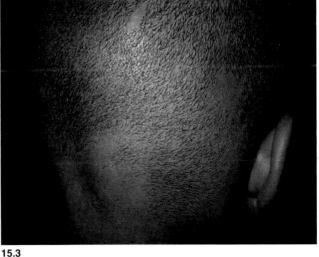

15.3

Figures 15.2 and 15.3 Typical, circumscribed lesions of alopecia areata.

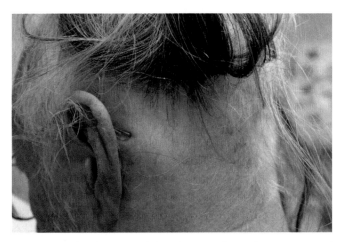

Figure 15.6 Ophiasis pattern of alopecia areata. *Source*: Image courtesy of Brett King M.D., Ph.D.

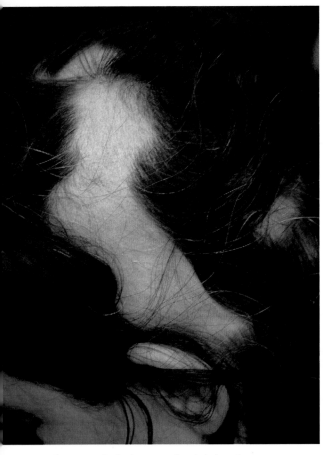

Figure 15.4 Coalescing areas of typical alopecia areata.

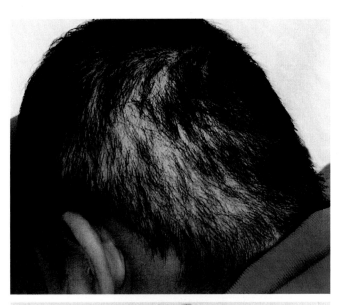

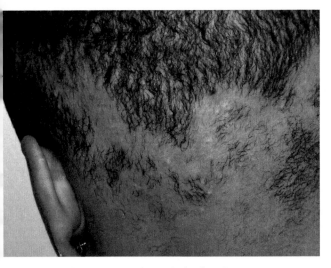

Figures 15.5 Mosaic or reticular alopecia areata.

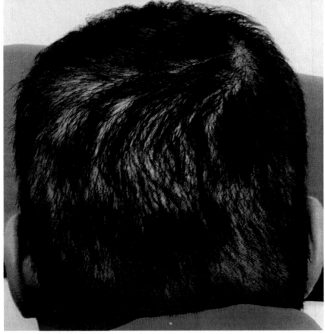

in evolution is more appropriate than a form of diffuse AA (Fig. 15.8). Even in alopecia totalis or universalis, isolated hairs or tufts of hairs may continue to grow.

The involved scalp in AA is usually normal in color but may show slight erythema, edema, or a peachy-orange discoloration (18). Short hairs that taper as they approach the scalp are called "exclamation point hairs," and if present are very characteristic of AA (Fig. 15.9). Because of shaft narrowing and hypopigmentation near the scalp surface (Fig. 15.10), exclamation point hairs appear to "float" on the

Figure 15.7 Diffuse alopecia areata (alopecia areata incognita) in an adolescent Caucasian boy.

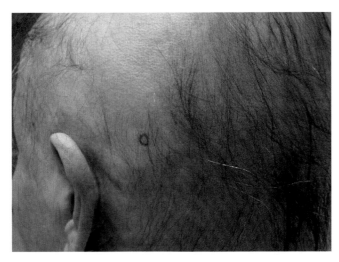

Figure 15.8 Alopecia totalis in evolution. This patient had rapid, diffuse hair loss progressing over a period of just a few months without subsequent regrowth.

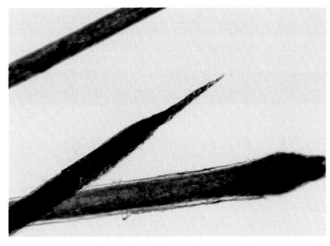

Figure 15.11 Tapered, "pencil point" hair gently extracted from a patient with alopecia totalis in evolution.

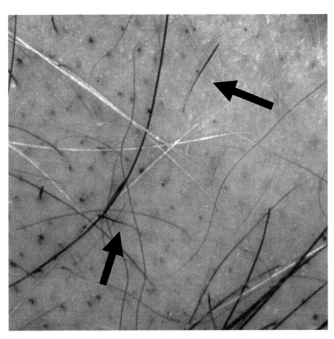

Figure 15.9 Patch of alopecia areata with exclamation point hairs as indicated by the arrows.

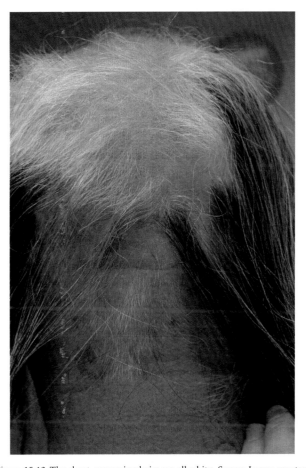

Figure 15.12 The short, regrowing hairs are all white. *Source*: Image courtesy of Brett King, M.D., Ph.D.

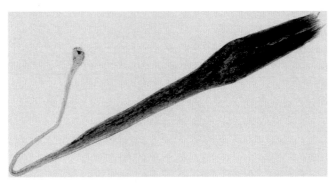

Figure 15.10 Exclamation point hair. This hair was easily pulled from the scalp. The wider, distal end (right side) shows a fracture, and the proximal end is narrow and hypopigmented. Most exclamation mark hairs are in the telogen phase.

scalp surface. When gentle pulling pressure is applied to hairs at the edges of an expanding lesion of AA, many telogen hairs and/or tapered "pencil point shafts" can be easily extracted (Fig. 15.11). This is most prominent in patients with rapidly progressive disease. AA seems to preferentially affect pigmented hairs, and the onset of diffuse AA in a person with salt-and-pepper hair could potentially explain sudden whitening of the hair described in some historical accounts (19). Hair regrowth also frequently initiates with depigmented hairs (Fig. 15.12).

Dermoscopy has gained traction in recent years as an aid in the diagnosis of alopecia. Yellow dots (Fig. 15.13), thought to represent collections of keratinaceous debris within the dilated infundibula of nanogen and catagen/telogen hairs, are reported to be relatively specific for AA and can provide additional evidence in favor of the diagnosis when the diffuse type raises the differential diagnoses of telogen effluvium or androgenetic alopecia (17,20,21).

There are numerous treatment options for AA; a recent review details a practical approach to the treatment of adult and pediatric populations (22). The treatment choice(s) should be selected with the clinical type and severity of disease progression in mind. Options include topical mid- or high-potency steroids (more commonly used in children who do not tolerate injections), intralesional triamcinolone injections (for localized disease), irritants such as topical anthralin or topical retinoids, and immunotherapy with diphenylcyclopropenone or squaric acid dibutyl ester. Further study of topical capsaicin is warranted (23). Systemic therapies are typically reserved for severe disease given higher side effect (and often relapse) profiles, and include systemic (often pulsed) corticosteroids and cyclosporine. Topical minoxidil is helpful as an adjuvant agent coupled with the above treatments. Patients should be directed to the National Alopecia Areata Foundation (www.naaf.org) for additional resources and support, including information on hair prostheses.

HISTOLOGICAL FINDINGS
Very early AA or cases with rapidly progressive hair loss present a very different histological picture than longstanding, well-established disease. The histopathology of AA can be divided into three stages. These stages, *acute, subacute, and chronic,* reflect the evolution of the disease with the passage of time (24). Different "stages" of disease may coexist at different sites on the same scalp. In any given patient, separate lesions of AA may begin, evolve, remit, and recur independently of one another.

The *acute* stage is seen in rapidly progressive disease or disease of recent onset, as in evolving alopecia totalis or at the advancing margin of an enlarging bald spot. The total number of follicles appears normal. The majority of hairs are still terminal anagen follicles, with bulbs in the fat or deep dermis. However, within a matter of weeks after onset, several follicles will enter the catagen/telogen phase (24) or miniaturize (Fig. 15.14).

Some (especially miniaturizing) anagen phase and early catagen phase hairs demonstrate a peribulbar mononuclear cell inflammatory infiltrate. Both CD4+ and CD8+ T cells are found, with CD4+ cells typically dominating (25,26) (Figs. 15.15 and 15.16). CD8+ cells, however, are more likely to invade the epithelium than CD4+ cells (27). In some cases, peribulbar inflammation may be very subtle or even absent, and other histological features are required to establish the diagnosis. The presence of peribulbar inflammation is very

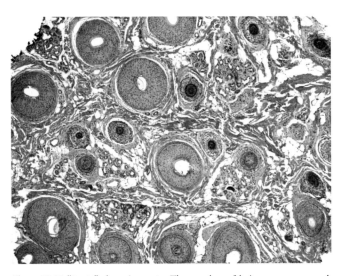

Figure 15.14 "Acute" alopecia areata. The number of hairs appears normal, but there is an increase in the number of miniaturized hairs. The bulbs of true vellus hairs should not be visible at the level of the eccrine glands.

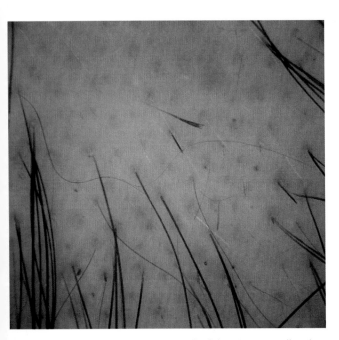

Figure 15.13 Trichoscopy of an alopecic patch of alopecia areata. Yellow dots, thought to represent keratinaceous debris within the dilated follicular infundibula, and exclamation point hairs are visible. *Source:* Image courtesy of Antonella Tosti, M.D.

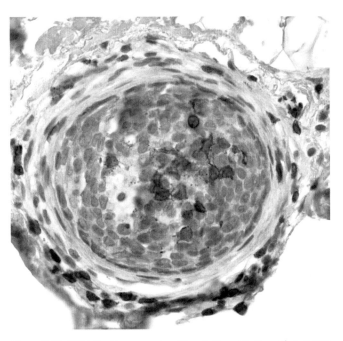

Figure 15.15 CD3+ T cells surround and invade the epithelium of an anagen hair.

helpful *but not essential* to making the diagnosis of AA. In the active phase of recurrent disease, the peribulbar lymphocytes may be found around the miniaturized bulbs situated in the reticular dermis. Variable numbers of eosinophils may also be present (28,29), but plasma cells are unusual in AA (30) (Figs. 15.17 and 15.18).

The infiltrate may invade the follicular papilla and hair matrix, resulting in damage to matrical cells. This can result in a "blurry" or "disorganized" appearance of the hair matrix (Figs. 15.19 and 15.20). While the exocytosis of inflammatory cells contributes to this appearance, the alteration of the matrical cells is frequently present even without exocytosis (31). Edema, both intercellular (spongiosis) and intracellular, may also be present; it can be subtle or quite prominent, and can affect the suprabulbar as well as the bulbar zone. Like the matrix, the outer root

sheath can also assume a disorganized appearance as a result of the inflammation (Figs. 15.21 and 15.22).

Some anagen follicles may display necrosis of matrical cells and vacuole formation just above the upper pole of the follicular papilla, corresponding to the site of early hair cortex formation (Fig. 15.23). This can result in small cystic spaces filled with acantholytic, necrotic cells. Focal matrix cell vacuolization and necrosis is a characteristic feature of AA, but it affects relatively few follicles and is found in only a minority of cases. Nuclear pyknosis and apoptosis occur not only in matrical

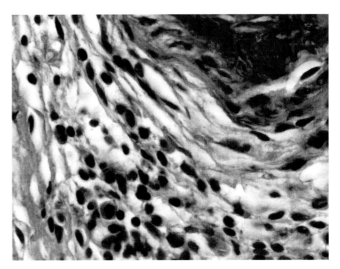

Figure 15.18 Eosinophils are admixed with the peribulbar lymphocytic infiltrate.

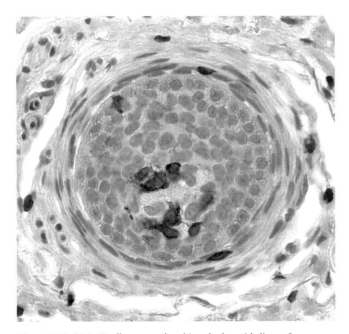

Figure 15.16 CD4+ T cells surround and invade the epithelium of an anagen hair. The density is similar to that seen in the same specimen stained for CD3 in the preceding figure.

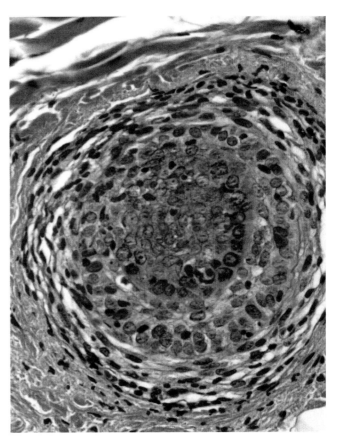

Figure 15.19 The hair matrix of this inflamed bulb appears blurry and disorganized.

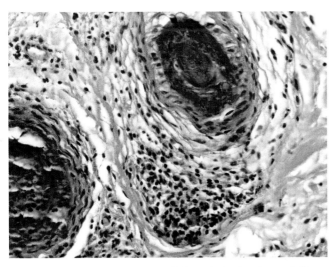

Figure 15.17 Eosinophils are admixed with the peribulbar lymphocytic infiltrate.

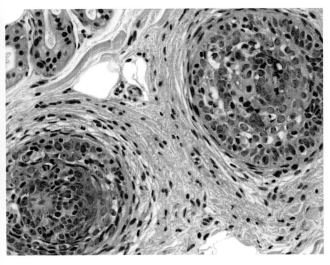

Figure 15.20 Despite the scanty peribulbar infiltrate, the epithelia of these two bulbs appear blurry and somewhat disorganized. Exocytosis of a few lymphocytes and apoptosis of a few epithelial cells, contribute to the impression.

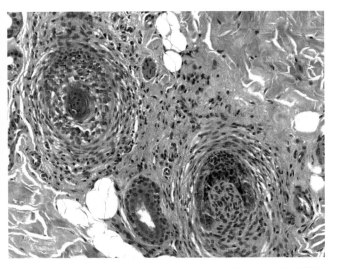

Figures 15.21 To the left of the image is the suprabulbar zone of a follicle showing blurring of the outer root sheath. To the right is a rim of disorganized-appearing matrical epithelium hugging the follicular papilla.

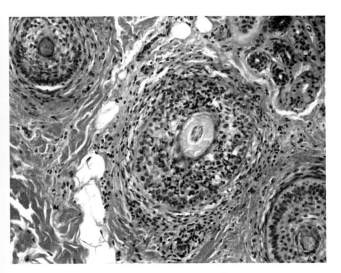

Figure 15.22 Another example of lymphocytes invading the outer root sheath, which appears blurry and disorganized as a result.

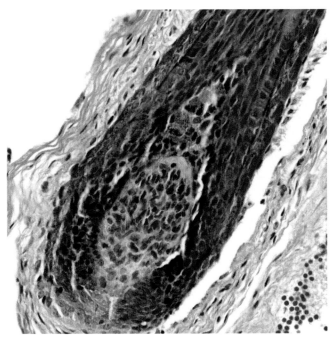

Figure 15.23 Several necrotic matrical cells lie just above the upper pole of the hair papilla. Destruction of these keratinocytes (and occasional melanocytes) leads to clumps of melanin pigment visible within the epithelium, and pigment incontinence within the papilla.

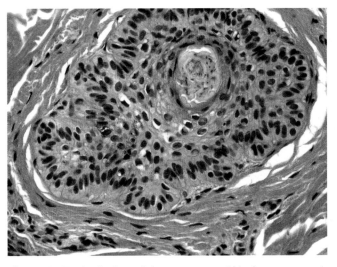

Figure 15.24 Focal collections of pigment are seen within the outer root epithelium of this follicle.

keratinocytes, but also in the bulbar melanocytes and the outer root sheath cells.

Amorphous collections of pigment are occasionally found within the follicular epithelium as a byproduct of hair matrix degeneration (Fig. 15.24). More significant inflammatory damage leads to larger collections of pigment, which can be found in the epithelium, the follicular papilla (Figs. 15.25 and 15.26), and the follicular sheath or stela (Fig. 15.27) of affected hairs. Aggregates of pigment can also be seen within the infundibular ostia (Fig. 15.28), reminiscent of the pigment casts of trichotillomania.

The second or *subacute* stage of AA is the one most commonly encountered by pathologists. Although the transition between stages is fluid, the subacute stage roughly correlates

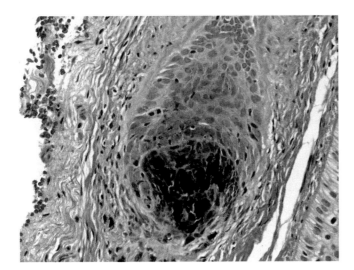

Figure 15.25 Vertical section showing a dense clump of incontinent pigment within the follicular papilla.

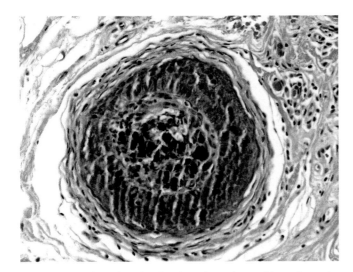

Figure 15.26 Horizontal section showing a dense clump of incontinent pigment within the follicular papilla.

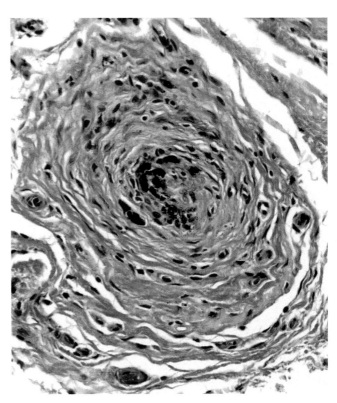

Figure 15.27 Clumps of pigment within a stela.

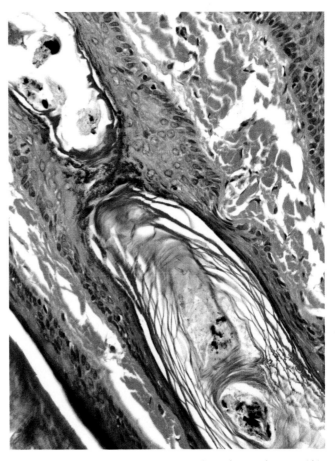

Figure 15.28 Clumps of pigment, en route to the surface, can be seen within the canal of the follicular infundibulum.

with a period 2–3 months after the initiation of disease (24). When all follicles are counted (which requires the examination of transverse sections at both deep and superficial levels), the total number of follicles appears normal. However, in virtually all cases, there is a striking increase in the percentage of catagen/telogen hairs, often exceeding 50% of total follicles (Figs. 15.29 and 15.30). Some of the catagen/telogen hairs are still terminal (large) hairs and some terminal anagen hairs may also be seen; however, the terminal:vellus (T:V) hair ratio has started to decrease, indicating miniaturization. Peribulbar inflammation tends to subside after the hair has entered the catagen phase; as a result, late catagen and telogen hairs are usually free of inflammation (Fig. 15.31). A few inflammatory cells may nevertheless persist near the lower portion of some catagen/telogen follicles, as well as within the collapsed sheaths (Figs. 15.32 and 15.33).

Despite the peribulbar inflammation and matrix injury, some anagen hairs continue to produce hair shafts. Some of these shafts show *trichomalacia*, and are smaller, incompletely

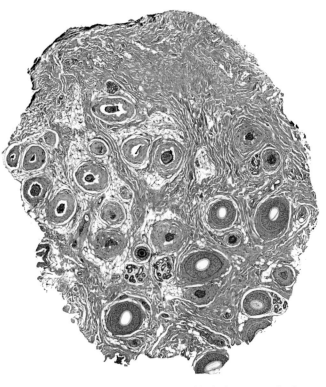

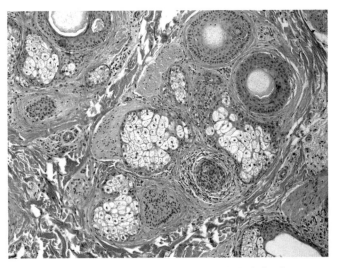

Figure 15.31 Inflammation predominantly surrounds the bulb of an anagen hair (follicle just right and below center). Late catagen/telogen follicles (the surrounding five follicles) are spared from inflammation.

Figure 15.29 This specimen shows aspects of both the acute and subacute stages. The majority of the hairs in the upper part of this biopsy are terminal (large) and nearly all are in the catagen phase (subacute). Several of the hairs in the lower right aspect of the specimen appear unaffected and are terminal anagen, but their bulbs (seen at another level) show heavy lymphocytic inflammation (acute disease). Some hairs have miniaturized as well.

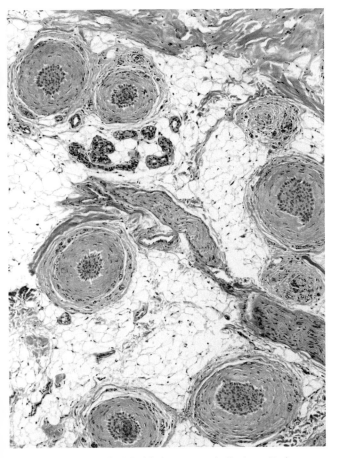

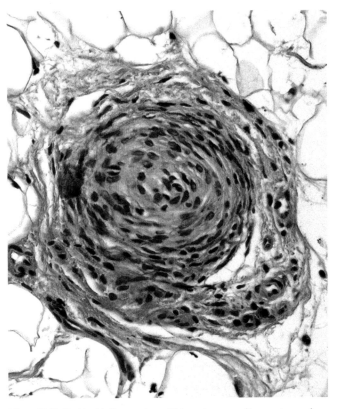

Figure 15.32 Residual inflammation within and surrounding a catagen phase hair bulb.

cornified and distorted in shape. Many follicles produce shafts that become progressively smaller in volume and cross-sectional dimension as the diseased follicles are progressively less able to generate shafts. These hairs gradually taper down to a point (Figs. 15.34–15.36), resulting in an extremely fragile constriction. They represent the "pencil point hairs," which fall from the scalp in great numbers. A transverse section through the site of constriction may show a minute or absent hair shaft. The term *anagen arrest* (or *anagen effluvium*) has been applied to those forms of alopecia characterized by the rapid cessation of shaft formation, leading to tapering and shedding of large

Figure 15.30 Within this field all of the hairs are terminal in size and in the catagen phase. There are two streamers representing hairs that have already miniaturized.

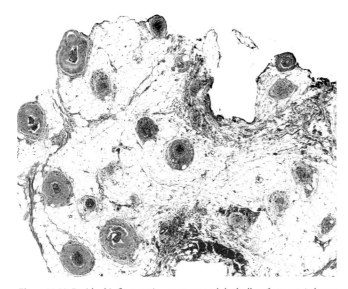

Figure 15.33 Residual inflammation seen around the bulbs of catagen/telogen hairs. Several of the stelae also show residual inflammation; observed with this magnification, the impression is that of a "busy streamer."

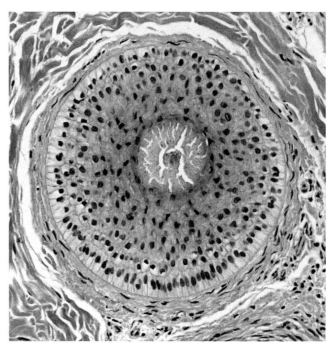

Figure 15.35 This terminal anagen hair has only a few cornified cells centrally in place of a normal shaft.

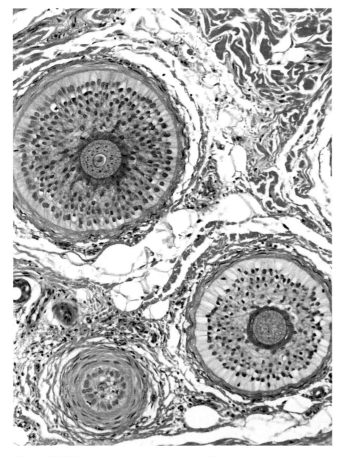

Figure 15.34 The anagen hair in the upper left of the photograph is producing a minute shaft that is smaller than the width of the inner root sheath that surrounds it. Once the inner root sheath has desquamated, the shaft easily fractures to form a "pencil point hair." The anagen hair in the lower right of the photograph has produced a cornified inner root sheath, but no cortex/shaft formation has occurred.

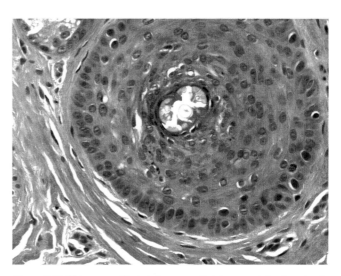

Figure 15.36 This anagen-like hair has a cornified inner root sheath and only a miniscule central shaft; the amount of surrounding epithelium is out of proportion to the tiny shaft.

numbers of anagen hairs. Anagen arrest is characteristic of chemotherapy-induced alopecia, but the initial stages of AA (when terminal hairs are still present) also have features of anagen arrest. However, after producing a dystrophic (or no) shaft for a period of time, these anagen hairs eventually enter the catagen/telogen phase.

After remaining in the telogen phase for a period of time (about 100 days in a normal follicle, an unknown length of time in AA), hair follicles re-enter the anagen phase. Unless the disease has spontaneously subsided, an inflammatory infiltrate again confronts the newly forming anagen hairs. This results in a repetition of the pathologic process: peribulbar inflammation, disturbance of anagen hair growth, and a precipitous shift into the catagen/telogen phase (Fig. 15.37). As this process repeats itself, the duration of anagen becomes ever briefer.

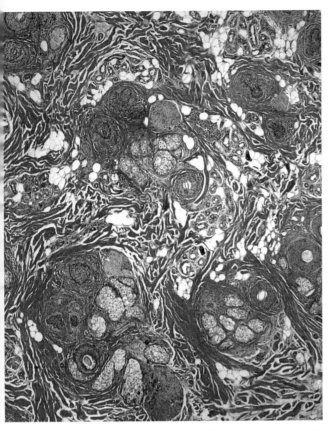

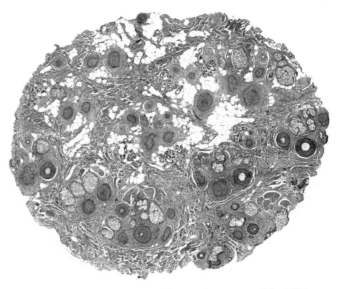

Figure 15.38 Alopecia areata, "chronic" stage. The majority of the follicles are in the telogen phase. Only two terminal anagen hairs are present, and peribulbar inflammation may be difficult or impossible to identify.

Figure 15.37 The percentage of telogen hairs in "subacute" disease is >50% and approaches 100% with ongoing chronicity. Many of the follicles are miniaturized, and the remaining terminal follicles will follow with time.

Along with this, the anagen hairs miniaturize, and an increasingly large percentage of hairs will be found in the catagen/telogen phase, sometimes approaching 100% of the total as the disease moves into the chronic phase.

The third histological stage, which we will refer to as *chronic*, is found in stable, longstanding, bald patches and in well-established alopecia totalis or universalis. Terminal anagen hairs, with or without a surrounding mononuclear infiltrate, are rare. Thus the most familiar histological finding of AA may be absent. In addition, all or most of the follicles may become miniaturized (the T:V ratio can reach 1:10), although the total number of follicles remains normal (Figs. 15.38–15.40). This remains true for years or even decades, but eventually follicular dropout may occur (an example of the "biphasic" pattern of permanent alopecia). When follicles are miniaturized, they are often missed on a routine vertical sectioning. Transverse sections are necessary to examine and count all follicles.

The miniaturized anagen follicles found in "chronic" disease are situated in the mid-to-lower dermis, usually slightly deeper than nonminiaturized vellus hairs (Fig. 15.41). Normally, anagen hairs develop through a series of stages named Anagen I–VI. The majority of the diseased, miniaturized follicles in AA develop to a stage resembling Anagen III or IV, but no further. These small, abnormal follicles have been called "nanogen hairs" (*nanos*, Greek for "dwarf"), and are a distinctive feature of longstanding AA (Fig. 15.42) (32). Nanogen hairs are not merely small—their rapid and distorted life cycle leads to mixed morphologies, making them difficult to categorize as anagen, catagen, or telogen hairs.

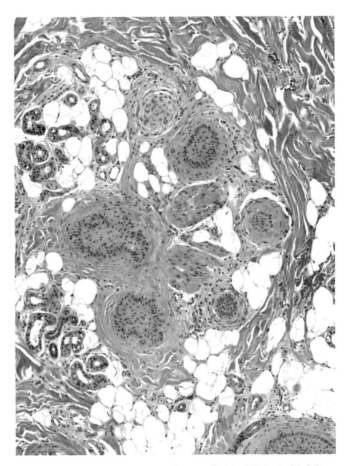

Figure 15.39 Alopecia areata, "chronic" stage. All of the follicles in this follicular unit have shifted into the telogen phase.

Nanogen hairs have an epithelial matrix that is small relative to the size of the follicular papilla, which is also reduced in volume. The nuclei of the papilla become rounder and the cells more compact, much as they do in the catagen/telogen phase (Fig. 15.43). Nanogen hairs can be identified in transverse section because they frequently have thin inner and outer root sheaths (as little as two or three cell layers), but most importantly

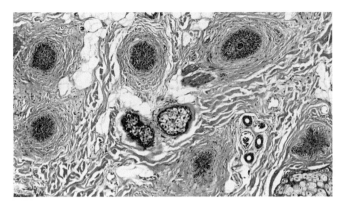

Figure 15.40 Alopecia areata, "chronic" stage. All of the follicles in this field are in the telogen phase.

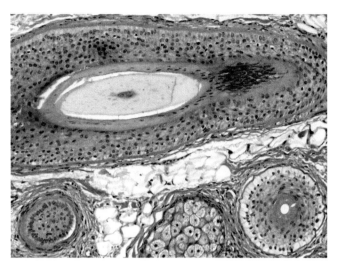

Figure 15.42 A terminal hair (*superior*) stands in marked contrast to the two tiny nanogen hairs (*inferior*), a catagen-like nanogen (*left*) and an anagen-like nanogen (*right*).

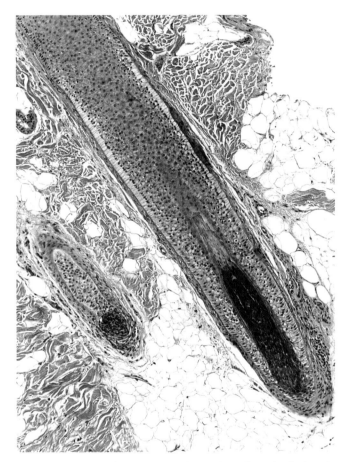

Figure 15.41 The bulb of this miniaturized anagen hair is located at the dermal–subcutaneous junction, deeper than would be seen in the case of a normal vellus hair. A terminal anagen hair is present for comparison. There is active inflammation around the bulb of the anagen hair, and mild residual inflammation adjacent to the bulb of the miniaturized hair.

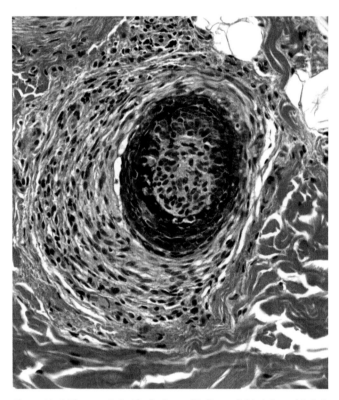

Figure 15.43 Nanogen hair. The bulbar epithelium of this inflamed hair is only a few cells in thickness, and is thin relative to the diameter of the papilla.

they have no central hair shaft, or at most an extremely fine, incompletely cornified shaft (Figs. 15.44–15.53).

Furthermore, they may simultaneously demonstrate morphologic features of both the anagen and catagen/telogen phases. The bulb may resemble that of an anagen hair (basophilic cells with mitotic activity), whereas the suprabulbar portion shows features of a catagen hair. Conversely, the bulb may show features typical of a catagen hair, whereas the suprabulbar zone possesses an anagen-like inner root sheath with trichohyaline granules. Nanogen hairs with "anagen-like"

bulbs may have some matrix cells in mitosis, while others are undergoing apoptosis (Fig. 15.54). Thus, features of active growth (mitosis) and involution (apoptosis) are seen simultaneously. The strange histological characteristics of nanogen hairs signify a profound disorder of cell cycling that is unique to AA. In most cases, the majority of nanogen hairs will be found in the catagen/telogen phase, so that "anagen-like" nanogen hairs may be difficult to find (Figs. 15.55 and 15.56).

Nanogen hair bulbs may be surrounded and sometimes invaded by inflammatory cells, but generally the degree of inflammation is mild and often subtle (Fig. 15.57). The most inflamed nanogen bulbs are those with "anagen-like" and early "catagen-like" bulbs (Figs. 15.43, 15.44, 15.49 and 15.50).

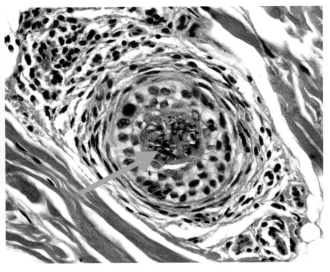

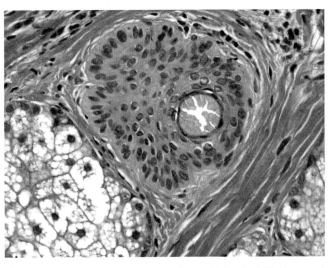

Figure 15.44 Nanogen hair, transverse section in the suprabulbar zone. The outer root sheath is diminished, and is only a few cells in thickness. The central, eosinophilic zone (*arrow*) represents the inner root sheath. Formation of the hair shaft, expected at this level, is not seen.

Figure 15.46 Nanogen hair, transverse section at a higher level. The inner root sheath has cornified, but there is no shaft.

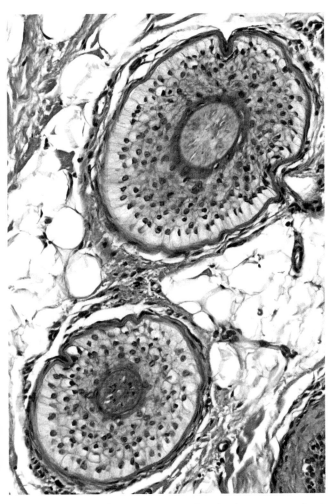

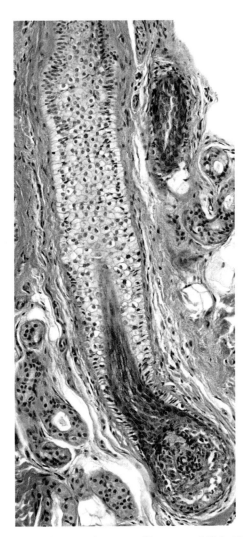

Figure 15.45 Nanogen hairs. Transverse section showing outer root sheath and inner sheath formation without formation of the hair shaft.

Figure 15.47 Vertical section of an anagen-like nanogen follicle. The adjacent eccrine glands give a sense of the small size of this nanogen follicle. The bulbar epithelium, inner and outer root sheaths are all quite thin. Formation of a shaft is not seen.

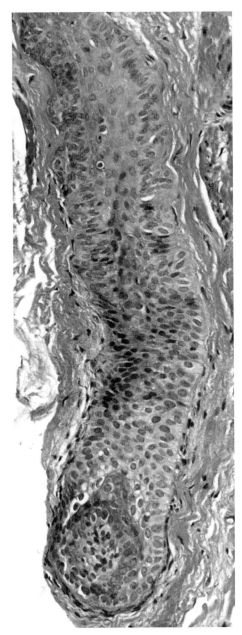

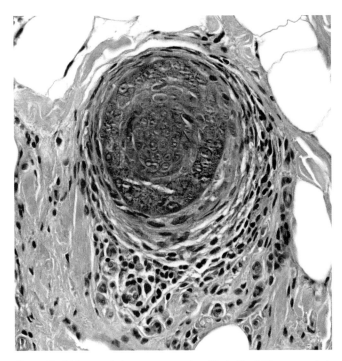

Figure 15.49 Nanogen hair, transverse section. The bulb of this nanogen hair shows anagen-like features. The beginnings of thin inner and outer root sheaths are visible. There are peribulbar lymphocytes.

Figure 15.48 Vertical section of a catagen-like nanogen follicle. Keratinocyte apoptosis identifies this follicle as a catagen-like follicle. The size of the papilla, the bulbar epithelium and overlying outer root sheath are all reduced in volume.

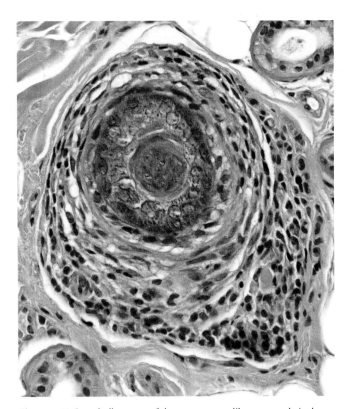

Figure 15.50 Suprabulbar zone of the same anagen-like nanogen hair shown in Figure 15.49, with the abnormally thin outer root sheath, trichohyaline granules of the inner root sheath and central cortex. There is surrounding inflammation.

When inflammation is seen in the chronic/recurrent stage of AA, it is typically seen surrounding the anagen or early catagen bulbs of miniaturized or nanogen hairs in the reticular dermis; as in the acute stage, the telogen follicles are relatively spared from an inflammatory infiltrate. In the chronic phase, the majority (or all) of the follicles in a specimen may be in the catagen/telogen phase, and so inflammation can be entirely absent, and is not required to make a diagnosis (Fig. 15.58). This results in a picture of "non-inflammatory" AA, a surprising finding in patients who may have very severe disease with a dramatic clinical presentation. Deep to each miniaturized follicle is a collapsed fibrous root sheath (*stela*). In acute disease the stelae are more likely to appear loose, with numerous capillaries (Fig. 15.59), residual inflammatory cells, and clumps of melanin. With time, the stelae become more fibrotic, the inflammation decreases, the melanin is scavenged,

and the number of capillaries slowly diminishes. Unless they are inflamed, these collapsed sheaths appear identical to the "fibrous streamers" described in androgenetic alopecia and telogen effluvium. Typical of the majority of noncicatricial alopecias, atrophy of sebaceous glands is not seen in AA (Fig. 15.60).

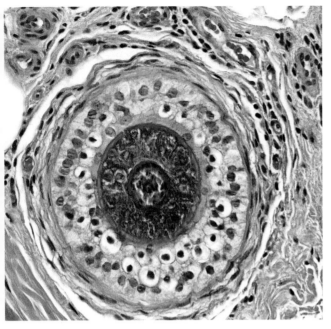

Figure 15.51 A more superficial level within the suprabulbar region of the same nanogen hair seen in Figures 15.49 and 15.50. It shows anagen-like features of inner root sheath and cortex formation, however, a well-developed shaft (expected at this level) is not present.

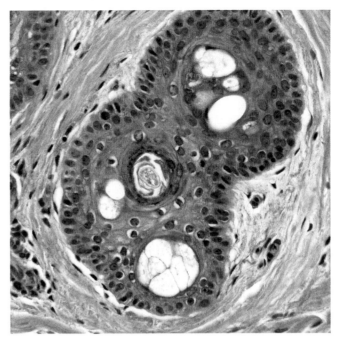

Figure 15.53 Superficial (infundibular) level of the nanogen hair shown in Figures 15.49–15.52. The rudimentary shaft is visible. There is a single apoptotic keratinocyte, atypical for anagen epithelium.

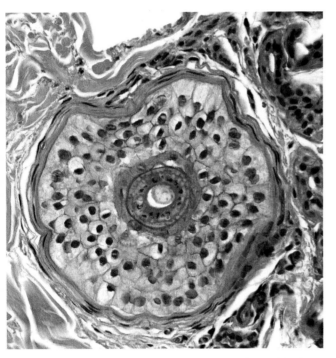

Figure 15.52 A more superficial level of the same nanogen hair seen in Figures 15.49–15.51, with the formation of a tiny, rudimentary shaft.

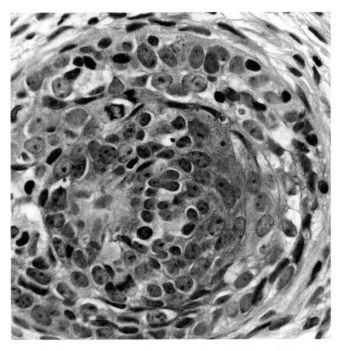

Figure 15.54 This greatly magnified nanogen hair bulb shows both mitotic and apoptotic cells.

Dilated follicular infundibula, filled with residual keratinaceous debris, may be seen at any stage of the disease (Fig. 15.61). This finding has been coined the "follicular Swiss-cheese pattern" (for the appearance of the dilated infundibula on horizontal sections) and has been suggested as the histopathological correlate to the yellow dots seen on dermoscopy (Fig. 15.13) (33).

Rarely (in our experience about 10% of the time), focal follicular destruction with hair shaft extrusion and/or localized granulomatous inflammation can be seen in AA (Figs. 15.62 and 15.63). Although this finding is suggestive of a cicatricial alopecia, when present only focally and in conjunction with other characteristic features, this finding should not dissuade the pathologist from making a diagnosis of AA.

Biopsies are rarely taken from the recovering scalp, but if performed they will show a gradual reversal of the above cycle, with an increasing number of anagen hairs and a trend toward normalization of the T:V hair ratio. Inflammation is absent (24).

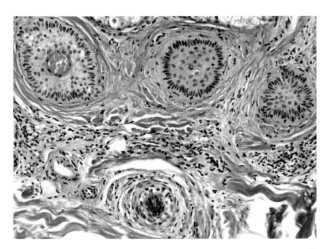

Figure 15.55 Three catagen-like nanogen follicles are seen (*superior*) within the same field as one anagen-like nanogen follicle (*right*).

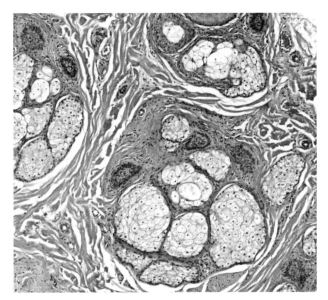

Figure 15.56 In this field alone, seven catagen/telogen-like nanogen follicles are seen.

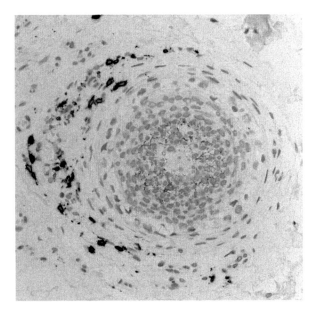

Figure 15.57 An immunoperoxidase stain for CD3+ cells highlights the lymphocytes surrounding the bulb of a nanogen hair. This stain may be helpful in cases where inflammation is scant.

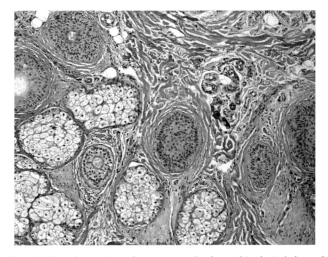

Figure 15.58 In this specimen demonstrating the chronic histological phase of alopecia areata, the majority of the miniaturized follicles are in the telogen phase; their bulbs (visible in deeper sections) are not inflamed.

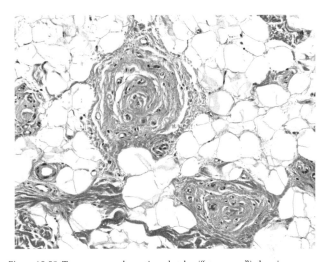

Figure 15.59 Two transversely sectioned stelae ("streamers") showing numerous capillaries in a patient with alopecia areata.

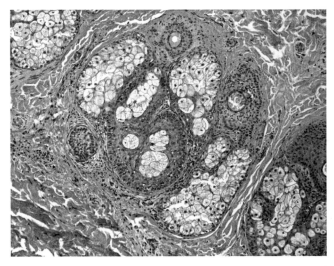

Figure 15.60 Normal sebaceous glands appear outsized for the miniaturized follicles in the follicular unit.

The histological diagnosis of AA may be difficult to make with confidence in the absence of clinical correlation because AA has some histological mimics. These include syphilitic alopecia, the patchy, noncicatricial alopecia seen in systemic lupus erythematosus, and very early lesions of "discoid" lupus erythematosus. In most cases, the biopsy specimens of patients with these mimics provide subtle clues as to the correct diagnosis. However, when we are not provided with a history typical of AA, it is our practice to add the following proviso to the tissue examination report: "Similar histological findings can sometimes be seen in syphilitic alopecia, and in the patchy, noncicatricial alopecia of systemic lupus erythematosus; these should be excluded by history, physical findings, and appropriate serologies, as clinically indicated." Few patients will be done a disservice by receiving a more careful review of systems, physical examination, or serologic screening for occult systemic disease.

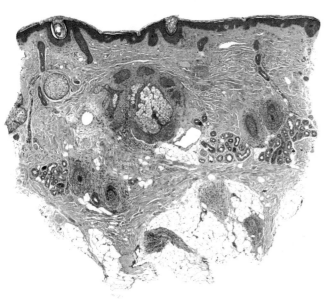

Figure 15.61 Dilated follicular infundibula containing keratinaceous debris can be seen opening to the epidermal surface in this case of early subacute disease. There is active inflammation with evidence of miniaturization and catagen/telogen shift.

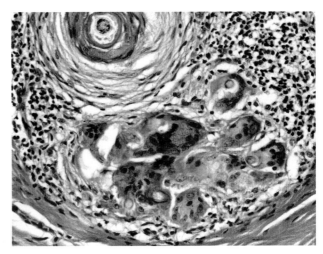

Figure 15.63 An otherwise typical biopsy of alopecia areata showed this focus of granulomatous inflammation with fragments of hair shaft within multinucleated giant cells.

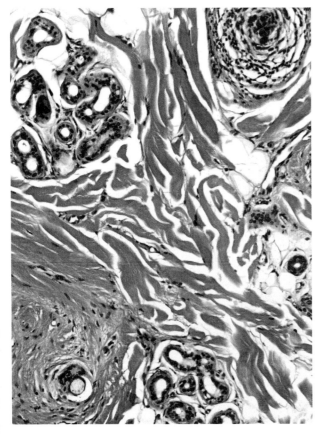

Figure 15.62 An inflamed miniaturized bulb is visible in the upper right corner. In the lower left corner is a free hair shaft with an adjacent multinucleated giant cell.

Alopecia Areata in Summary

Clinical correlation: A classic AA patient presents with patchy, circumscribed, or rarely diffuse hair loss without evidence of inflammation and may develop total scalp, or scalp and body alopecia. Lesions appear suddenly and may expand rapidly. "Exclamation mark hairs" may sometimes be seen, especially at the active (advancing) margins of the alopecic patches where they can be easily extracted for examination. Broken-off hairs, fine regrowing hairs and yellow dots can be seen on dermoscopy. Pigmented hairs may be shed first, leaving behind grey or white hairs. Regrowth is often hypopigmented initially.

Histological findings:
Early, severe, or progressive disease ("acute" and "subacute"):
❖ Normal *total* number of hairs
❖ Increased number of miniaturized hairs
❖ Increased number of terminal catagen and telogen hairs (may be moderately increased in acute disease, and may exceed 50% in subacute disease)
• Peribulbar, mononuclear cell infiltrate (with occasional eosinophils), predominantly affecting terminal anagen and catagen hair bulbs
• Occasional exocytosis of inflammatory cells into bulbar epithelium

- Degenerative changes (nuclear pyknosis, inter- and intracellular edema, vacuole formation) of the hair matrix, especially the lower, central matrix
- Trichomalacia and marked narrowing of hair shafts

Longstanding and stable disease ("chronic"):

❖ Majority of hairs are in catagen/telogen phase (can approach 100%)

❖ Numerous miniaturized, aberrant hairs (nanogen hairs) with hybrid morphologies of anagen, catagen, and telogen

- Mild peribulbar, mononuclear cell infiltrate around those miniaturized or nanogen hairs having anagen-like or catagen-like bulbs
- When telogen-like hairs dominate, inflammation may be absent

Histological differential diagnosis:

- **"Essential" syphilitic alopecia:** closely mimics AA but occasional peribulbar plasma cells (not a feature of AA) can be a distinguishing clue. Confirmatory serologies should be performed.
- **Noncictricial alopecia of systemic lupus erythematosus:** may be differentiated by the presence of increased mucin, perivascular, and periadnexal lymphocytes and plasma cells, and vacuolar interface changes; eosinophils are rare in lupus but are often seen in AA. Direct immunofluorescence can be helpful to distinguish the entities when the specific features of lupus are not present.
- **Psoriatic alopecia:** can be distinguished by the significant atrophy of sebaceous glands, which are unaffected by AA. Psoriatic changes to the interfollicular epidermis are telling, but may be absent in partially treated disease.

⚠ **Pitfalls**

Clinical correlation along with serologic testing and direct immunofluorescence may be required to reliably differentiate between the above three entities. Rarely, focal follicular destruction with granulomatous inflammation can be seen in AA. Total absence of peribulbar inflammation may be found in longstanding lesions.

Abbreviation: AA, alopecia areata.

REFERENCES

1. Safavi K. Prevalence of alopecia areata in the First National Health and Nutrition Examination Survey. Arch Dermatol 1992; 128: 702.
2. Safavi KH, Muller SA, Suman VJ, Moshell AN, Melton LJ. 3rd. Incidence of alopecia areata in Olmsted County, Minnesota, 1975 through 1989. Mayo Clin Proc 1995; 70: 628–33.
3. Price VH. Alopecia areata: clinical aspects. J Invest Dermatol 1991; 96: 68S.
4. Tosti A, Bellavista S, Iorizzo M. Alopecia areata: a long term follow-up study of 191 patients. J Am Acad Dermatol 2006; 55: 438–41.
5. Kang H, Wu WY, Lo BK, et al. Hair follicles from alopecia areata patients exhibit alterations in immune privilege-associated gene expression in advance of hair loss. J Invest Dermatol 2010; 130: 2677–80.
6. Gilhar A. Collapse of immune privilege in alopecia areata: coincidental or substantial? J Invest Dermatol 2010; 130: 2535–7.
7. Gilhar A, Paus R, Kalish RS. Lymphocytes, neuropeptides, and genes involved in alopecia areata. J Clin Invest 2007; 117: 2019–27.
8. Petukhova L, Duvic M, Hordinsky M, et al. Genome-wide association study in alopecia areata implicates both innate and adaptive immunity. Nature 2010; 466: 113–7.
9. Rebora A. Alopecia areata incognita: a hypothesis. Dermatologica 1987; 174: 214–8.
10. Quercetani R, Rebora AE, Fedi MC, et al. Patients with profuse hair shedding may reveal anagen hair dystrophy: a diagnostic clue of alopecia areata incognita. J Eur Acad Dermatol Venereol 2011; 25: 808–10.
11. Molina L, Donati A, Valente NS, Romiti R. Alopecia areata incognita. Clinics (Sao Paulo) 2011; 66: 513–5.
12. Rebora A. Alopecia areata incognita. J Am Acad Dermatol 2011; 65: 1228.
13. Rebora A. Acute diffuse and total alopecia of the female scalp: a new subtype of diffuse alopecia areata that has a favorable prognosis–a reply. Dermatology 2003; 207: 339; author reply 340.
14. Sato-Kawamura M, Aiba S, Tagami H. Acute diffuse and total alopecia of the female scalp. A new subtype of diffuse alopecia areata that has a favorable prognosis. Dermatology 2002; 205: 367–73.
15. Lew BL, Shin MK, Sim WY. Acute diffuse and total alopecia: a new subtype of alopecia areata with a favorable prognosis. J Am Acad Dermatol 2009; 60: 85–93.
16. Choi HJ, Ihm CW. Acute alopecia totalis. Acta Dermatovenerol Alp Panonica Adriat 2006; 15: 27–34.
17. Inui S, Nakajima T, Itami S. Significance of dermoscopy in acute diffuse and total alopecia of the female scalp: review of twenty cases. Dermatology 2008; 217: 333–6.
18. Alkhalifah A, Alsantali A, Wang E, McElwee KJ, Shapiro J. Alopecia areata update: part I. Clinical picture, histopathology, and pathogenesis. J Am Acad Dermatol 2010; 62: 177–88; quiz 189–190.
19. Jelinek JE. Sudden whitening of the hair. Bull N Y Acad Med 1972; 48: 1003–13.
20. Tosti A, Whiting D, Iorizzo M, et al. The role of scalp dermoscopy in the diagnosis of alopecia areata incognita. J Am Acad Dermatol 2008; 59: 64–7.
21. Ardigo M, Tosti A, Cameli N, et al. Reflectance confocal microscopy of the yellow dot pattern in alopecia areata. Arch Dermatol 2011; 147: 61–4.
22. Gupta LK, Khare A, Garg A, Mittal A. Congenital triangular alopecia: a close mimicker of alopecia areata. Int J Trichol 2011; 3: 40–1.
23. Ehsani AH, Toosi S, Seirafi H, et al. Capsaicin vs. clobetasol for the treatment of localized alopecia areata. J Eur Acad Dermatol Venereol 2009; 23: 1451–3.
24. Whiting DA. Histopathologic features of alopecia areata: a new look. Arch Dermatol 2003; 139: 1555–9.
25. Todes-Taylor N, Turner R, Wood GS, Stratte PT, Morhenn VB. T cell subpopulations in alopecia areata. J Am Acad Dermatol 1984; 11(2 Pt 1): 216–23.
26. Bodemer C, Peuchmaur M, Fraitaig S, et al. Role of cytotoxic T cells in chronic alopecia areata. J Invest Dermatol 2000; 114: 112–6.
27. Gilhar A, Landau M, Assy B, et al. Mediation of alopecia areata by cooperation between CD4+ and CD8+ T lymphocytes: transfer to human scalp explants on Prkdc(scid) mice. Arch Dermatol 2002; 138: 916–22.
28. Elston DM, McCollough ML, Bergfeld WF, Liranzo MO, Heibel M. Eosinophils in fibrous tracts and near hair bulbs: a helpful diagnostic feature of alopecia areata. J Am Acad Dermatol 1997; 37: 101–6.
29. El Darouti M, Marzouk SA, Sharawi E. Eosinophils in fibrous tracts and near hair bulbs: A helpful diagnostic feature of alopecia areata. J Am Acad Dermatol 2000; 42(2 Pt 1): 305–7.
30. Lee JY, Hsu ML. Alopecia syphilitica, a simulator of alopecia areata: histopathology and differential diagnosis. J Cutan Pathol 1991; 18: 87–92.
31. Sperling LC, Lupton GP. Histopathology of non-scarring alopecia. J Cutan Pathol 1995; 22: 97–114.
32. Headington J, Mitchell A, Swanson N. New histopathologic findings in alopecia areata studied in transverse section. 42nd Annual Meeting of the Society for Investigative Dermatology Vol. 76. San Francisco, CA. USA J Investig Dermatol 1981; 325.
33. Muller CS, El Shabrawi-Caelen L. 'Follicular Swiss cheese' pattern–another histopathologic clue to alopecia areata. J Cutan Pathol 2011; 38: 185–9.

16 Psoriatic alopecia

Psoriatic alopecia, long an overlooked diagnosis, has received increased attention in recent years. Clinically apparent psoriatic alopecia among patients with a history of psoriasis is uncommon; however, given the relatively high prevalence of scalp psoriasis in the general population, this form of alopecia is clearly under-recognized and underdiagnosed. It is not understood why some patients have hair loss within their scalp psoriasis, whereas others do not, despite having longstanding disease.

CLINICAL FINDINGS

Many patients have a personal or family history of plaque-type psoriasis preceding the development of psoriatic alopecia (1). The severity and body surface area of involvement of pre-existing psoriasis do not appear to be predictive factors for the development of psoriatic alopecia. The typical presentation (seen in approximately three quarters of patients (1)) is alopecia associated with a psoriatic plaque (erythema with overlying silvery scale); within that plaque, the alopecic area may be patchy or relatively well circumscribed (1–4) (Figs. 16.1 and 16.2). Less commonly, diffuse thinning can be seen when the entire scalp is involved (Fig. 16.3) (1,2,4). Onset of psoriatic alopecia in patients with a history of scalp sebopsoriasis or seborrheic dermatitis also occurs, and *de novo* onset of scalp-only disease is also surprisingly common (34% of patients in the largest series) (1). The clinical course has been reported to be acute in 51% of patients, chronic in 36%, and chronic-recurrent in 13% (1).

Treatment with standard antipsoriatic agents such as high-potency topical steroids, tar or salicylic acid-based products will often lead to resolution of seborrheic dermatitis-like

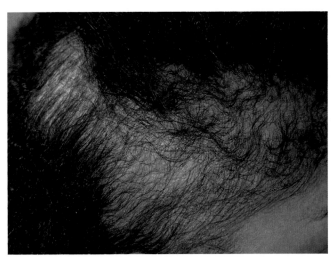

Figure 16.2 Alopecia in a 17-year-old African-American woman (without a prior history of psoriasis) who had presented a month earlier to the clinician with new red, scaly scalp plaques with associated hair loss. She was treated for one month with clobetasol and an antiseborrheic shampoo and returned with vast improvement of the eruption but residual alopecia in the same distribution. A biopsy done at this time showed the typical features of psoriatic alopecia, with mild epidermal features consistent with partial treatment effect. *Source*: Image courtesy of Ronald Savin, M.D. and Gregory Rau, P.A.

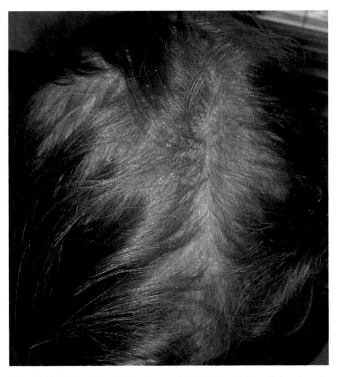

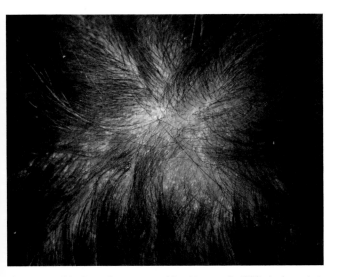

Figure 16.1 This Caucasian woman with a history of mild/limited psoriasis vulgaris on the body presented with alopecia associated with scalp erythema and scale. This photograph was taken after the patient was treated with topical steroids and antipsoriatic shampoos and represents an 80% improvement in scaling, with persistent erythema and alopecia.

Figure 16.3 Diffuse alopecia in a 9-year-old girl with a history of chronic scalp and body psoriasis. This photograph was taken after extended use of class I topical steroids and antiseborrheic shampoos. There is persistent erythema of the scalp, mild scaling, and diminished hair density. *Source*: Image courtesy of Richard Antaya, M.D.

patches and relatively thin plaques. Thicker plaques have responded well to intralesional triamcinolone. More diffuse and severe cases may require systemic antipsoriatic medications such as cyclosporine, methotrexate, or biologic agents. Clinical scarring has been reported (1–8), but appears to occur in a minority of cases; in the largest published series, scarring was seen in approximately 12% of the 41 cases after 7 years of followup (1). Hair growth resumes after the resolution of the inflammatory eruption in the vast majority of patients. Since the duration and intensity of inflammation in active alopecic plaques are suspected to contribute to scarring, prompt treatment is preferred (1,5,8).

HISTOLOGICAL FINDINGS
Perhaps the most striking feature on initial examination is the abnormally high percentage of follicles that have shifted into the catagen and telogen phases (Figs. 16.4–16.6), a finding which has also been reported in hair pull tests (1,9). Eighty percent or more of the follicles can be in the catagen/telogen phase (1).

A variable degree of miniaturization of follicles can also be seen (Figs. 16.7 and 16.8), making a precise terminal anagen: catagen/telogen ratio difficult to calculate due to the small number of

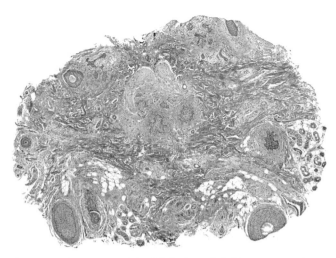

Figure 16.6 The majority of the follicles have shifted into catagen/telogen. A terminal anagen hair is present in the lower right corner for comparison.

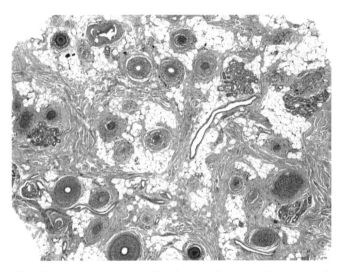

Figure 16.4 A section at the level of the dermal–subcutaneous junction reveals numerous follicles shifted into catagen/telogen including many fibrovascular stelae sitting deep to the regressing epithelia of shifted follicles. There is a mild lymphocytic infiltrate around some of the bulbs and within some of the stelae.

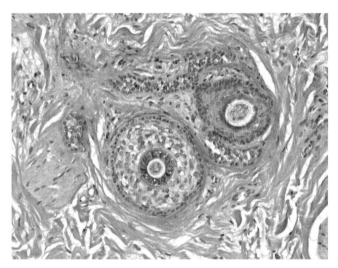

Figures 16.7 The small shafts of two miniaturized hairs in psoriatic alopecia.

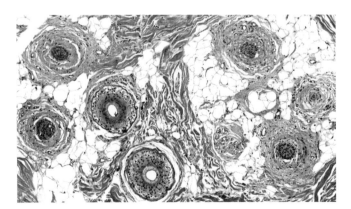

Figure 16.5 A higher magnification image at the level of the dermal–subcutaneous junction shows four follicles shifted into the catagen/telogen phase and two stelae underlying shifted follicles.

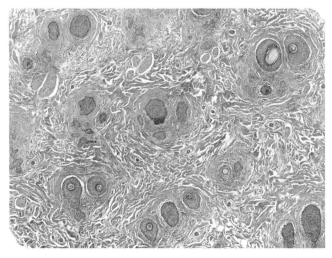

Figure 16.8 A section through the level of the isthmus shows miniaturization and a majority of follicles in catagen/telogen.

remaining terminal hairs. However, it is usually obvious in cases of psoriatic alopecia that 50% or more of the hairs are shifted into catagen/telogen phase.

The overall number of follicles is typically normal or slightly reduced. When viewed in a deep plane, the number of bulbs and hairs may initially appear to be reduced, but when miniaturized and shifted follicles visible at more superior levels are accounted for, the numbers are generally approximately normal. The presence of fibrovascular stelae within the fat is a clue to the miniaturized and shifted follicles that can be found superiorly in the tissue (Figs. 16.4 and 16.5).

Changes of psoriasis are typically present in the interfollicular epidermis. These include psoriasiform hyperplasia, intracorneal (and sometimes intraepidermal) neutrophils, parakeratosis, hypogranulosis, and thinning of the suprapapillary plates (Fig. 16.9). Slight spongiosis and lymphocyte exocytosis may be present. Occasionally, the epidermal features resemble seborrheic dermatitis more than psoriasis, with parakeratosis localized to the lips of follicular ostia (Fig. 16.10), and focal collections of neutrophils within the stratum corneum. The epidermal findings may be mild or even absent if the patient has been treated (particularly with steroids) before biopsy. This may be the case if the scalp appears normal except for alopecia at the biopsy site.

Capillary loops in the papillary dermis are typically dilated (Fig. 16.11). A superficial perivascular, peri-infundibular, and/or peri-isthmic lymphocytic inflammatory infiltrate is present (Fig. 16.12); occasional plasma cells or eosinophils may also be seen in the same compartment. The focal presence of lymphocytes surrounding follicular bulbs (or the stelae left in their place after the shift into catagen) can be identified in approximately one third of cases in the authors' experience (Figs. 16.13–16.15). Multiple sections may need to be examined to identify foci of inflammation. Deep eosinophils are uncommonly seen (Figs. 16.13 and 16.14), and deep plasma cells are rare.

Peribulbar lymphocytes, a dramatically elevated catagen/telogen percentage, and miniaturization are also found in alopecia areata, a potential diagnostic pitfall. Unlike alopecia

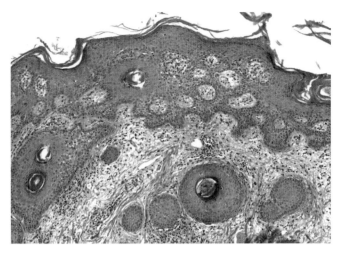

Figure 16.10 The epidermal changes can be more subtle, in some cases resembling seborrheic dermatitis. In this case of psoriatic alopecia there is mild spongiosis, hypogranulosis, thinning of the suprapapillary plates, and focal parakeratosis abutting the two follicular ostia in this image.

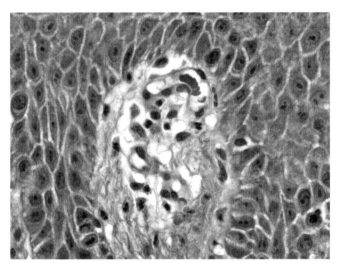

Figure 16.11 Dilated and tortuous vessels are visible within a dermal papillary tip.

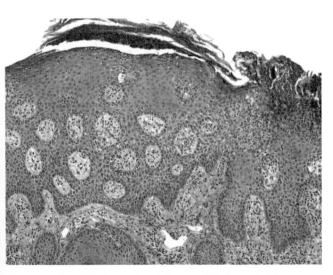

Figures 16.9 Interfollicular epidermal features of classic psoriasis in a case of psoriatic alopecia. There is psoriasiform epidermal hyperplasia, parakeratosis with neutrophils within the stratum corneum, and hypogranulosis.

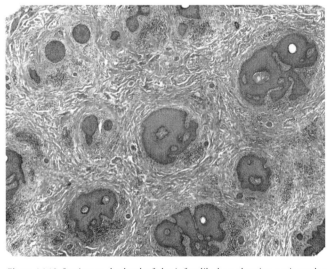

Figure 16.12 Section at the level of the infundibulum showing perivascular and focally perifollicular lymphocytes. The shafts of many of the follicles are small, a result of miniaturization.

areata, however, psoriatic alopecia also demonstrates dramatic atrophy or apparent absence of sebaceous glands (Figs. 16.16–16.18). Although this is typically regarded as a feature of cicatricial alopecias, atrophy of sebaceous glands is a distinctive feature seen in psoriatic alopecia, and in this case does not connote a scarring outcome (10–12). In fact, biopsies from patients with scalp psoriasis but *without* alopecia also show atrophy of sebaceous glands (10). The sebaceous glands are shrunken down to a basophilic remnant (Fig. 16.19), which can at times take on an irregular outline that mimics the shape of the telogen germ unit.

Premature desquamation of the inner root sheath has been seen in some cases of psoriatic alopecia (Fig. 16.20). The significance of this finding is unclear and will require further study. Follicular destruction and hair shaft extrusion can be

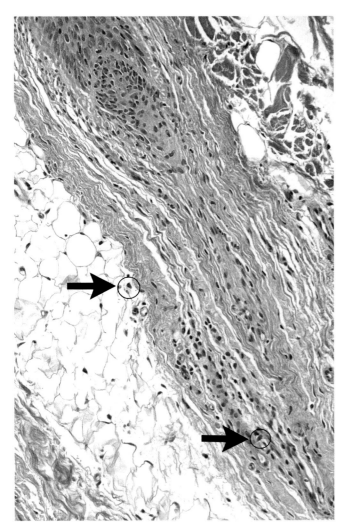

Figure 16.13 Lymphocytes and two eosinophils (circled with arrows) are seen surrounding the regressing bulb of this catagen follicle; they are also seen around and within the stela below the bulb.

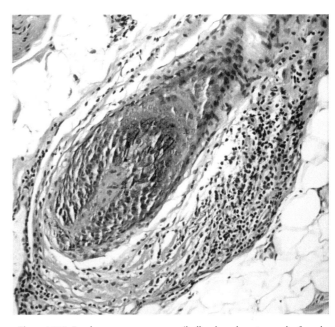

Figure 16.15 Rarely, more numerous peribulbar lymphocytes can be found.

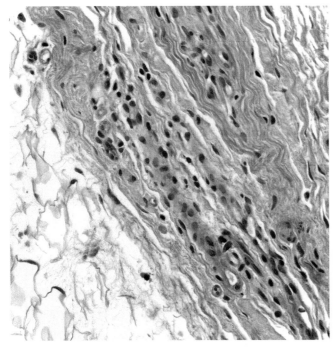

Figure 16.14 A higher power view of the same stela shown in Fig. 16.13. There are multiple lymphocytes and two eosinophils.

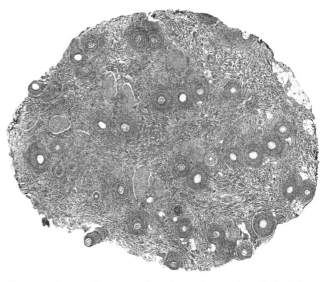

Figure 16.16 A scanning power view of a section cut through the isthmus shows dramatic atrophy of the sebaceous glands. Smooth muscle is seen, but the sebaceous lobules expected at the same level are not visible at this magnification.

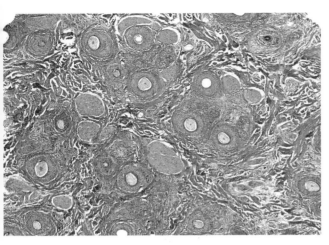

Figure 16.17 A section at the level of the isthmus shows atrophy of the sebaceous glands. Similar findings can be seen in Figures 16.7 and 16.8.

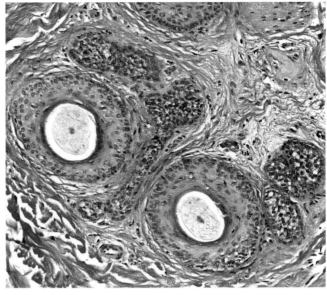

Figure 16.19 A higher magnification view of a section cut through the isthmus shows the atrophy of the sebaceous glands, which are reduced to basophilic remnants. Similar findings can be seen in Figure 16.7. At times, these shrunken glands can resemble (and potentially can be mistaken for) the asterisk-like structures of the telogen–germ unit.

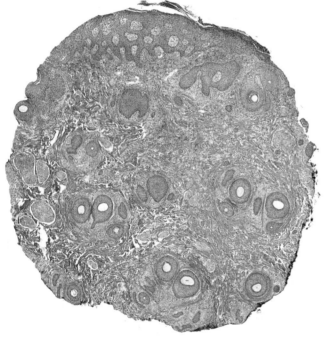

Figure 16.18 A low magnification view of an oblique section shows many of the features of psoriatic alopecia: psoriasiform epidermis, follicles shifted into the catagen/telogen phase, and atrophic sebaceous lobules.

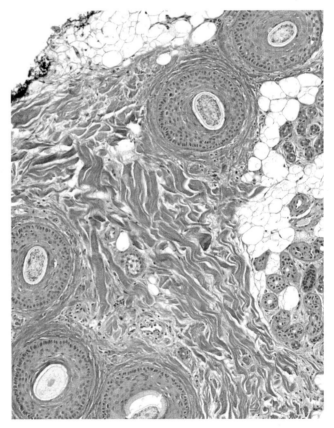

Figure 16.20 Premature desquamation has been noted in some cases of psoriatic alopecia; the significance of this finding is as of yet unclear. Four of the five follicles in this section, photographed at the level of the dermal–subcutaneous junction, show premature desquamation of the inner root sheath. The only follicle that has not yet shed its inner root sheath is at the *bottom center* of the image.

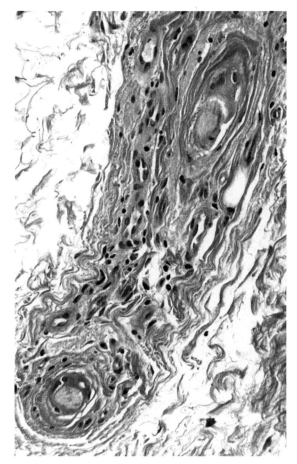

Figure 16.21 Isolated follicular destruction resulting in fragments of a free hair shaft within the dermis. There is a giant cell response and residual lymphocytic inflammation. A limited focus of follicular destruction can be seen in many cases of otherwise clinically noncicatricial psoriatic alopecia.

seen in a minority of cases of psoriatic alopecia and typically very few follicles are affected (Fig. 16.21).

Many of the histological features of psoriatic alopecia are shared by the drug-associated variants (e.g., TNF-alpha inhibitor associated psoriasiform alopecia), the subject of the subsequent chapter.

Psoriatic Alopecia in Summary

Clinical correlation: pink, scaly plaques consistent with psoriasis with superimposed alopecia. A seborrheic dermatitis-like presentation is also not uncommon, with scalp erythema and scale; weeping/crusting has been reported. The alopecia can be patchy or diffuse. Regrowth of hair typically occurs when the scalp is treated with standard antipsoriatic regimens, although permanent hair loss can occur rarely.

Histological findings:
❖ Preserved or slightly diminished follicular density
❖ Many or most hairs in catagen or telogen phases
❖ Extensive follicular miniaturization
❖ Dramatic sebaceous gland atrophy
• Typical psoriatic changes in the interfollicular epidermis or changes resembling seborrheic dermatitis may also be seen

• Mild, focal peribulbar lymphocytic infiltrates with occasional eosinophils
• Patchy peri-infundibular and peri-isthmic lymphocytic inflammation
• Occasional destruction of isolated follicles
• Premature desquamation of the inner root sheath

Histological differential diagnosis:
• **Alopecia areata:** shares the dramatic catagen/telogen shift, miniaturization, and peribulbar lymphocytes (occasionally seen in psoriatic alopecia), but the sebaceous glands are retained and epidermal psoriatic changes are absent in alopecia areata.
• **TNF-alpha inhibitor associated psoriasiform alopecia:** shares the epidermal changes, catagen/telogen shift, and diminished sebaceous glands but shows increased superficial and deep inflammation, including numerous plasma cells and eosinophils as compared with psoriatic alopecia.
• **Tinea capitis:** can present similarly clinically and show the psoriasiform epidermal changes; however, the anagen:catagen/telogen ratio is not dramatically increased, and the sebaceous glands are intact in the noncicatricial phase. The presence of fungal spores or hyphae can frequently be demonstrated by special stains

⚠ **Pitfalls**

Patients frequently receive treatment before their first biopsy, and therefore, epidermal changes of psoriasis may be subtle or no longer present. Epidermal changes are not required to make a diagnosis of psoriatic alopecia in the presence of the major features listed above and a supportive clinical history.

REFERENCES

1. Runne U, Kroneisen-Wiersma P. Psoriatic alopecia: acute and chronic hair loss in 47 patients with scalp psoriasis. Dermatology 1992; 185: 82–7.
2. Shuster S. Psoriatic alopecia. Br J Dermatol 1972; 87: 73–7.
3. van de Kerkhof PC, Chang A. Scarring alopecia and psoriasis. Br J Dermatol 1992; 126: 524–5.
4. Bardazzi F, Fanti PA, Orlandi C, Chieregato C, Misciali C. Psoriatic scarring alopecia: observations in four patients. Int J Dermatol 1999; 38: 765–8.
5. Wright AL, Messenger AG. Scarring alopecia in psoriasis. Acta Derm Venereol 1990; 70: 156–9.
6. Cockayne SE, Messenger AG. Familial scarring alopecia associated with scalp psoriasis. Br J Dermatol 2001; 144: 425–7.
7. Schon MP, Reifenberger J, Gantke B, Megahed M, Lehmann P. [Progressive cicatricial psoriatic alopecia in AIDS]. Hautarzt 2000; 51: 935–8.
8. Kretzschmar L, Bonsmann G, Metze D, Luger TA, Schwarz T. [Scarring psoriatic alopecia]. Hautarzt 1995; 46: 154–7.
9. Schoorl WJ, van Baar HJ, van de Kerkhof PC. The hair root pattern in psoriasis of the scalp. Acta Derm Venereol 1992; 72: 141–2.
10. Headington JT, Gupta AK, Goldfarb MT, et al. A morphometric and histologic study of the scalp in psoriasis. Paradoxical sebaceous gland atrophy and decreased hair shaft diameters without alopecia. Arch Dermatol 1989; 125: 639–42.
11. Werner B, Brenner FM, Boer A. Histopathologic study of scalp psoriasis: peculiar features including sebaceous gland atrophy. Am J Dermatopathol 2008; 30: 93–100.
12. Wilson CL, Dean D, Lane EB, Dawber RP, Leigh IM. Keratinocyte differentiation in psoriatic scalp: morphology and expression of epithelial keratins. Br J Dermatol 1994; 131: 191–200.

17 Tumor necrosis factor-alpha inhibitor associated psoriasiform alopecia (drug-induced psoriasiform alopecia)

Psoriasiform alopecia arising in patients on tumor necrosis factor-alpha inhibitors (anti-TNFs) is a newly described entity with a recognizable histopathological correlate. The manifestation of TNF-alpha inhibitor associated psoriasiform alopecia (TAIAPA) is perhaps not surprising given the well-recognized phenomenon of paradoxical psoriasiform eruptions, especially palmoplantar pustular psoriasis, as well as scalp psoriasis, seborrheic dermatitis, guttate psoriasis, and plaque-type psoriasiform eruptions, in patients treated with anti-TNFs (1–3).

Alteration of the cytokine balance between TNF-alpha and interferon-alpha (INF-alpha) is thought to cause the psoriasiform eruption seen with the anti-TNF biologic agents. The primary producer of INF-alpha is the plasmacytoid dendritic cell (PDC), which ceases to produce INF-alpha when fully mature (4). TNF-alpha simultaneously limits INF-alpha production in two ways: it (*i*) antagonizes the generation of immature PDCs from their hematopoietic progenitors, and (*ii*) promotes the maturation of existing PDCs (4,5). Inhibiting TNF-alpha allows for increased production of INF-alpha by PDCs. These cells, which are found in early lesions of psoriasis, have been shown to be key effectors in the promotion of cutaneous psoriasis by INF-alpha production and a complex downstream autoimmune T-cell cascade (6).

Two reported cases of this form of alopecia arose after the use of adalimumab for Crohn's disease (7). One of the patients had a psoriasiform eruption on the body in addition to scalp involvement, and one of the two patients showed evidence of cicatricial alopecia on biopsy (7). Another report of three patients with Crohn's disease included one on adalimumab and two on infliximab (8). Two of these patients developed psoriasiform lesions on the body in addition to the scalp eruption. Regrowth of hair was achieved in all three patients (8).

Children treated with anti-TNFs are also reported to develop this form of alopecia. A recent report describes the histories of five children (two boys and three girls), three with Crohn's disease, and one each with ulcerative colitis and juvenile inflammatory arthritis (9). Four of the patients were on infliximab and one on adalimumab. The authors emphasize the need for increased awareness of this entity in children as three of the five were empirically treated with antifungals under the assumption that the diagnosis was tinea capitis. Delayed treatment can lead to permanent hair loss.

Recent reports of alopecia following the use of epidermal growth factor-inhibitors (such as erlotinib) bear some resemblance to the TNF-alpha inhibitor-associated cases (10–13). Reports describe an increased catagen/telogen ratio (10,11,13) and a superficial and deep lymphoplasmacytic infiltrate (10–13), including eosinophils or neutrophils (11–13). A clinical report of cicatricial alopecia resulting in a tufted folliculitis pattern (a marker of late-stage cicatricial alopecia) has been reported with trastuzumab, a human epidermal receptor-2

(HER2) inhibitor (14). Histopathological findings were not reported. Additional study of these various immunomodulatory drug associated alopecias will be required and comparison with the findings in TAIAPA to determine whether or not they can be grouped under a shared rubric.

Finally, there is abundant literature supporting anti-TNF medications as a cause of alopecia areata (alopecia totalis and alopecia universalis) (15–29). Although there are a number of shared histological findings between alopecia areata (and its clinical variants) and TAIAPA, there are also key differences, and the clinical presentations of these two entities are distinctive. The distinction is especially important in cases where alopecia areata-like patches and cutaneous psoriasiform plaques appear simultaneously (28).

CLINICAL FINDINGS

Patients can have a variety of underlying diseases, ranging from inflammatory bowel disease and rheumatoid arthritis to psoriasis itself, for which the anti-TNF agent may have been prescribed. The majority of patients who develop this reaction (those reported in the literature combined with those that we have seen) have a history of Crohn's disease. Whether or not patients with Crohn's disease have a predisposition to develop this reaction has yet to be elucidated. The majority of patients do not have a personal or family history of psoriasis (excepting those that are using the anti-TNF specifically for psoriasis) (8,9). The most commonly implicated agents have been infliximab and adalimumab. Onset of the eruption has been reported from 2 months to 2 years after initiation of the medication (7–9). The authors have seen this type of alopecia present up to 5 years after initiation of an anti–TNF-alpha agent.

Patients typically present with crusted psoriasiform plaques involving various areas of the scalp with associated alopecia (Fig. 17.1). If the psoriasiform plaque is not very thick, erythema of the scalp can be seen (Fig. 17.2). Erosion may be present. Rarely the plaques take on a boggy, dissecting cellulitis-like consistency (9). The scalp may be asymptomatic or patients may complain of pruritus or pain. The majority of patients have some evidence of cutaneous involvement, even if it is only postauricular scaling. Nail involvement in the TNF-alpha inhibitor associated psoriasiform eruptions may occur, manifesting as yellowing, onycholysis, and subungual hyperkeratosis (1). A careful total body skin examination can often provide additional supporting clinical findings.

Treatment typically consists of the use of class I topical steroids or intralesional triamcinolone with or without an antiseborrheic shampoo. In many, this approach will achieve adequate results (8). In some, the eruption (and alopecia) is severe enough to consider withholding, discontinuing, or changing anti-TNF therapy (7). The decision to withdraw the anti-TNF agent is a risk/benefit calculation that must be made

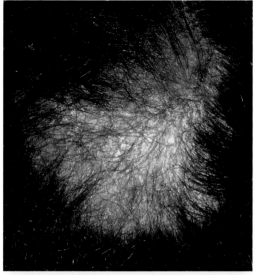

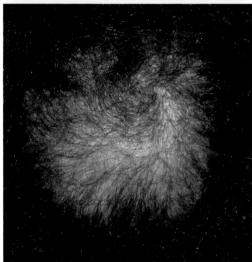

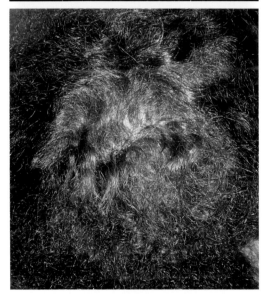

Figure 17.1 A 13-year-old Caucasian girl with a history of Crohn's disease, well-controlled on the TNF-alpha inhibitor, infliximab, for a number of years, developed this psoriasiform eruption on her scalp associated with alopecia over a one-month period (*top panel*). She responded well to clobetasol ointment, even with continuation of infliximab, with subsequent full regrowth of hair (*middle panel*, resolution of the scale after one month of treatment; *bottom panel*, regrowth of hair after three months). The patient later developed psoriasiform plaques again on the scalp, this time without alopecia. *Source:* Image courtesy of Richard Antaya, M.D.

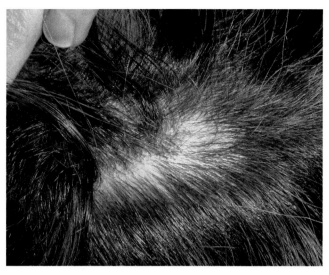

Figure 17.2 A Caucasian woman being treated with etanercept developed focal alopecia of the vertex scalp associated with a scaly plaque. She was treated with intralesional triamcinolone with resolution of the plaque before this photograph was obtained. There is mild residual erythema still visible in the alopecic scalp. *Source:* Image courtesy of Stephanie Dietz, M.D.

on the basis of severity of underlying disease *versus* severity of the scalp eruption and alopecia. This decision is ultimately guided by the patient's priorities. After being treated with class I topical steroids, one of the author's patients was able to achieve enough plaque resolution and hair regrowth to permit the continuation of infliximab for Crohn's disease. Two patients who discontinued their anti-TNF agents while treating their scalp eruption with class I topical steroids were able to resume the same anti-TNF at a later date, without adverse sequelae. Scarring appears to occur more commonly in anti-TNF alopecia than in psoriatic alopecia. Prompt treatment is advocated to limit progression to cicatricial alopecia.

HISTOLOGICAL FINDINGS

The findings are similar to those seen in psoriatic alopecia, but with a significantly greater degree of inflammation in the superficial and deep compartments. Typically, the majority of follicles are shifted into the catagen/telogen phase (Fig. 17.3). If the specimen is examined at the level of the subcutis, there is a reduced number of bulbs with streamers indicating the presence of catagen/telogen follicles that have retreated to the dermis. Another feature TAIAPA shares in common with psoriatic alopecia is the marked atrophy of sebaceous glands. The sebaceous glands are reduced in volume, often present only as a basophilic remnant (Figs. 17.4 and 17.5).

Peribulbar inflammation is a prominent feature of TAIAPA (Fig. 17.6). Inflammation is also frequently seen around stelae (Fig. 17.7). The presence of peribulbar plasma cells is characteristic of this entity (they are not ordinarily seen in psoriatic alopecia) (Figs. 17.8–17.10). Deep eosinophils and lymphocytes are also much more commonly seen in TAIAPA than in psoriatic alopecia (Fig. 17.10).

The epidermis displays psoriasiform acanthosis, hypogranulosis, and parakeratosis with mounds of intracorneal neutrophils, and often frank pustulation (Fig. 17.11). Both dilated papillary dermal vessels and thinned suprapapillary plates may

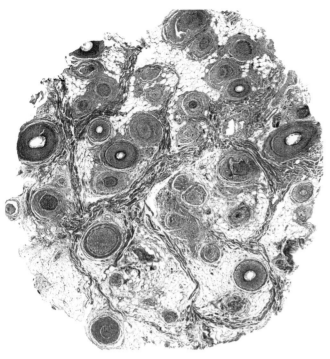

Figure 17.3 This image from a patient on infliximab shows a majority of follicles in the catagen/telogen phase. Within the subcutaneous fat there are numerous stelae underlying follicles that have already shifted and regressed upward into the dermis. There is inflammation surrounding bulbs and stelae.

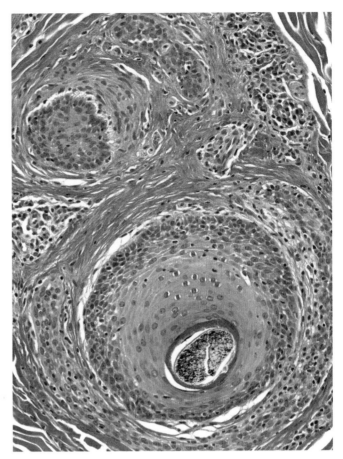

Figure 17.5 A higher power image of the image shown in Fig. 17.4 showing the atrophic sebaceous gland adjacent to the follicle. There is plasmacytic inflammation.

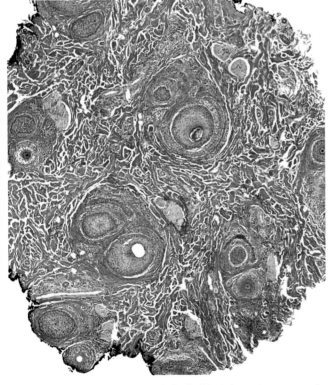

Figure 17.4 This image captured at the level of the isthmus demonstrates the sebaceous gland atrophy seen in TAIAPA. The sebaceous glands in this image are thin basophilic structures adjacent to the follicles. There is perivascular and focally perifollicular inflammation. Arrector pili muscles are present to help identify the level of this section within the dermis.

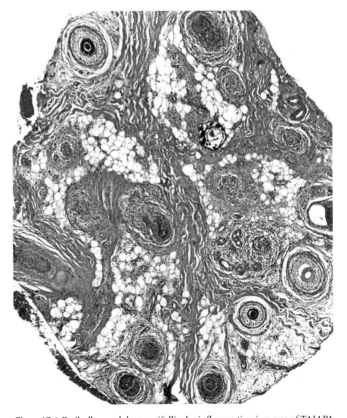

Figure 17.6 Peribulbar and deep perifollicular inflammation in a case of TAIAPA due to infliximab. Many of the follicles are shifted into the catagen/telogen phase.

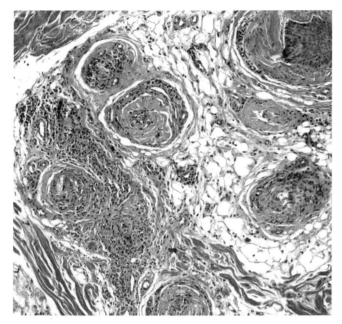

Figure 17.7 There is ample lymphoplasmacytic inflammation surrounding the stelae (and shifting follicles) in this image.

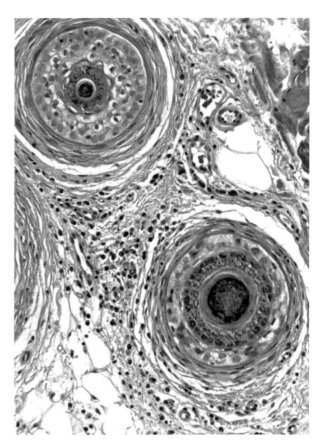

Figure 17.9 A higher power image of the section shown in Fig. 17.8. The majority of the inflammatory cells are plasma cells. There are occasional eosinophils.

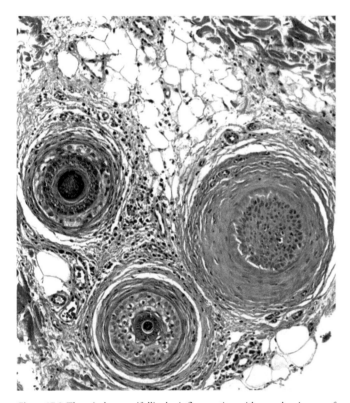

Figure 17.8 There is deep perifollicular inflammation with a predominance of plasma cells. There is a terminal catagen hair and miniaturization of the adjacent follicle showing a hair shaft of the same diameter as the inner root sheath.

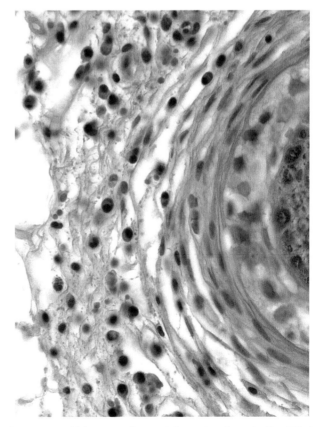

Figure 17.10 A higher power image of the section shown in Fig. 17.9. An eosinophil is seen with the plasma cells.

be seen. The sometimes marked perivascular, perifollicular, and interstitial inflammation may include lymphocytes, plasma cells, eosinophils, and neutrophils (Fig. 17.12). There may be prominent exocytosis of lymphocytes into the epidermis or follicular epithelium with some associated spongiosis (Fig. 17.13). Spongiosis and a lichenoid infiltrate are more commonly seen in anti–TNF-alpha psoriasiform eruptions

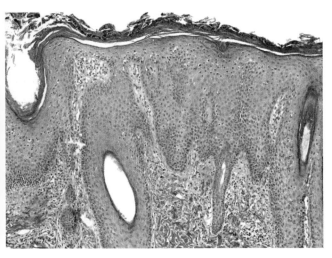

Figure 17.11 This view of the epidermis of a patient on infliximab shows psoriasiform acanthosis, hypogranulosis, thinning of the suprapapillary plates, and neutrophils within the stratum corneum. There are perivascular lymphocytes.

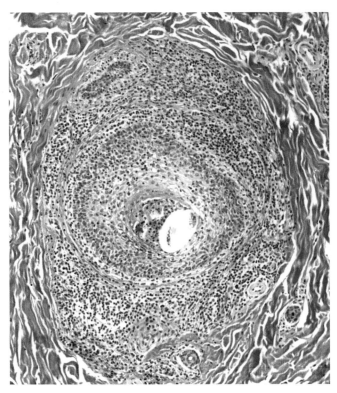

Figure 17.13 A section at the level of the infundibulum shows marked perifollicular inflammation with exocytosis of lymphocytes and associated spongiosis in the follicular epithelium. There are neutrophils within the central cavity.

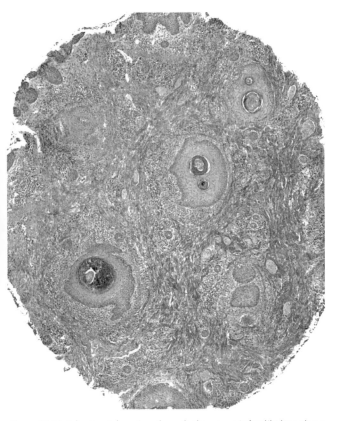

Figure 17.12 A horizontal section through the upper infundibulum shows marked perifollicular and perivascular inflammation; lymphocytes are predominant, but there is a mix of plasma cells, neutrophils, and occasional eosinophils as well. There is neutrophilic microabscess formation within a follicle.

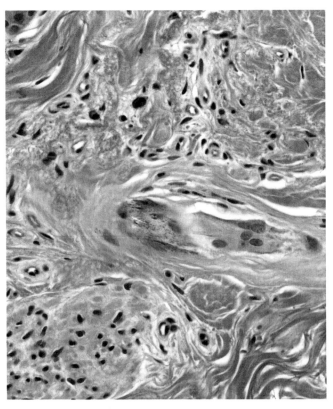

Figure 17.14 A destroyed follicle has resulted in a free hair shaft that is surrounded by multinucleated giant cells.

than in psoriasis itself (5). When compared with typical psoriasis, the cutaneous psoriasiform lesions in these patients also tend to have a denser inflammatory infiltrate that includes plasma cells and eosinophils (8).

Follicular destruction resulting in free hair shafts within the dermis or subcutis (Fig. 17.14) is more commonly seen in this highly inflammatory alopecia than in classic psoriatic alopecia.

TNF-alpha Inhibitor Associated Psoriasiform Alopecia (Drug-Induced Psoriasiform Alopecia) in Summary

Clinical correlation: psoriasiform, frequently crusted plaques with associated alopecia presenting in a patient on anti-TNF therapy, or perhaps other biologic agents. Both scarring and nonscarring outcomes have been described.

Histological findings:
- ❖ Preserved or slightly diminished follicular density
- ❖ Many or most hairs in catagen/telogen phase
- ❖ Follicular miniaturization
- ❖ Dramatic sebaceous gland atrophy
- ❖ Brisk superficial and deep perifollicular inflammation, specifically with peribulbar lymphocytes and prominent plasma cells with variable numbers of eosinophils
- Psoriasiform changes in the interfollicular epidermis, often with significant inflammation, including lymphocyte exocytosis
- Focal follicular destruction

Histological differential diagnosis:
- **Psoriatic alopecia:** shares the epidermal changes, catagen/telogen shift and diminished sebaceous glands, but is typically far less inflamed superficially and has very limited deep inflammation without plasma cells and eosinophils
- **Alopecia areata:** shares the dramatic catagen/telogen shift and peribulbar lymphocytes with occasional eosinophils; the epidermal psoriasiform changes, intense superficial inflammatory infiltrates, and peribulbar plasma cells are absent, and the sebaceous glands are retained
- **Tinea capitis:** can present similarly clinically and show psoriasiform epidermal changes, however, the anagen: catagen/telogen ratio is not dramatically increased and the sebaceous glands are intact in the noncicatricial phase of tinea capitis; the presence of fungal spores or hyphae can frequently be demonstrated by special stains. Culture may be necessary to rule out infection in these already immune-suppressed patients

⚠ **Pitfalls**
- Alopecia areata may also be triggered by anti-TNF medications. The clinical picture and a careful examination of the histopathology should allow for a clear distinction between this and the drug-induced psoriasiform alopecia.

REFERENCES

1. Sfikakis PP, Iliopoulos A, Elezoglou A, Kittas C, Stratigos A. Psoriasis induced by anti-tumor necrosis factor therapy: a paradoxical adverse reaction. Arthritis Rheum 2005; 52: 2513–18.
2. Ko JM, Gottlieb AB, Kerbleski JF. Induction and exacerbation of psoriasis with TNF-blockade therapy: a review and analysis of 127 cases. J Dermatolog Treat 2009; 20: 100–8.
3. Grinblat B, Scheinberg M. The enigmatic development of psoriasis and psoriasiform lesions during anti-TNF therapy: a review. Semin Arthritis Rheum 2008; 37: 251–5.
4. Palucka AK, Blanck JP, Bennett L, Pascual V, Banchereau J. Cross-regulation of TNF and IFN-alpha in autoimmune diseases. Proc Natl Acad Sci USA 2005; 102: 3372–7.
5. Seneschal J, Milpied B, Vergier B, et al. Cytokine imbalance with increased production of interferon-alpha in psoriasiform eruptions associated with antitumour necrosis factor-alpha treatments. Br J Dermatol 2009; 161: 1081–8.
6. Nestle FO, Conrad C, Tun-Kyi A, et al. Plasmacytoid predendritic cells initiate psoriasis through interferon-alpha production. J Exp Med 2005; 202: 135–43.
7. El Shabrawi-Caelen L, La Placa M, Vincenzi C, et al. Adalimumab-induced psoriasis of the scalp with diffuse alopecia: a severe potentially irreversible cutaneous side effect of TNF-alpha blockers. Inflamm Bowel Dis 2010; 16: 182–3.
8. Doyle LA, Sperling LC, Baksh S, et al. Psoriatic alopecia/alopecia areata-like reactions secondary to anti-tumor necrosis factor-alpha therapy: a novel cause of noncicatricial alopecia. Am J Dermatopathol 2011; 33: 161–6.
9. Perman MJ, Lovell DJ, Denson LA, Farrell MK, Lucky AW. Five cases of anti-tumor necrosis factor alpha-induced psoriasis presenting with severe scalp involvement in children. Pediatr Dermatol 2011.
10. Pongpudpunth M, Demierre MF, Goldberg LJ. A case report of inflammatory nonscarring alopecia associated with the epidermal growth factor receptor inhibitor erlotinib. J Cutan Pathol 2009; 36: 1303–7.
11. Graves JE, Jones BF, Lind AC, Heffernan MP. Nonscarring inflammatory alopecia associated with the epidermal growth factor receptor inhibitor gefitinib. J Am Acad Dermatol 2006; 55: 349–53.
12. Donovan JC, Ghazarian DM, Shaw JC. Scarring alopecia associated with use of the epidermal growth factor receptor inhibitor gefitinib. Arch Dermatol 2008; 144: 1524–5.
13. Hepper DM, Wu P, Anadkat MJ. Scarring alopecia associated with the epidermal growth factor receptor inhibitor erlotinib. J Am Acad Dermatol 2011; 64: 996–8.
14. Rosman IS, Anadkat MJ. Tufted hair folliculitis in a woman treated with trastuzumab. Target Oncol 2010; 5: 295–6.
15. Lee HH, Song IH, Friedrich M, et al. Cutaneous side-effects in patients with rheumatic diseases during application of tumour necrosis factor-alpha antagonists. Br J Dermatol 2007; 156: 486–91.
16. Chaves Y, Duarte G, Ben-Said B, et al. Alopecia areata universalis during treatment of rheumatoid arthritis with anti-TNF-alpha antibody (adalimumab). Dermatology 2008; 217: 380.
17. Posten W, Swan J. Recurrence of alopecia areata in a patient receiving etanercept injections. Arch Dermatol 2005; 141: 759–60.
18. Fabre C, Dereure O. Worsening alopecia areata and de novo occurrence of multiple halo nevi in a patient receiving infliximab. Dermatology 2008; 216: 185–6.
19. Pelivani N, Hassan AS, Braathen LR, Hunger RE, Yawalkar N. Alopecia areata universalis elicited during treatment with adalimumab. Dermatology 2008; 216: 320–3.
20. Le Bidre E, Chaby G, Martin L, et al. [Alopecia areata during anti-TNF alpha therapy: Nine cases]. Ann Dermatol Venereol 2011; 138: 285–93.
21. Garcia Bartels N, Lee HH, Worm M, et al. Development of alopecia areata universalis in a patient receiving adalimumab. Arch Dermatol 2006; 142: 1654–5.
22. Kirshen C, Kanigsberg N. Alopecia areata following adalimumab. J Cutan Med Surg 2009; 13: 48–50.
23. Ettefagh L, Nedorost S, Mirmirani P. Alopecia areata in a patient using infliximab: new insights into the role of tumor necrosis factor on human hair follicles. Arch Dermatol 2004; 140: 1012.
24. Tosti A, Pazzaglia M, Starace M, et al. Alopecia areata during treatment with biologic agents. Arch Dermatol 2006; 142: 1653–4.
25. Hernandez MV, Nogues S, Ruiz-Esquide V, et al. Development of alopecia areata after biological therapy with TNF-alpha Blockers: description of a case and review of the literature. Clin Exp Rheumatol 2009; 27: 892–3.
26. Pan Y, Rao NA. Alopecia areata during etanercept therapy. Ocul Immunol Inflamm 2009; 17: 127–9.
27. Katoulis AC, Alevizou A, Bozi E, et al. Biologic agents and alopecia areata. Dermatology 2009; 218: 184–5.
28. Nakagomi D, Harada K, Yagasaki A, et al. Psoriasiform eruption associated with alopecia areata during infliximab therapy. Clin Exp Dermatol 2009; 34: 923–4.
29. Ferran M, Calvet J, Almirall M, Pujol RM, Maymo J. Alopecia areata as another immune-mediated disease developed in patients treated with tumour necrosis factor-alpha blocker agents: report of five cases and review of the literature. J Eur Acad Dermatol Venereol 2011; 25: 479–84.

18   Syphilitic alopecia

Syphilitic alopecia is an uncommon manifestation of secondary syphilis, occurring in only 4% of such patients (1). As always, syphilis is "the great imitator," capable of causing alopecia with several clinical and histological patterns.

CLINICAL FINDINGS

Alopecia found in secondary syphilis may be associated with other cutaneous lesions, or may be the only external manifestation of syphilis. The pattern of hair loss can be patchy ("moth-eaten"), diffuse (as in a telogen effluvium), or a combination of the two (Figs. 18.1 and 18.2) (1). Hair loss in the *absence* of papulosquamous lesions of the scalp is termed "essential" syphilitic alopecia.

HISTOLOGICAL FINDINGS

When papulosquamous lesions of secondary syphilis are found on the scalp in association with alopecia ("symptomatic" syphilitic alopecia), the histological findings are usually those typically associated with lesions of secondary syphilis. These findings include a perivascular and perifollicular infiltrate of lymphocytes, histiocytes, and often numerous plasma cells; involvement of both superficial and deep dermal vascular plexuses; vascular dilation and prominent, swollen endothelial cells; and frequent epidermal involvement with epidermal hyperplasia, spongiosis, neutrophilic infiltration, and interface inflammation (2).

As one cause of telogen effluvium and diffuse hair loss, syphilis can present with a histological pattern that is typical of telogen effluvium (Fig. 18.3). However, more often the histological pattern is an inflammatory, predominantly peribulbar and suprabulbar, noncicatricial process closely mimicking alopecia areata (AA) (Figs. 18.4–18.6) (3–5). Catagen/telogen follicles are increased in number, initially as terminal hairs but eventually as miniaturized follicles. A mononuclear cell infiltrate surrounds the inferior segment of the follicle or involves the fibrous tracts below catagen/telogen hairs. A minority of specimens exhibit a solitary peribulbar lymphoid aggregate, and in some cases large numbers of lymphocytes infiltrate the outer root sheath at the level of the isthmus.

In well-established syphilitic alopecia, nearly all of the follicles have miniaturized (Figs. 18.6 and 18.7). The peribulbar infiltrate tends to be scanty and plasma cells may be difficult to find (Fig. 18.8). Because so many follicles are miniaturized, finding and counting involved hairs are best achieved with transverse sectioning. Eosinophils in the infiltrate are uncommonly seen, but in many cases plasma cells are present in small numbers. Histochemical stains for spirochetes (such as the Warthin–Starry stain) do not reveal organisms. However, a recent study using specific immunohistochemical stains directed against spirochetal antigens showed the presence of organisms limited to the peribulbar region and penetrating into the follicular matrix (6).

Syphilitic alopecia and AA may have the following features in common: (*i*) no epidermal changes; (*ii*) a lymphocytic infiltrate with or without a few scattered eosinophils

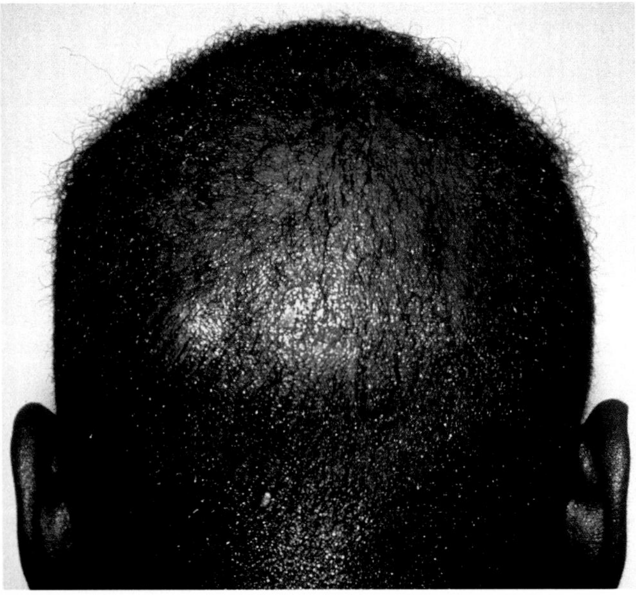

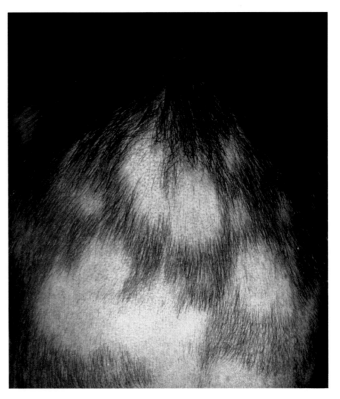

Figures 18.1 Syphilitic alopecia can be diffuse (affecting the entire scalp) as seen here, or patchy.

Figure 18.2 A combination of diffuse *and* patchy can also be seen in syphilitic alopecia. *Source:* Figure 18.2 courtesy of William D. James, M.D.

around the lower segment of follicles, in fibrous tracts, or within the deepest follicular epithelium; (*iii*) the presence of miniaturized anagen hairs; and (*iv*) markedly increased numbers of catagen/telogen follicles. Plasma cells and lymphocytic infiltration of the outer root sheath are more likely to be seen in syphilitic alopecia than in AA. Serologic tests for syphilis and a prompt and complete response to antitreponemal antibiotics help to confirm the diagnosis. A positive antispirochetal immunohistochemical stain would, of course, be helpful.

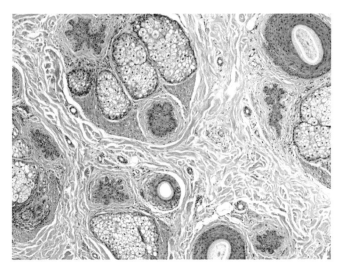

Figure 18.3 A patient with secondary syphilis and diffuse hair loss, showing typical histological changes of telogen effluvium (see also chap. 10).

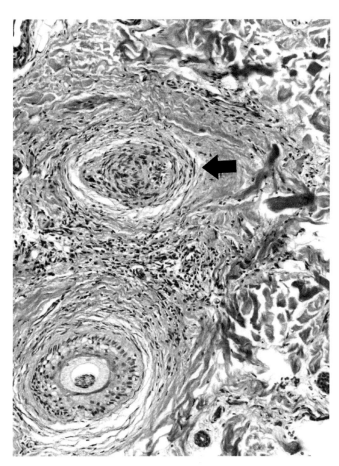

Figure 18.5 Residual inflammation surrounds the papilla of a catagen hair (*arrow*). The anagen follicle below has become miniaturized.

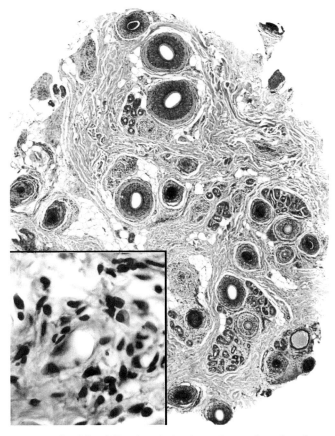

Figure 18.4 "Early" syphilitic alopecia showing an increased number of catagen hairs. A relatively mild lymphocytic infiltrate with occasional plasma cells (inset) surrounds the lower portion of several follicles.

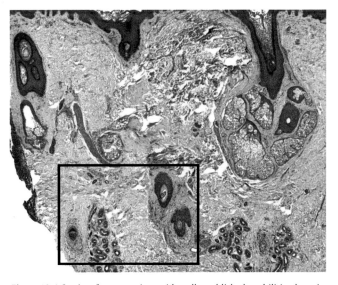

Figure 18.6 Section from a patient with well-established syphilitic alopecia. The follicles are very small and inflammation is scanty. The boxed area in this figure is magnified in the lower panel of Figure 18.7.

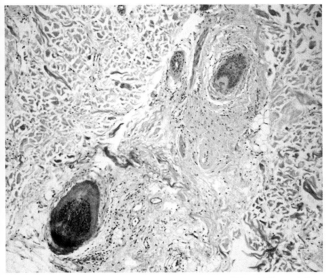

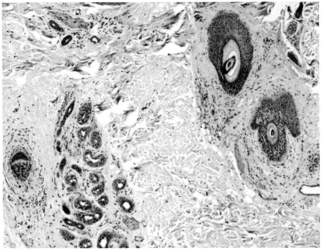

Figure 18.7 Greatly magnified view of miniaturized follicles in two different patients with syphilitic alopecia.

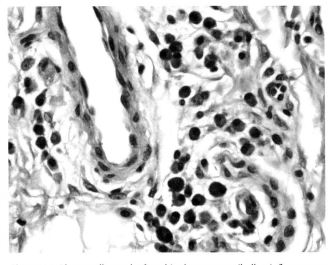

Figure 18.8 Plasma cells may be found in the sparse peribulbar inflammatory infiltrate of syphilitic alopecia. Plasma cells are very unusual in alopecia areata.

Syphilitic Alopecia in Summary

Clinical correlation: a diffuse (resembling telogen effluvium) or a diffuse but "moth-eaten" alopecia. Other signs and symptoms of syphilis may be present, and there should be a positive serologic test for syphilis and a favorable response to antibiotics

Histological findings:
"Symptomatic" alopecia (associated with papulosquamous lesions)
❖ Similar to typical papulosquamous lesions of secondary syphilis
❖ Superficial and deep perivascular and perifollicular infiltrate composed of plasma cells, lymphocytes, and histiocytes
• Vascular dilation and endothelial cell prominence

Diffuse alopecia secondary to telogen effluvium
❖ Identical to *telogen effluvium*, as discussed chapter 10

"Essential" alopecia, moth-eaten or diffuse, inflammatory
❖ Resembles AA, with a peribulbar mononuclear cell infiltrate, miniaturization of hairs, increased number of catagen/telogen hairs (approaching 100% in some cases)
• Occasional plasma cells in contradistinction to AA
• Perifollicular and outer root sheath inflammation may extend up to the follicular isthmus
• Most histological findings associated with typical lesions of secondary syphilis are absent

Histological differential diagnosis:
• **Telogen effluvium:** TE will not show miniaturization or peribulbar inflammation
• **Alopecia areata:** AA will not show peribulbar plasma cells

⚠ **Pitfall**
Syphilitic alopecia is much less common than AA, which it closely mimics. Therefore, a high index of suspicion may be required to make the diagnosis.

Abbreviation: AA, alopecia areata.

REFERENCES

1. Bi MY, Cohen PR, Robinson FW, Gray JM. Alopecia syphilitica-report of a patient with secondary syphilis presenting as moth-eaten alopecia and a review of its common mimickers. Dermatol Online J 2009; 15: 6.
2. Jeerapaet P, Ackerman A. Histologic patterns of secondary syphilis. Arch Dermatol 1973; 107: 373.
3. Jordaan HF, Louw M. The moth-eaten alopecia of secondary syphilis. A histopathological study of 12 patients. Am J Dermatopathol 1995; 17: 158–62.
4. Lee JY-Y, Hsu M-L. Alopecia syphilitica, a simulator of alopecia areata: histopathology and differential diagnosis. J Cutan Pathol 1991; 18: 87–92.
5. Sperling L, Lupton G. The histopathology of non-scarring alopecia. J Cutan Pathol 1995; 22: 97–114.
6. Nam-Cha SH, Guhl G, Fernandez-Pena P, Fraga J. Alopecia syphilitica with detection of *Treponema pallidum* in the hair follicle. J Cutan Pathol 2007; 34(Suppl 1): 37–40.

19 Noncicatricial alopecia from systemic lupus erythematosus

Hair loss in systemic lupus erythematosus (SLE) is common (1) and can produce several patterns. The most familiar form of alopecia to both clinicians and dermatopathologists is the cicatricial alopecia of chronic cutaneous lupus erythematosus, which is discussed in detail in chapter 28. Noncicatricial patterns of alopecia may also be encountered in SLE. Because patients can be severely ill for long periods of time, a diffuse noncicatricial pattern of hair loss due to telogen effluvium may occur. This pattern is further described in chapter 10.

A third pattern of hair loss in SLE that is fairly common (2) but has received little attention in the literature (3). It begins as a patchy, noncicatricial alopecia. This form of alopecia occurs in patients with severe disease, in whom the underlying diagnosis of SLE has already been established or is suspected. However, very early lesions in patients with strictly cutaneous disease can show similar features.

CLINICAL FINDINGS
Clinically, there are patches of partial or total hair loss scattered on the scalp (Fig. 19.1). These are associated with mild erythema without evidence of scarring (follicular ostia and surface texture appear normal). The residual hairs in the balding patches are almost all telogen hairs (Fig. 19.2) or dystrophic "pencil-point" anagen hairs, a finding diagnostic of an "anagen arrest" (described in chap. 15). If the underlying disease is controlled promptly, complete hair regrowth occurs. In inadequately treated patients, however, these noncicatricial patches can evolve into plaques of cicatricial alopecia. Noncicatricial alopecia from SLE can therefore be classified as one of the biphasic alopecias. The following discussion is a description of the early, noncicatricial process that is most often found in association with active SLE.

HISTOLOGICAL FINDINGS
A peribulbar mononuclear cell infiltrate is found adjacent to anagen hair bulbs, many of which become miniaturized over time (Figs. 19.3 and 19.4). The inflammatory infiltrate may be denser than that found in alopecia areata (Fig. 19.5). The percentage of catagen and telogen hairs is greatly increased, and may approach 100% (Fig. 19.6). Pigment incontinence and a mild inflammatory infiltrate are often found in the collapsed root sheaths (stelae) below telogen hairs.

These histological findings are very similar to those found in alopecia areata and "essential" syphilitic alopecia, and a diagnosis of lupus erythematosus may not be possible on histological grounds alone. Clinical findings and serologic testing may be required to reliably differentiate between these three forms of noncicatricial, reversible, inflammatory alopecia. However, some additional histological features may help to distinguish SLE from its histological mimics. For example, an increase in dermal mucin is often present (Fig. 19.7). Although

mucin may be visible with routine staining, colloidal iron or similar stains can accentuate the mucin (Fig. 19.8). Lymphocytic inflammation around eccrine glands and dermal vasculature is often seen in the alopecia of SLE (Fig. 19.9). When inflammation involves dermal blood vessels, extravasated red blood cells are sometimes found. An especially dense inflammatory infiltrate supports a diagnosis of lupus erythematosus (as seen in Fig. 19.9). Finally, focal areas of basal vacuolar degeneration affecting the infundibula of follicles may be found (Fig. 19.10).

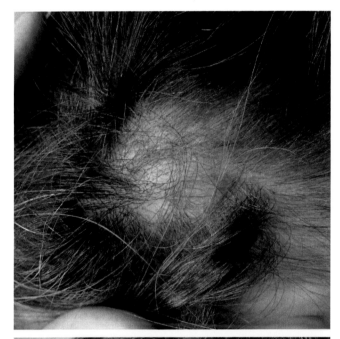

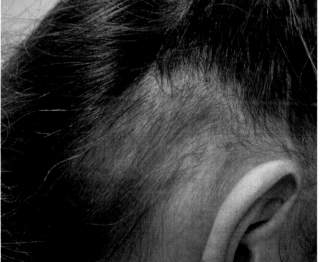

Figure 19.1 Young woman with active systemic lupus erythematosus and patchy, noncicatricial hair loss.

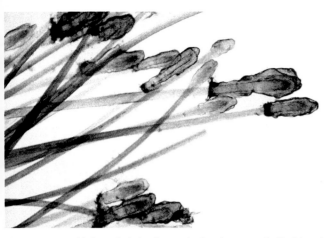

Figure 19.2 Forcible hair pluck (trichogram) taken from a markedly thinned patch of scalp in a patient with active systemic lupus erythematosus. Since the anagen hair shafts have already shed, these hairs are all telogen hairs.

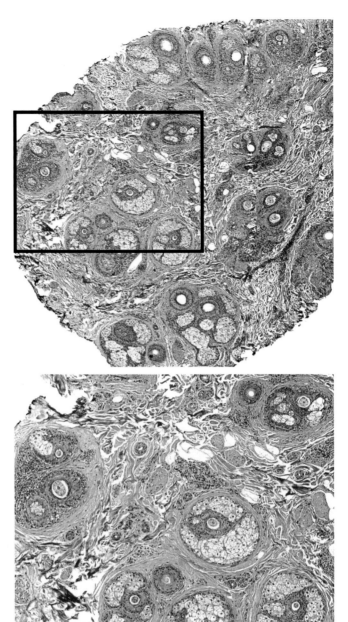

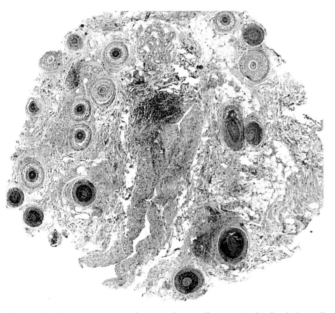

Figure 19.3 Numerous terminal anagen hairs still persist in this "early lesion" of patchy, noncicatricial alopecia of systemic lupus erythematosus. A moderately dense lymphocytic infiltrate surrounds the lower segments of several anagen hairs, involving interfollicular blood vessels as well. The perivascular infiltrate contains some plasma cells. Many hairs are missed at this level, but in more superficial sections will be found as miniaturized or telogen hairs.

Figure 19.4 This is the same biopsy specimen as pictured in Figure 19.3, but sectioned at a more superficial level. The lower panel represents a magnified view of the boxed area in the top panel. The total number of hairs is normal, but many hairs have miniaturized. Lymphocytic inflammation is concentrated in the vicinity of some follicular units, but the persistence of sebaceous glands indicates that inflammatory, follicular destruction has not yet occurred.

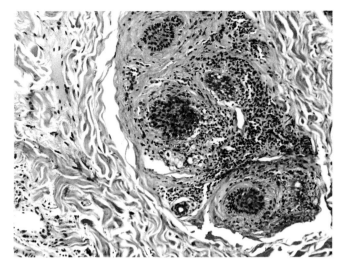

Figure 19.5 Deep, perifollicular inflammation is quite dense as compared with alopecia areata.

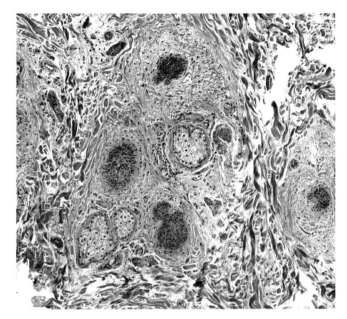

Figure 19.6 In this lesion of patchy, noncicatricial alopecia in a patient with SLE, the majority of hairs are miniaturized and in the catagen/telogen phases.

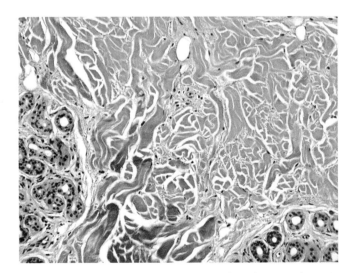

Figure 19.7 Even without special stains, interstitial dermal mucin is obvious in this specimen from a patient with the patchy, noncicatricial alopecia of systemic lupus erythematosus.

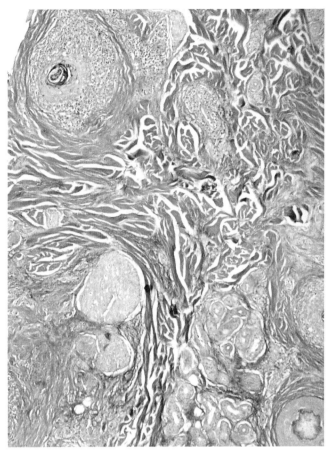

Figure 19.8 Deep dermal mucin is highlighted with a colloidal iron stain.

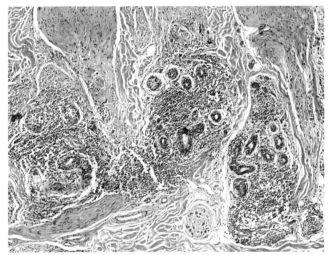

Figure 19.9 Dense perieccrine inflammation in a patient with noncicatricial alopecia of systemic lupus erythematosus.

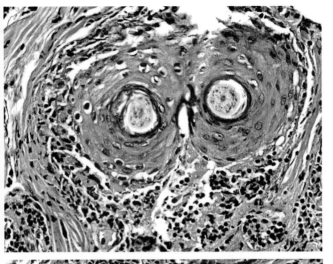

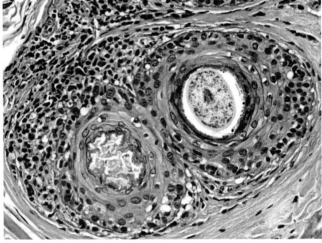

Figure 19.10 Brisk vacuolar interface change affecting the infundibula of one follicular unit in a patient with patchy, noncicatricial systemic lupus erythematosus alopecia.

Patchy, Noncicatricial Alopecia of SLE, in Summary

Clinical correlation: The patient is usually a young adult with severe systemic disease, in whom the underlying diagnosis of SLE has already been established or is suspected. Patches of partial or total hair loss are scattered on the scalp. Mild erythema of the scalp may be present.

Histological findings:
- ❖ Miniaturization of follicles
- ❖ Increased catagen/telogen percentage in affected areas (may approach 100%)
- ❖ Peribulbar mononuclear cell infiltrate, often more dense than in alopecia areata
- • Increased dermal mucin
- • Basal vacuolar degeneration of the infundibular epithelium
- • Perieccrine and perivascular lymphoplasmacytic inflammation
- • Extravasated red blood cells around inflamed blood vessels

Histological differential diagnosis:
- • **Alopecia areata:** shows less inflammation overall. Perieccrine inflammation, vacuolar interface change, and increased mucin are not found.
- • **Syphilitic alopecia:** more closely resembles alopecia areata, except that peribulbar plasma cells may be seen.
- • **Psoriatic alopecia:** may show epidermal changes typical of psoriasis and shows atrophy of sebaceous lobules. Other changes resemble alopecia areata.

Abbreviation: SLE, systemic lupus erythematosus.

REFERENCES

1. Wysenbeek AJ, Leibovici L, Amit M, Weinberger A. Alopecia in systemic lupus erythematosus. Relation to disease manifestations. J Rheumatol 1991; 18: 1185–6.
2. Yun SJ, Lee JW, Yoon HJ, et al. Cross-sectional study of hair loss patterns in 122 Korean systemic lupus erythematosus patients: a frequent finding of non-scarring patch alopecia. J Dermatol 2007; 34: 451–5.
3. Sperling LC, Lupton GP. Histopathology of non-scarring alopecia. J Cutan Pathol 1995; 22: 97–114.

20 Loose anagen hair syndrome

Although loose anagen hair syndrome (LAHS) was not described until 1984 (1) and 1989 (2,3), it is a fairly common form of noncicatricial hair loss. Lack of familiarity with the condition is the major obstacle to establishing the diagnosis.

CLINICAL FINDINGS

Most patients are first diagnosed at the age of 2–5 years when they are brought to a physician with the complaint of thin, uneven hair with an abnormal texture (4). Parents often state that the child's hair "won't grow." LAHS is most frequently diagnosed in girls, but it is not clear if the disorder actually has a propensity for females or is underreported in boys, who usually keep their hair short (5). Most cases of LAHS occur in individuals with light-colored hair, although cases in dark brown–haired persons have been reported (Figs. 20.1 and 20.2) (4,6,7). In some cases there is an autosomal dominant pattern of inheritance (6). The hair loss may be diffuse or patchy but there is no increase in hair fragility. In some cases the hair has a "sticky" or "tacky" feel (7). Usually the hair is thin, dry, somewhat unmanageable with a windblown appearance. (Fig. 20.3). The degree of unruliness is generally mild, but cases resembling uncombable hair syndrome have been reported (8,9).

Anagen hairs can be easily and painlessly extracted from the scalp by gentle traction. However, even in the same patient the ease of extraction will vary considerably from one evaluation to the next; therefore, a negative pull test for anagen hairs does not exclude the diagnosis (10). Using trichograms (forcible hair plucks), some authors have found an increased telogen count (27%) in patients with LAHS, (2) but others have found a *decreased* count (2%) (3). This issue will require more careful study in large numbers of patients. We believe that the diagnostic value of the telogen count in the evaluation of LAHS is uncertain. Regardless of the telogen count, when trichograms

are performed at least 50% of hairs should be "dystrophic" loose anagen hairs (as depicted in Fig. 20.4) (7,10,11).

In most cases, LAHS spontaneously improves with age, (6) and therapy is unnecessary. However, even in adulthood, evidence of the condition may persist if patients are carefully examined.

Hair Shaft Microscopic Examination

Extracted anagen hairs show a characteristic ruffling of the hair shaft cuticle where it separates from the inner root sheath (Fig. 20.4). The hair matrix and adjacent suprabulbar zone,

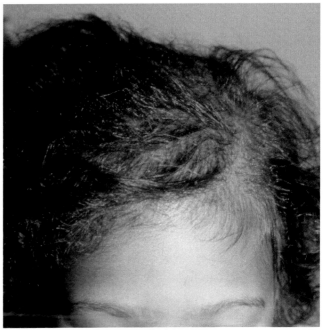

Figure 20.2 Dark-skinned, dark haired, LAHS patient—a 4-year-old boy.

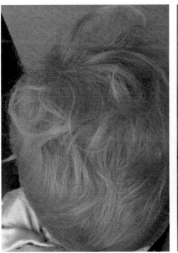
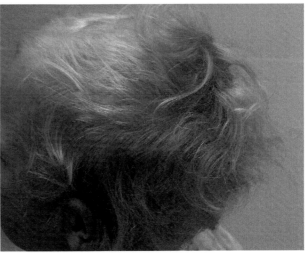

Figure 20.1 Typical LAHS patient—a 2-year-old blond girl. *Source:* Photographs courtesy of Walter Lamar, M.D.

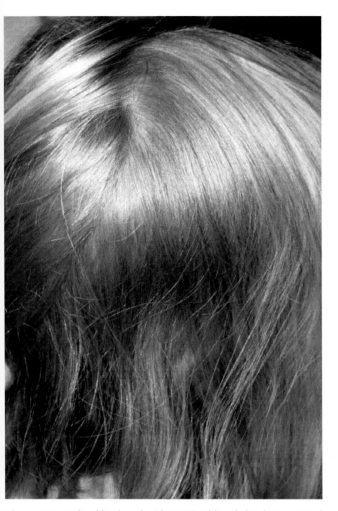

Figure 20.3 Another blonde girl with LAHS. Although her hair remained fairly thick, it had a persistent unruliness and windblown appearance.

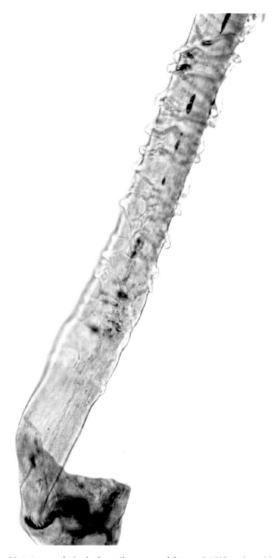

Figure 20.4 Anagen hair shaft, easily extracted from a LAHS patient. Note the ruffling of the hair shaft cuticle and the bent, squared-off anagen bulb.

which are not yet cornified, are prone to kinking during extraction, resulting in a "hockey stick" appearance. This appearance is often referred to in the literature as "dystrophic anagen hairs." In fact, the dysmorphic appearance is an artifact of plucking that can also be seen in trichograms from normal scalps and is simply more common and prominent in LAHS. The inner and outer root sheaths are left behind in the scalp when LAHS anagen hairs are extracted.

HISTOLOGICAL FINDINGS

The existing literature on the subject of histological findings is sparse and consists of brief descriptions of a few isolated cases and small case series. In a series of 5 patients with LAHS, there were no obvious morphologic abnormalities of the hair follicles besides a high incidence of fragmentation ("crumbling degeneration") and premature cornification of the inner root sheath (IRS) (11). Some authors have also noted marked cleft formation within the root sheaths (3). Other authors noted that the keratinized Henle cell layer showed a tortuous and irregular swelling, with irregular keratinization of the cuticle cells of the inner root sheath and a swollen appearance of Huxley cells (12). There are no reports of inflammation in biopsy specimens from LAHS patients.

With electron microscopy, the major pathological changes consist of intercellular edema, vacuolization in the prekeratinized Huxley cell zone, and dyskeratosis of Henle cells and cuticle cells of the inner root sheath.

We too have found numerous fractures within the cornified inner root sheath (Fig. 20.5, *top panel*). This probably corresponds to the "crumbling degeneration" referred to elsewhere in the literature. Varying degrees of unusual artifactual separation can also occur between layers of the inner root sheath (IRS) (Fig. 20.5, *bottom panel*, and Fig. 20.6) and between the inner and outer root sheaths (Fig. 20.7). These fractures and clefts are an artifact of processing and can also be seen in normal specimens, albeit to a lesser degree. Although not specific for LAHS, IRS fragmentation in particular appears to be a more common, prominent, and consistent feature of LAHS. We have also seen specimens from clinically typical cases of LAHS that to our eyes look histologically normal. It must be emphasized that the ubiquitous clefting found between the hair shaft and the cornified IRS is an artifact of processing that occurs in almost *all* normal as well as abnormal follicles. It is

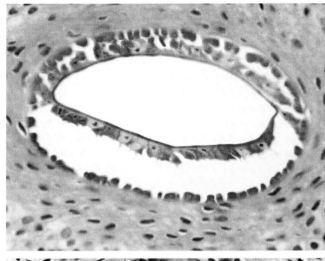

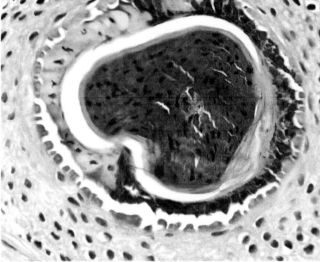

Figure 20.5 Numerous fractures within and between layers of the inner root sheath are commonly found in LAHS (*top panel*). A fragmented inner root sheath surrounds a grooved hair shaft (*lower panel*).

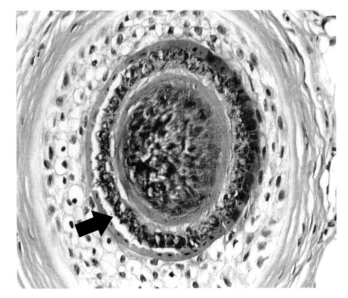

Figure 20.6 A circumferential cleft (*arrow*) has occurred within the inner root sheath between the cornified Henle's and noncornified Huxley's layer.

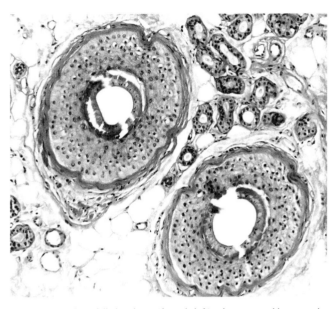

Figure 20.7 In these follicles, the artifactual clefting has occurred between the inner root sheath and the outer root sheath, as well as within the inner root sheath.

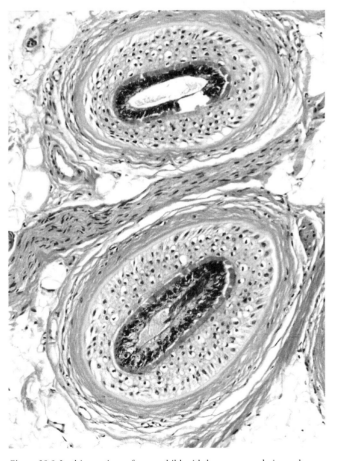

Figure 20.8 In this specimen from a child with loose anagen hair syndrome, hair shafts have been previously extracted from two follicles, and the inner root sheaths have collapsed inward. *Source*: Slide courtesy of Jeffrey Miller, M.D.

therefore of no diagnostic value and should be ignored. Occasionally, incomplete follicular anatomy resembling trichotillomania is found. When this occurs, only the hair shaft is absent, and the residual inner and outer root sheaths are collapsed (Fig. 20.8). This finding is hardly surprising as the shafts can be easily and painlessly extracted in children with LAHS, and sites of recent depilation may be chosen for biopsy.

Although most hair shafts in LAHS retain the normal oval or circular shape, some shafts have unusual polygonal shapes (Fig. 20.9). This corresponds to the grooving of hair shafts that can often be found in LAHS, and to some extent accounts for the slight unruliness of the hair. A few patients with LAHS have more prominent hair shaft grooving, affecting most hairs.

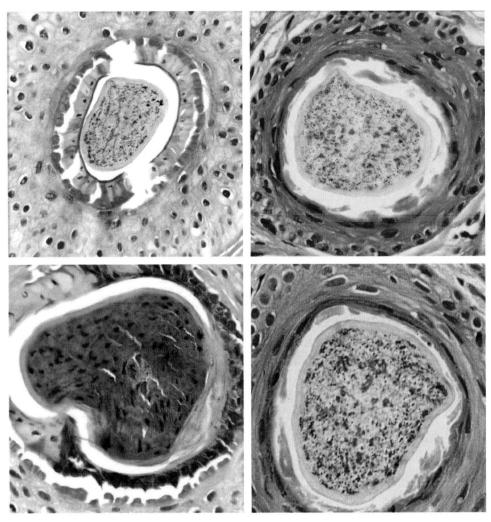

Figure 20.9 In transverse section, grooved hair shafts from LAHS patients are seen as polygonal and irregularly shaped.

Loose Anagen Hair Syndrome in Summary

Clinical correlation: Child with areas of slightly thinned, somewhat unruly hair. Parents complain that the child's hair "won't grow."

Histological findings:
❖ A hair pull showing bent or squared off anagen shafts with ruffled cuticles
❖ Marked fragmentation of the cornified inner root sheath
❖ Frequent clefting within the inner root sheath and between the inner and outer root sheaths
• Absent hair shafts with collapsed root sheaths and unusual hair shaft shapes in some specimens
• No significant inflammation

Histological differential diagnosis:
• **Telogen effluvium**: lacks hair shaft abnormalities
• **Trichotillomania**: may show loss of both shaft and inner root sheath, as well as trichomalacia, pigment casts, and intrafollicular hemorrhage

⚠ Pitfalls

Inner root sheath fragmentation is a common artifact of processing. Without good clinical correlation LAHS may not be distinguishable histologically from normal scalp.

REFERENCES

1. Zaun H. Syndrome of loosely attached hair in children. In: Happle R, Grosshans E, eds. Pediatric Dermatology: Advances in Diagnosis and Treatment. New York: Springer Verlag, 1984: 64–5.
2. Price VH, Gummer CL. Loose anagen syndrome. J Am Acad Dermatol 1989; 20(2 Pt 1): 249–56.
3. Hamm H, Traupe H. Loose anagen hair of childhood: the phenomenon of easily pluckable hair. J Am Acad Dermatol 1989; 20(2 Pt 1): 242–8.
4. O'Donnell BP, Sperling LC, James WD. Loose anagen hair syndrome. Int J Dermatol 1992; 31: 107–9.
5. Baden H, Kvedar J, Magro C. Loose anagen hair as a cause of hereditary hair loss in children. Arch Dermatol 1992; 128: 1349.
6. Li VW, Baden HP, Kvedar JC. Loose anagen syndrome and loose anagen hair. Dermatol Clin 1996; 14: 745–51.
7. Chapalain V, Winter H, Langbein L, et al. Is the loose anagen hair syndrome a keratin disorder? A clinical and molecular study. Arch Dermatol 2002; 138: 501–6.
8. Boyer JD, Cobb MW, Sperling LC, Rushin JM. Loose anagen hair syndrome mimicking the uncombable hair syndrome. Cutis 1996; 57: 111–2.
9. Lee AJ, Maino KL, Cohen B, Sperling L. A girl with loose anagen hair syndrome and uncombable, spun-glass hair. Pediatr Dermatol 2005; 22: 230–3.
10. Chong AH, Sinclair R. Loose anagen syndrome: a prospective study of three families. Australas J Dermatol 2002; 43: 120–4.
11. Tosti A, Peluso AM, Misciali C, et al. Loose anagen hair. Arch Dermatol 1997; 133: 1089–93.
12. Mirmirani P, Uno H, Price VH. Abnormal inner root sheath of the hair follicle in the loose anagen hair syndrome: An ultrastructural study. J Am Acad Dermatol 2011; 64: 129–34.

21 Central, centrifugal, cicatricial alopecia

This condition was first described in 1968 as "hot comb alopecia" (1), a name that has since been abandoned. The term *central, centrifugal, cicatricial alopecia* (CCCA; formerly known as *central, centrifugal, scarring alopecia* and *follicular degeneration syndrome* (2,3)) was coined to incorporate several related variants of inflammatory, cicatricial alopecia (4,5). The entities grouped under CCCA include most cases of *folliculitis decalvans* (4) (see chap. 23) and so-called *tufted folliculitis* (6) (see chap. 24). The differences between the variants may be due to racial differences or the well-recognized variability in immune responses between individuals. However, as variants of CCCA, they share the following features: (*i*) they are chronic and progressive, with possible spontaneous "burn out" after years or decades; (*ii*) they are predominantly centered on the central vertex (crown) or posterior vertex (hair whorl zone); (*iii*) they progress in a roughly symmetrical fashion, with the most active disease occurring in a peripheral zone of variable width, surrounding a central, alopecic zone; and (*iv*) they show both clinical and histological evidence of inflammation in the active, peripheral zone.

CLINICAL FINDINGS

One reason that CCCA has accumulated different names is that the condition exhibits a spectrum of inflammation, resulting in variability in signs and symptoms. Highly inflammatory disease, evidenced by pustule formation, crusting, intense erythema, and bacterial superinfection, has typically been labeled "folliculitis decalvans." More indolent disease, characterized by perifollicular scaling and occasional papule formation, has been called "the follicular degeneration syndrome," and in recent years, CCCA. Some patients described in the older literature as having "pseudopelade" of the central vertex may actually have had CCCA. Clinically and especially histologically, the similarity of CCCA between racial groups and sexes far exceeds any differences.

Most patients with CCCA are dark-skinned persons of African descent CCCA is the most common form of cicatricial alopecia in any population that includes large numbers of African-American patients. Among African-Americans, CCCA is responsible for more cases of cicatricial alopecia than all other forms combined. The majority of African-American patients with CCCA are women, with a female:male ratio of about 4:1. The average age at presentation is 36 years for women and 31 years for men, although most patients have progressive disease for years or decades before they seek medical attention. The disease invariably begins and remains most severe on the vertex (either the central vertex = "crown" or the posterior vertex = "hair whorl zone") of the scalp, gradually expanding in a centrifugal fashion (Fig. 21.1). Even when the amount of hair loss is dramatic, symptoms may be mild or absent. Most patients note only mild, episodic pruritus or tenderness of involved areas. A "pins and needles" sensation is often described.

Virtually all African-American women with CCCA are using or have used chemical hair relaxers for styling purposes. Besides pomades, few men have used similar products. Untreated patients experience progression of the disease even after all chemical products are discontinued. Caustic cosmetics or the use of "hot combs" may aggravate the disease or hasten its progression but cannot fully explain its pathogenesis. Similarly, the notion that the condition is caused by traction (7) is not supported by objective evidence and is inconsistent with actual hair care practices in many patients.

Upon clinical examination, the central or posterior vertex of the scalp shows a symmetrical zone of partial or complete alopecia. When inflammation is subtle, CCCA may be incorrectly diagnosed as androgenetic alopecia (Fig. 21.2). Typical of cicatricial alopecia, the follicular ostia are obliterated, and the interfollicular scalp is smooth and shiny.

A few isolated hairs, some showing polytrichia (tufting), may be stranded in an otherwise denuded central zone. Early or mild disease may present as a partially bald patch only a few centimeters in diameter. Longstanding or severe disease can result in hair loss covering the entire crown of the scalp (Fig. 21.3). Moving peripherally from the center of the alopecic zone to its perimeter, a gradual increase in hair density is noted. The alopecic zone eventually merges with the surrounding normal scalp. In the transitional zone, perifollicular erythema and a few inflammatory, follicular papules (or depending on the severity of the disease, even pustules) may be found. When these resolve, the hair follicle may be permanently lost, although many lesions likely heal without sequelae. Even "normal" scalp skin may show small foci of alopecia and an occasional follicular papule or some perifollicular scaling.

Therapy is empiric (8), but is usually sufficient to halt or slow progression. Mild-to-moderate disease responds well to a combination of potent topical corticosteroids (e.g., clobetasol) applied daily and an oral, "anti-inflammatory" antibiotic such as doxycycline (100 mg daily) (3). This "maintenance therapy" should be continued until inflammation and hair loss is controlled, which can take years to achieve. Highly inflammatory disease (the "folliculitis decalvans" pattern) may require a 10-week course of rifampicin and clindamycin (both 300 mg twice daily) (9) followed by the aforementioned "maintenance therapy."

HISTOLOGICAL FINDINGS

If the central, bald zone is sampled, the histological findings will be those of a "burnt out" cicatricial alopecia (see chap. 31). The most productive area for biopsy is the peripheral, partially alopecic fringe, but even clinically "normal" scalp may be diseased at the microscopic level. Not every follicle in a given area is involved simultaneously. A 4 mm punch biopsy specimen may contain only one or two "diagnostic" follicles. This is because the *involved* follicles are selectively *destroyed*, with

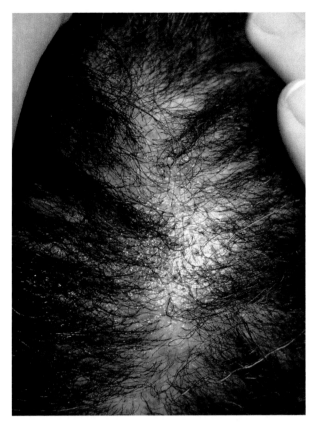

Figure 21.1 "Early" central, centrifugal, cicatricial alopecia emerges as a zone of partial hair thinning centered on the central (crown) or posterior (hair whorl zone) vertex. Permanent hair loss is evident by the loss of follicular ostia between the remaining follicles.

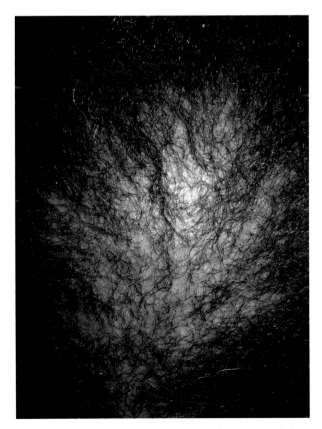

Figure 21.2 Even in fairly advanced central, centrifugal, cicatricial alopecia, evidence of clinical inflammation, such as papules and pustules may be absent. In such cases, the patient may be mislabeled as having androgenetic alopecia.

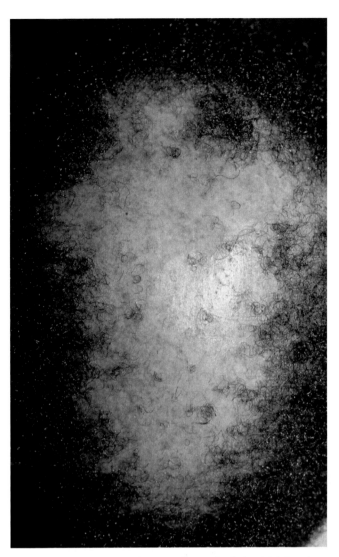

Figure 21.3 Severe, longstanding central, centrifugal, cicatricial alopecia.

sparing of the relatively normal follicles. Although an occasional vertical section may reveal an involved hair, in most cases transverse sections at several levels are required for a definitive diagnosis.

The word "distinctive" throws me since PDIRS is nonspecific as you state earliest histological finding is premature desquamation of the inner root sheath (PDIRS). This finding is most often noted in African-American patients but can be found in all races. Normally, the inner root sheath desquamates and disappears within the mid- to upper isthmus, which is usually located in the upper half of the dermis. In many cases of CCCA, the inner root sheath of an *involved* follicle desquamates in the lower half of the dermis, sometimes as low as (or deep to) the dermal/subcutaneous junction (Fig. 21.4). Desquamation of the IRS deep to the level of the eccrine coils can be regarded as "premature" because it is rarely found in a normal scalp. PDIRS can be observed in follicles that are otherwise normal, suggesting that it represents a very early phase of the disease. It can occasionally be seen in other conditions in which follicles are subject to marked inflammation and degenerative changes (10). However, as a manifestation of *early* disease, PDIRS appears to be distinctive of CCCA (11). This anatomical defect is probably an important component in the pathogenesis of the disease and may predispose the affected

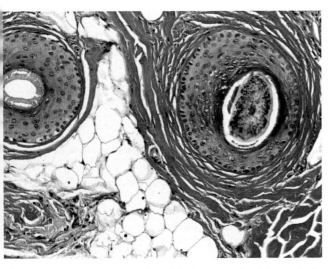

Figure 21.4 Premature desquamation of the inner root sheath is seen in the follicle on the right, as compared to a normal follicle (with inner root sheath) on the left.

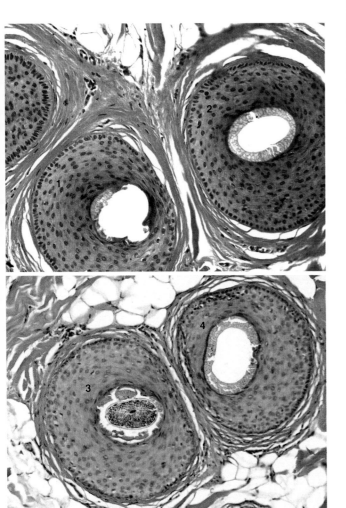

Figure 21.5 Early stages of PDIRS. Follicle "1" shows partial loss of the IRS. Follicle "2" is normal. Follicle "3" shows advanced loss of the IRS, and in "4" the IRS is intact, but the surrounding ORS cells are flattening, a sign of impending PDIRS. *Abbreviations*: IRS, inner root sheath; PDIRS, premature desquamation of the inner root sheath.

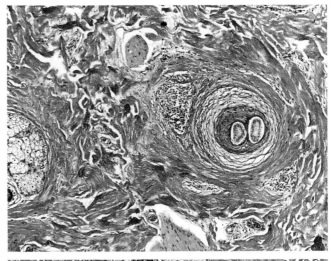

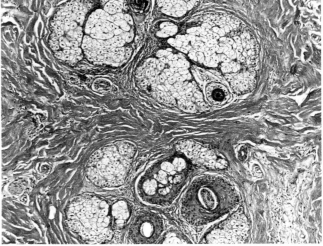

Figure 21.6 Two adjacent fields from the same tissue section demonstrate the selective loss of sebaceous glands in this case of "early" central, centrifugal, cicatricial alopecia. An inflamed follicular unit (*upper panel*) has lost its sebaceous gland, although the follicles are not yet destroyed; perifollicular fibrosis is also present. Two noninflamed units (*lower panel*) show the presence of sebaceous glands, expected at this level of the dermis.

follicles to injury. The inner root sheath serves as a biological gasket, sealing off the lower two thirds of the follicle from external antigens (bacteria, spores, cosmetics, and others). Loss of this seal deep within the dermis allows these antigens access to the lower portion of the follicle, including the bulge zone.

The ability to identify PDIRS is important for the diagnosis of CCCA. When follicles demonstrating clear-cut PDIRS are not found, the identification of *impending* PDIRS can often be seen. As the IRS is about to desquamate (Fig. 21.5), the surrounding outer root sheath (ORS) cells begin to flatten and their cytoplasm becomes brightly eosinophilic. This is a reliable clue that at a slightly more superficial level, the IRS will desquamate. As the disease evolves in clinically abnormal scalp skin, involved follicles also demonstrate some or all of the following histological features: (4,12) loss of sebaceous glands in inflamed follicular units (Fig. 21.6); eccentric epithelial atrophy (thinning) with hair shafts in close proximity to the dermis (Fig. 21.7); concentric lamellar fibroplasia (onion skin-like fibrosis) of affected follicles (Fig. 21.8); variably dense lymphocytic perifollicular inflammation, primarily at the level of the upper isthmus and lower infundibulum (Fig. 21.9); occasional

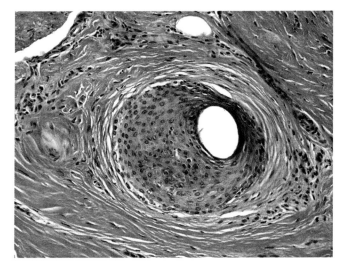

Figure 21.7 Once a follicle has undergone premature desquamation of the inner root sheath, it is prone to eccentric epithelial atrophy. In this image there is epithelial thinning with a hair shaft in close proximity to the dermis.

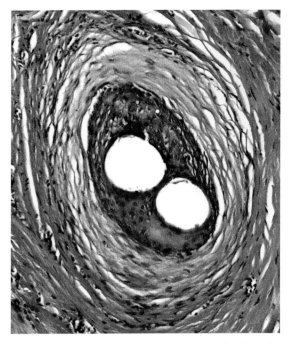

Figure 21.8 Concentric lamellar fibroplasia and epithelial atrophy

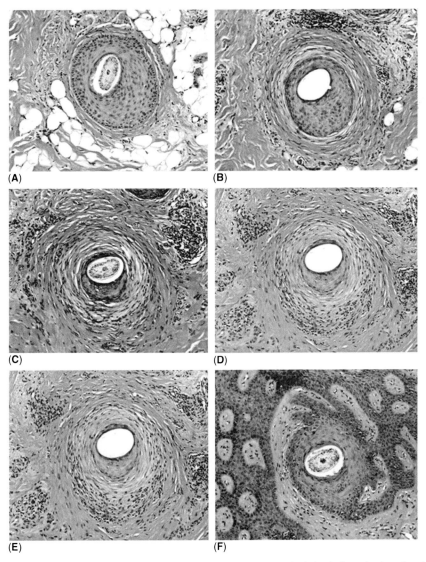

Figure 21.9 A follicle showing premature desquamation of the inner root sheath, sectioned at multiple levels from the deep dermis (A) up to the infundibular ostium (F); perifollicular lymphocytic inflammation is most intense at the level of the upper isthmus and lower infundibulum (C–E).

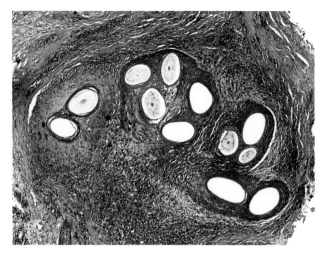

Figure 21.10 Polytrichia in a highly inflammatory example of central, centrifugal, cicatricial alopecia.

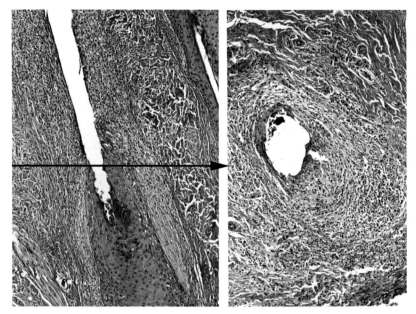

Figure 21.11 Epithelial destruction in a highly inflammatory example of central, centrifugal, cicatricial alopecia. The level of the arrow shown in the *left panel* (vertical section) is shown in transverse section on the right (in transverse section).

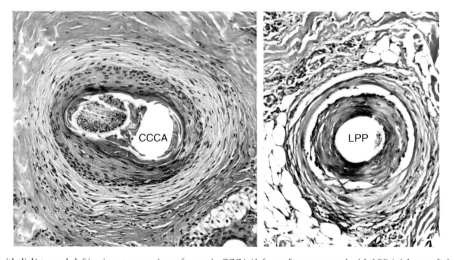

Figure 21.12 In general, epithelial/stromal clefting is not a prominent feature in CCCA (*left panel*) as compared with LPP (*right panel*). In CCCA, the stroma tends to cling to the squamatized epithelium, whereas the opposite is true in LPP. Unfortunately, there are many exceptions to this generalization. *Abbreviations*: CCCA, central, centrifugal, cicatricial alopecia; LPP, lichen planopilaris.

fusion of infundibula, with multiple hair shafts exiting a single infundibular orifice (polytrichia; Fig. 21.10); and in advanced lesions, total destruction of the follicular epithelium with retained hair shaft fragments and granulomatous inflammation (Fig. 21.11). Interface alteration of the follicular epithelium is not found, although in some cases "squamatization" of the infundibular epithelium can mimic a similar change seen in lichen planopilaris (LPP). A useful point of differentiation is that in the squamatized infundibulum of CCCA, the stroma tends to "cling" to the epithelium without much clefting; in contrast, the stroma in LPP will often show obvious clefting (Fig. 21.12). This feature, however, is nonspecific and must be placed in context with other histological findings. In addition, the frequent paucity of inflammation surrounding such obviously diseased follicles points to CCCA rather than LPP. To date, the immunofluorescent findings in patients with CCCA have not been critically studied.

As noted above, the most distinctive histological feature of CCCA is PDIRS in noninflamed follicles. The remainder of the histological features encountered in CCCA can also be found in other forms of inflammatory, cicatricial alopecia, and are therefore supportive but not conclusively diagnostic.

Central, Centrifugal, Cicatricial Alopecia in Summary

Clinical correlation: an adult, most often an African-American woman, with a progressive, permanent loss of scalp hair starting on the central crown or vertex. A spectrum of clinical inflammation exists, ranging from minimal to highly inflamed. The highly inflamed cases show marked erythema, pustules, and crusting ("folliculitis decalvans").

Histological findings:

❖ PDIRS may be found even when normal appearing scalp skin or perilesional skin is sampled. PDIRS may not be seen if all abnormal follicles have been destroyed
• Eccentric epithelial atrophy (thinning) with hair shafts in close proximity to the dermis
• Concentric lamellar fibroplasia (onion skin-like fibrosis) of affected follicles
• Variably dense lymphocytic perifollicular inflammation, primarily at the level of the upper isthmus and lower infundibulum

Late and end-stage histological findings include:

• Eventual destruction of the follicular epithelium with retained hair shaft fragments and granulomatous inflammation
• Replacement of the follicular epithelium by connective tissue (follicular scars)
• Occasional fusion of infundibula (polytrichia or "tufting")

Histological differential diagnosis:

• **Acne keloidalis**: can have the same histopathologic findings as CCCA; clinical correlation is required for differentiation (*Note*: clinical features of both diseases may be seen in a single patient)
• **Advanced LPP**: may show interface dermatitis or individually necrotic keratinocytes and prominent clefting between the follicular epithelium and the fibrotic dermis. *Unlikely* to show PDIRS in relatively noninflamed follicles.

⚠ **Pitfalls**

PDIRS may be found as a nonspecific feature in heavily inflamed follicles in any disease state, so it must be interpreted in the context of other clinical and histological findings

Abbreviations: LPP, lichen planopilaris; PDIRS, premature desquamation of the inner root sheath.

REFERENCES

1. LoPresti P, Papa C, Kligman A. Hot comb alopecia. Arch Dermatol 1968; 98: 234–8.
2. Sperling L, Sau P. The follicular degeneration syndrome in black patients: "hot comb alopecia" revisited and revised. Arch Dermatol 1992; 128: 68–74.
3. Sperling L, Skelton H, Smith K, Sau P, Friedman K. The follicular degeneration syndrome in men. Arch Dermatol 1994; 130: 763–9.
4. Sperling L, Solomon A, Whiting D. A new look at scarring alopecia. Arch Dermatol 2000; 136: 235–42.
5. Olsen EA, Bergfeld WF, Cotsarelis G, et al. Summary of North American Hair Research Society (NAHRS)-sponsored Workshop on Cicatricial Alopecia, Duke University Medical Center, February 10 and 11, 2001. J Am Acad Dermatol 2003; 48: 103–10.
6. Annessi G. Tufted folliculitis of the scalp: a distinctive clinicohistological variant of folliculitis decalvans. Br J Dermatol 1998; 138: 799–805.
7. Ackerman AB, Walton NW, Jones RE, Charissi C. Quandary resolved!: "hot comb alopecia"/"follicular degeneration syndrome" in African-American women is traction alopecia! Dermatopathology: Practical & Conceptual 2000; 6–4.
8. Whiting DA. Cicatricial alopecia: clinico-pathological findings and treatment. Clin Dermatol 2001; 19: 211–25.
9. Powell J, Dawber R, Gatter K. Folliculitis decalvans including tufted folliculitis: clinical, histological and therapeutic findings. Br J Dermatol 1999; 140: 328–33.
10. Horenstein MG, Simon J. Investigation of the hair follicle inner root sheath in scarring and non-scarring alopecia. J Cutan Pathol 2007; 34: 762–8.
11. Sperling LC. Premature desquamation of the inner root sheath is still a useful concept! J Cutan Pathol 2007; 34: 809–10.
12. Templeton S, Solomon A. Scarring alopecia: a classification based on microscopic criteria. J Cutan Pathol 1994; 21: 97–109.

22 Acne keloidalis (folliculitis keloidalis)

Often called *acne keloidalis nuchae*, this disorder typically affects young African-American men and occasionally young African-American women (1,2). AK is at least 10 times more common in African-Americans than in Caucasians and comprises nearly 0.5% of all dermatologic cases in the American black population (i.e., African-Americans), and even more elsewhere (0.7% in Benin (3) and almost 10% in Nigeria (4)). However, the condition can occur in Caucasian men and on rare occasion in Caucasian women.

CLINICAL FINDINGS

AK begins as small, smooth, firm papules with occasional pustules on the occipital scalp and posterior neck (Fig. 22.1). In a minority of cases lesions extend up to the vertex, and so it is best to use the term *acne keloidalis* without the modifier *nuchae*. Initially hairs can be seen exiting the papules, but the hair shafts are eventually shed (Fig. 22.2). With time, the papules resolve and leave small zones of alopecia within a field of papular lesions (Fig. 22.3). In many patients, the papules coalesce and form firm, hairless, keloid-like protuberant plaques (hence the term *keloidalis*) that can be painful and cosmetically disfiguring (Fig. 22.4). Abscesses and sinuses exuding pus can be present in advanced cases. Although AK may be asymptomatic, mild symptoms of burning and itching are often present.

The cause of AK remains unclear. The notion that lesions of AK are caused by "ingrown" hairs, analogous to the situation in pseudofolliculitis barbae, has been disproved (5). AK is frequently found in association with central, centrifugal, cicatricial alopecia (CCCA), suggesting a common or related pathogenesis. Occasionally, the papular lesions and hair loss of AK extend onto the vertex and crown of the scalp, producing a clinical "overlap" of AK and CCCA.

In the authors' experience, mild and moderate disease consisting of small papules and patches of hair loss responds well to an anti-inflammatory regimen consisting of potent topical corticosteroids (e.g., clobetasol) and oral doxycycline. A typical regimen includes topical clobetasol 0.05% ointment once daily and oral doxycycline 100 mg once daily. Treatment must be continued for a very prolonged period of time (often years) because the disease is chronic and progressive. Most articles that address treatment focus on the large, keloidal nodules that are common in advanced disease (6). For these patients, surgical treatment with excision and healing via secondary intention healing gives good results (Fig. 22.5) (7). Bulky lesions seldom achieve a sustained response with just intralesional corticosteroids or shave-debulking. After larger lesions have been excised, the same chronic, anti-inflammatory regimen used for milder disease must be instituted to avoid recurrence and progressive hair loss.

HISTOLOGICAL FINDINGS

Most descriptions of the pathology of AK are based on late-stage, nodular (keloid-like) lesions. When early papular lesions (or samples of perilesional skin) are studied (5,8), the findings are those of a chronic, lymphocytic folliculitis. AK is a primary form of cicatricial alopecia, and many of the findings closely resemble those found in certain other forms of cicatricial alopecia. The most common findings, in descending order of frequency, are as follows: perifollicular, chronic inflammation (lymphocytic and plasmacytic), most intense at the level of the isthmus and lower infundibulum; lamellar fibroplasia, most marked at the level of the isthmus; complete disappearance of sebaceous glands associated with inflamed or destroyed follicles; thinning of the follicular epithelium, especially at the level of the isthmus; polytrichia (several hairs sharing a common, fused infundibulum); premature desquamation of the inner root sheath; and total epithelial destruction (superficial and deep) with residual "naked" hair fragments (Figs. 22.6–22.11). Some of these retained shafts are slowly resorbed, resulting in a focal bald spot. Others, however, can serve as a nidus for

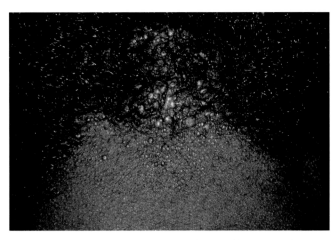

Figure 22.1 Patient with numerous papular lesions of AK. Some alopecia is already evident.

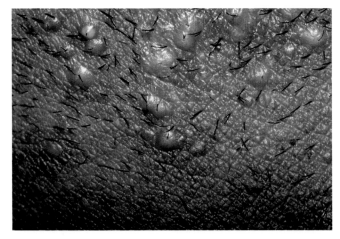

Figure 22.2 Several "early" papular or papulopustular lesions of AK with hair shafts still present. Small zones of alopecia can already be seen.

126

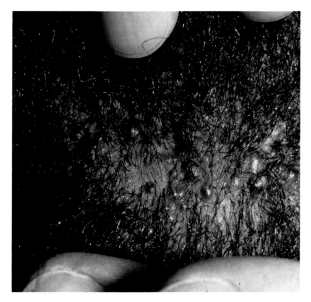

Figure 22.3 In well-established AK, small zones of cicatricial alopecia can be found between the papules.

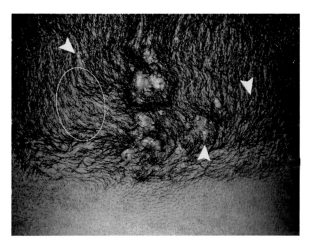

Figure 22.4 In this patient with AK, papules have coalesced into keloid-like nodules. However, papules (*arrow heads*) and zones of partial alopecia (*ellipse*) are also present.

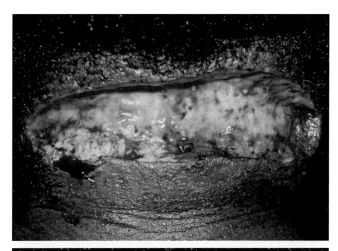

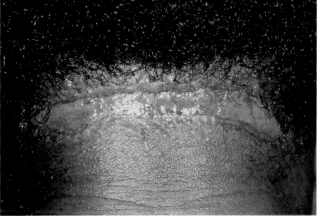

Figure 22.5 A bulky, keloidal nodule of AK was excised from this patient, resulting in this postoperative defect (*top panel*). Five weeks later (*bottom panel*), healing by secondary intention is almost complete.

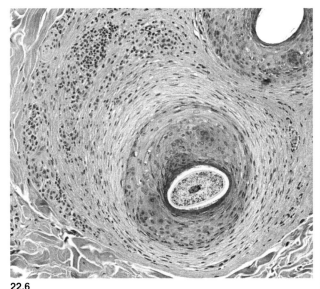

22.6

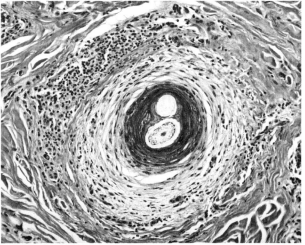

22.7

Figures 22.6 and 22.7 A specimen taken from perilesional skin in a patient with typical AK, demonstrating typical histological findings. In Figure 22.6, a follicle demonstrates perifollicular lymphocytic inflammation, lamellar fibroplasia, and loss of the sebaceous glands. A normal-appearing adjacent follicle (*upper right*) is present for comparison. Similarly inflamed follicles with fused infundibula are seen in Figure 22.7. Sections shown in both figures were taken at the level of the lower infundibulum.

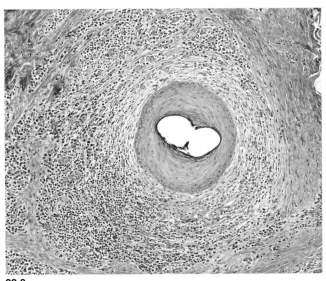

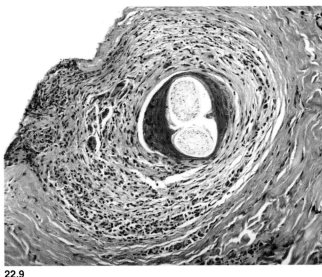

22.8   **22.9**

Figures 22.8 and 22.9 Specimens taken from erythematous, papular lesions in patients with typical papular AK demonstrate more advanced inflammatory changes. In Figure 22.8, the two fused follicles are surrounded by a dense infiltrate of predominantly chronic inflammation. In Figure 22.9, the epithelium is markedly attenuated, and surrounded by both chronic and granulomatous inflammation. In both figures, sections were taken at the level of the lower infundibulum.

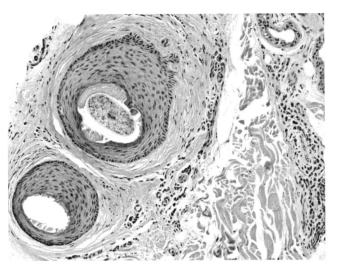

Figure 22.10 In a specimen taken from perilesional skin, two follicles demonstrate premature desquamation of the inner root sheath.

marked fibrosis, persistent inflammation, and bacterial superinfection. The resulting tissue hypertrophy traps adjacent follicles, and eventually leads to the "keloidal," hypertrophic scarring seen in some patients with AK (Figs. 22.12–22.17). Occasionally specimens from normal-appearing perilesional skin may contain true follicular scars, demonstrating subclinical disease (5). Special stains for bacteria demonstrate relatively few organisms, suggesting that bacterial overgrowth is not important in the pathogenesis of AK (5).

Many of the histological features of AK are shared by central, centrifugal, cicatricial alopecia (CCCA). This overlap of histological features suggests a common pathogenesis for AK and CCCA, a notion that is supported by the frequent occurrence of both conditions in the same patient. As mentioned above, clinical features sometimes overlap as well. However, the association between CCCA and AK has never been critically studied.

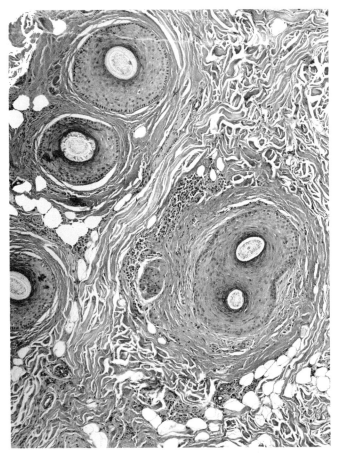

Figure 22.11 In a specimen taken from lesional skin, two follicles sharing a fused outer root sheath (*right side*) demonstrate premature desquamation of the inner root sheath. Surrounding follicles have intact inner root sheaths, as would be expected at a subisthmic level.

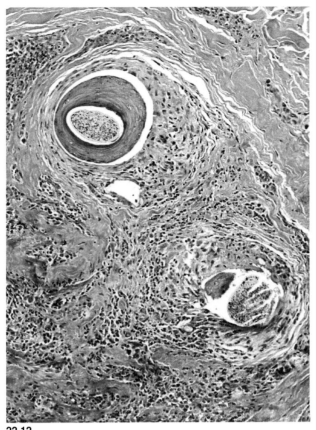
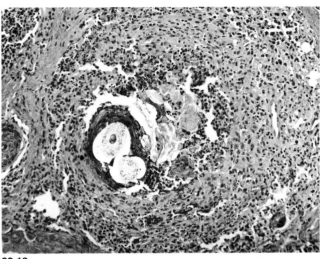

22.12   **22.13**

Figures 22.12 and 22.13 Figure 22.12 is from a papular lesion of AK and shows two follicles with advanced (end-stage) changes of AK. These include epithelial thinning and concentric lamellar fibroplasia (upper left follicle) and complete disintegration of the follicular epithelium (lower right follicle). Similar destructive changes are seen in Figure 22.13, a specimen taken from a "juicy" papular lesion of AK.

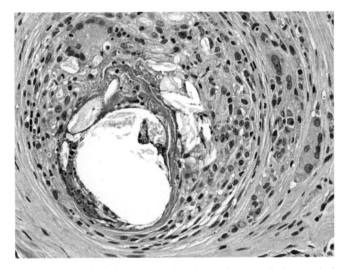

Figure 22.14 Papular lesions or small alopecic macules may only show residual "naked" hair shafts and/or foci of granulomatous inflammation at the sites of former follicles. The naked shaft in this specimen was lost during processing.

Histological findings:
❖ Perifollicular, chronic inflammation (lymphocytic and plasmacytic)
❖ Perifollicular, lamellar fibroplasia
❖ Complete disappearance of sebaceous glands associated with inflamed or destroyed follicles
❖ Thinning of the follicular epithelium, especially at the level of the isthmus
• Premature desquamation of the inner root sheath
• Eventual destruction of the follicular epithelium with retained hair shaft fragments and granulomatous inflammation
• Replacement of the follicular epithelium by connective tissue (follicular scars)

Histological differential diagnosis:
• **CCCA:** histological findings may be identical; clinical correlation required for diagnosis
• **Folliculitis decalvans:** histological findings may be identical; clinical correlation required for diagnosis

Acne Keloidalis in Summary

Clinical correlation: small, smooth, firm follicular papules with occasional pustules, eventually leading to partial hair loss. Most common on the nuchal region (occipital scalp and posterior neck). With advanced disease, there are coalescent papules forming firm, hairless, keloid-like protuberant plaques.

⚠ **Pitfalls**
If fibrotic nodules ("keloidal") are sampled, the findings will be those of a hypertrophic scar with retained hair shaft fragments, or simply an end-stage cicatricial alopecia.

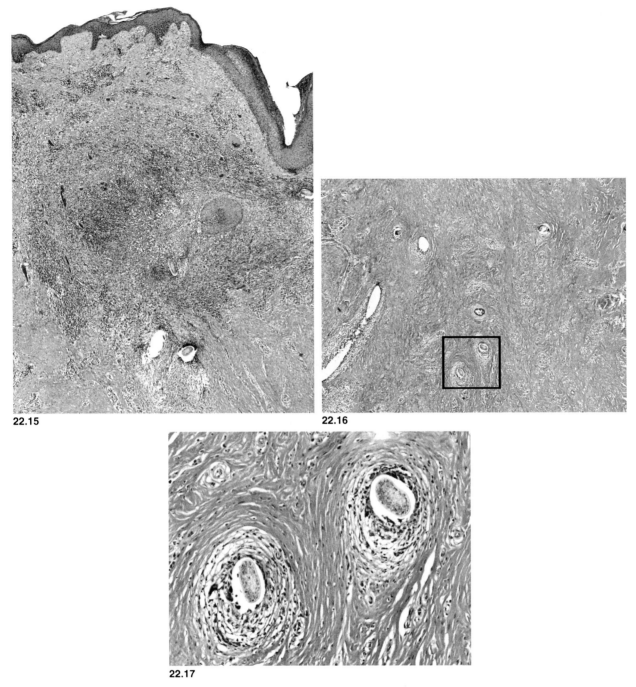

Figures 22.15, 22.16, 22.17 The hypertrophic scars of AK consist of a dense, fibrotic stroma with variable amounts of acute, chronic, and granulomatous inflammation (Fig. 22.15). Retained hair shaft fragments, trapped within zones of fibrosis, probably serve as a stimulus for persistent inflammation and reactive fibroplasia (Figs. 22.16 and 22.17). Figure 22.17 is a magnified view of the boxed area seen in Figure 22.16.

REFERENCES

1. Quarles FN, Brody H, Badreshia S, et al. Acne keloidalis nuchae. Dermatol Ther 2007; 20:128–32.
2. Ogunbiyi A, George A. Acne keloidalis in females: case report and review of literature. J Natl Med Assoc 2005; 97: 736–8.
3. Adegbidi H, Atadokpede F, do Ango-Padonou F, Yedomon H. Keloid acne of the neck: epidemiological studies over 10 years. Int J Dermatol 2005; 44(Suppl 1): 49–50.
4. Salami T, Omeife H, Samuel S. Prevalence of acne keloidalis nuchae in Nigerians. Int J Dermatol 2007; 46: 482–4.
5. Sperling LC, Homoky C, Pratt L, Sau P. Acne keloidalis is a form of primary scarring alopecia. Arch Dermatol 2000; 136: 479–84.
6. Gloster HM Jr. The surgical management of extensive cases of acne keloidalis nuchae. Arch Dermatol 2000; 136: 1376–9.
7. Bajaj V, Langtry JA. Surgical excision of acne keloidalis nuchae with secondary intention healing. Clin Exp Dermatol 2008; 33: 53–5.
8. Herzberg AJ, Dinehart SM, Kerns BJ, Pollack SV. Acne keloidalis. Transverse microscopy, immunohistochemistry, and electron microscopy. Am J Dermatopathol 1990; 12: 109–21.

23 Folliculitis decalvans

Many, if not most, textbooks and review articles (1) discuss folliculitis decalvans as a distinct condition, but depending on the author, different definitions have been applied. Therefore, the term needs to be defined each time it is used. We define *folliculitis decalvans* as a clinical pattern of highly inflammatory cicatricial alopecia characterized by frequent perifollicular papules and pustules, almost always most severe on the posterior vertex. For the term to apply, distinctive features of well-accepted and specific diagnoses [such as lichen planopilaris (LPP) and discoid lupus erythematosus] must be absent. We believe that most cases of folliculitis decalvans represent the "highly inflammatory" end of the central, centrifugal, cicatricial alopecia (CCCA) spectrum. Therefore, folliculitis decalvans represents one clinical pattern seen in CCCA, and not a separate disease. This does not exclude the possibility of other conditions causing a folliculitis decalvans pattern of inflammation, and indeed we have seen unusual cases of tinea capitis and LPP as occasional culprits.

CLINICAL FINDINGS

In the more inflammatory cases of CCCA (i.e., the "folliculitis decalvans" pattern), pustular lesions come and go during the course of the disease (Fig. 23.1). These pustules are often (but not invariably) culture-positive for *Staphylococcus aureus*. Some authors have argued that "folliculitis decalvans" is a primary staphylococcal infection (2,3). We believe, however, that the pustules represent a manifestation of bacterial superinfection and/or an immune response of the patient to degenerating follicular components in CCCA, rather than the driving cause of the alopecia. Inflamed lesions can be multifocal, but eventually merge into one larger patch on the crown or vertex (Fig. 23.2). An expanding zone of alopecia with peripheral pustules and crusting is not diagnostic of CCCA, and can be seen in tinea capitis (kerion) and presumably in true bacterial infections of the scalp. When these latter conditions are excluded, the majority of patients will prove to have CCCA.

Tinea capitis and bacterial folliculitis require appropriate antimicrobial therapy. The treatment of most cases of the "folliculitis decalvans" pattern of hair loss is similar to the management of a severe or refractory case of CCCA. Therapy is empirical, but is usually sufficient to reduce or eliminate symptoms and slow progression of disease. Usually, a short course of antibiotics or systemic corticosteroids can temporarily eliminate the purulent component of CCCA. A combination of potent topical corticosteroids (e.g., clobetasol 0.05% ointment) applied daily and an oral, anti-inflammatory antibiotics, such as doxycycline (100 mg daily) (4), can be tried as the first step on the "therapeutic ladder." This can be considered to be the long-term maintenance therapy. A short course of oral corticosteroids, such as prednisone is often effective in "cooling off" the inflammatory component of the disease, and might be considered. Refractory or severe disease may require

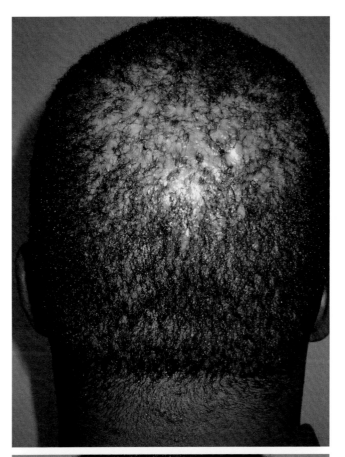

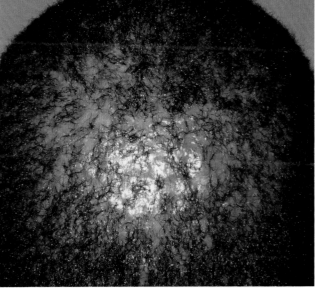

Figure 23.1 Folliculitis decalvans: a highly inflammatory and destructive cicatricial alopecia, centered on the posterior vertex. This photograph was taken several weeks following the initiation of therapy. There had been numerous perifollicular pustules and crusts until anti-inflammatory treatment with topical clobetasol and oral doxycycline was initiated.

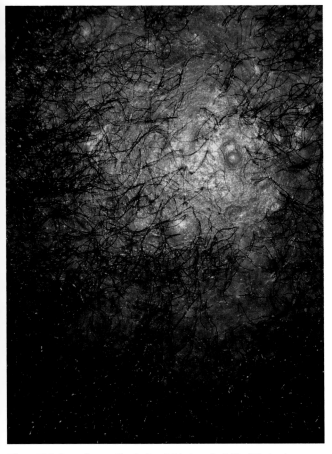

Figure 23.2 Central, centrifugal, cicatricial alopecia, folliculitis decalvans pattern. Papulopustules were distributed in a broad zone of cicatricial alopecia centered on the central vertex.

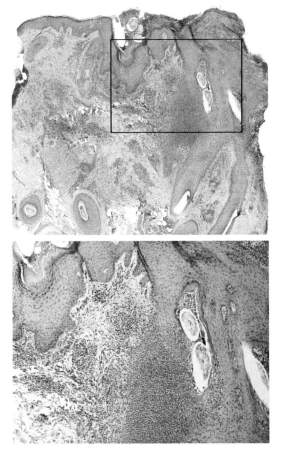

Figure 23.3 Vertical section of a papulopustular lesion in a patient with folliculitis decalvans. The clinical pattern of hair loss was typical of severe central, centrifugal, cicatricial alopecia. The boxed area in the upper panel is magnified in the lower panel.

a 10-week course of rifampicin and clindamycin (both 300 mg twice daily) (2). We have found this potent combination of antibiotics to be very helpful, but not curative. It must be followed by long-term maintenance therapy.

HISTOLOGICAL FINDINGS

The microscopic findings in pustular lesions include intrafollicular and perifollicular infiltrates rich in neutrophils as well as lymphocytes and plasma cells. Inflammation is generally most intense around the upper portion of affected follicles, especially at the level of the lower infundibulum. The epithelium of such follicles is often markedly thinned, the epithelial cells flattened and "squamatized" (Figs. 23.3 and 23.4). Polytrichia (fused infundibula) is often a prominent feature, with a cluster of hairs surrounded by a zone of fibroplasia and inflammation (Fig. 23.5). If nonpustular lesions at the active periphery are sampled, or if the biopsy is performed during a period of suppressive therapy, the histological picture of folliculitis decalvans is usually identical to less inflammatory forms of CCCA.

When CCCA is *not* responsible for a case showing the folliculitis decalvans histopathologic pattern, there may be obvious clinical clues (such as a distinctive pattern of hair loss) or subtle histological clues that allow for an alternative diagnosis. However, a biopsy sample from an "early," less inflamed lesion may be required to arrive at a definitive diagnosis.

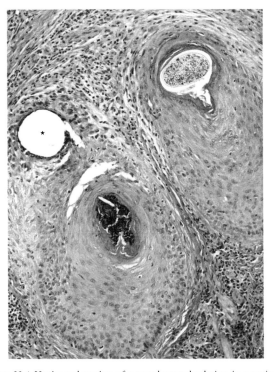

Figure 23.4 Horizontal section of a papulopustular lesion in a patient with folliculitis decalvans (same patient as Figure 23.3). The follicle on the left shows that the hair shaft (*) has migrated through the thinned and inflamed epithelium and is lying free in the dermis (the actual shaft was displaced during processing, but the space it occupied is visible). The clinical pattern of hair loss was typical of severe central, centrifugal, cicatricial alopecia.

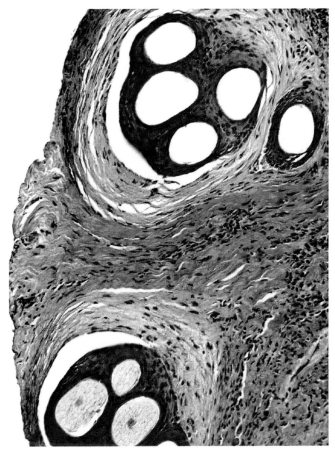

Figure 23.5 Folliculitis decalvans. Polytrichia is a prominent feature in this specimen.

Histological findings:

❖ Pustular lesions include intrafollicular and perifollicular infiltrates rich in neutrophils as well as lymphocytes and plasma cells. Inflammation is generally most intense around the upper portion of affected follicles, especially at the level of the lower infundibulum

❖ Flattened and "squamatized" follicular epithelium surrounded by a zone of fibroplasia and inflammation

❖ Polytrichia (fused infundibula)

• Nonpustular lesions at the active periphery show changes identical to those seen in less inflammatory forms of CCCA

Histological differential diagnosis:

• All forms of highly inflammatory and destructive alopecias can result in the *folliculitis decalvans* pattern

• Folliculitis decalvans and tufted folliculitis are terms that are sometimes used interchangeably because they both represent non-specific patterns found in highly inflammatory and destructive alopecias.

⚠ **Pitfalls**

A biopsy from a pustular or papular area is less likely to provide useful histopathological information than one from a peripheral area of "early" disease.

Folliculitis Decalvans in Summary

Clinical correlation: a clinical pattern of highly inflammatory cicatricial alopecia characterized by frequent perifollicular papules and pustules, almost always most severe on the posterior vertex. Most cases of folliculitis decalvans represent the "highly inflammatory" end of the central centrifugal cicatricial alopecia (CCCA) spectrum.

REFERENCES

1. Brooke RC, Griffiths CE. Folliculitis decalvans. Clin Exp Dermatol 2001; 26: 120–2.
2. Powell J, Dawber R, Gatter K. Folliculitis decalvans including tufted folliculitis: clinical, histological and therapeutic findings. Br J Dermatol 1999; 140: 328–33.
3. Powell J, Dawber RP. Folliculitis decalvans and tufted folliculitis are specific infective diseases that may lead to scarring, but are not a subset of central centrifugal scarring alopecia. Arch Dermatol 2001; 137: 373–4.
4. Sperling LC, Skelton HG 3rd, Smith KJ, Sau P, Friedman K. Follicular degeneration syndrome in men. Arch Dermatol 1994; 130: 763–9.

24 Tufted folliculitis

The term tufted folliculitis appears to date back to 1978, when Smith (1) used the term to describe distinctive tufting of hairs in an occipital lesion of longstanding cicatricial alopecia. Another name for this phenomenon is *polytrichia*. It has become evident since then that the tufting seen in this *pattern* of hair disease can result from different causes of cicatricial alopecia (Figs. 24.1–24.3). (2) Thus "tufted folliculitis" is not a specific disease, but an end-stage of several different conditions. Despite this recognition, "tufted folliculitis" continues to be applied as a diagnostic label in the medical literature, a usage that is incorrect and misleading.

CLINICAL FINDINGS

Tufting in the setting of cicatricial alopecia occurs most commonly in the occipital region (2). In both Caucasians and African-Americans, central, centrifugal, cicatricial alopecia (CCCA) is the most common cause of tufting. In patients with CCCA, the upper occipital region appears to be a favored site for tuft formation, even when the disease also affects the vertex and crown. Although tufting is fairly common in cases of CCCA, it can occasionally be seen in a wide variety of other disorders, including dissecting cellulitis, inflammatory tinea capitis,(3) pemphigus vulgaris, (4–6) acne keloidalis (folliculitis keloidalis) (7), and after use of biologic chemotherapeutic agents (8,9). We have also seen tufting in patients with lichen planopilaris and discoid lupus erythematosus (Fig. 24.3).

The highly inflammatory and destructive "folliculitis decalvans" pattern of CCCA commonly eventuates in follicular tufting (10,11). If the clinical pattern of hair loss is that of a slowly progressive cicatricial alopecia centered on or near the posterior vertex (hair whorl zone), then CCCA is the most likely culprit.

Appropriate treatment hinges upon making a specific diagnosis. An optimal biopsy technique as detailed below can help to pinpoint the underlying disease process. A fungal culture should be done to exclude tinea capitis. Bacterial cultures will often reveal *Staphylococcus aureus* colonization, but therapy directed solely against this organism will only provide short-term improvement. For the majority of patients whose tufted folliculitis ultimately proves to be a variant of CCCA, treatment for this disease (as discussed in chap. 21) can be used.

HISTOLOGICAL FINDINGS

The histological features in zones of cicatricial alopecia showing tufting are very advanced, nonspecific, end-stage changes. Just as the *clinical* pattern of tufting can be found in several

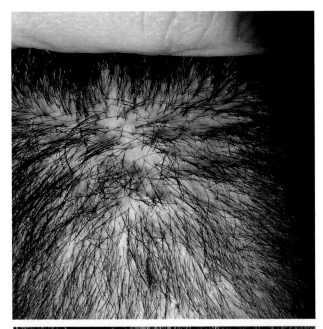

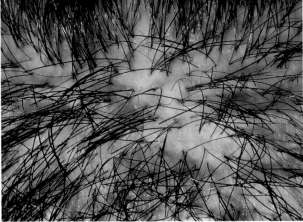

Figure 24.2 Focal tufting is seen in another patient with central, centrifugal, cicatricial alopecia. The area of interest in the top panel is magnified in the lower panel.

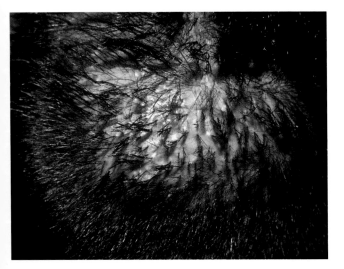

Figure 24.1 This image portrays a dramatic example of polytrichia ("tufting") in a patient with central, centrifugal, cicatricial alopecia.

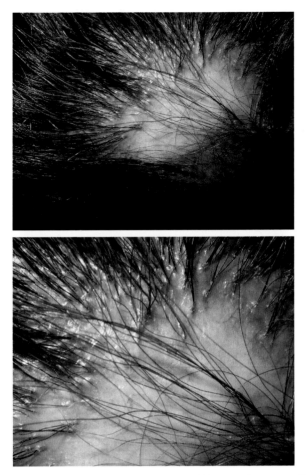

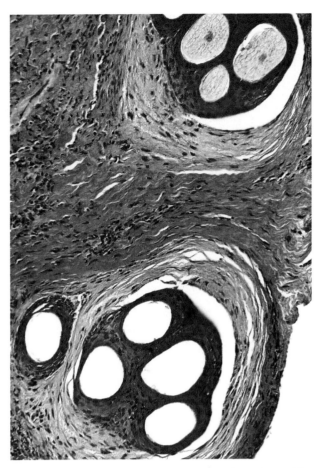

Figure 24.3 Focal tufting in a patient with discoid lupus erythematosus. The area of interest in the top panel is magnified in the lower panel.

Figure 24.6 Two tufts of hairs are separated by a circumferential ring of dense connective tissue and residual chronic inflammation.

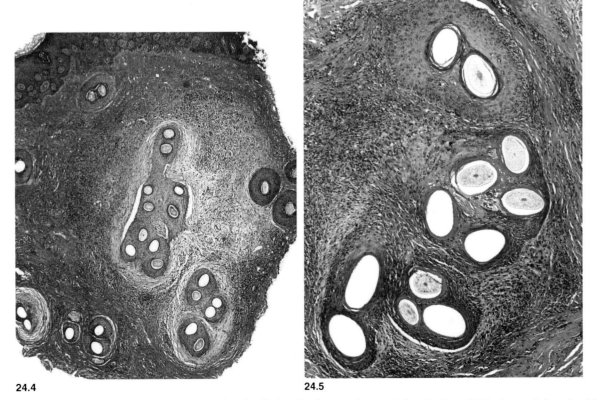

24.4

24.5

Figures 24.4 and 24.5 A scanning and higher power view of polytrichia ("tufting"). Whenever the upper halves of adjacent follicles become inflamed and damaged, a large, common infundibulum may form.

different diseases, so too can the *histological* pattern be found in various conditions. To establish a more precise diagnosis, biopsy specimens must be taken from "early disease" near the peripheral border of the involved scalp, where inflammation and follicular destruction are more subtle. Unfortunately, clinicians often choose to biopsy the more dramatic, tufted zones.

Tufting occurs because the infundibular epithelia of inflamed, damaged follicles often heal with the formation of a large, common infundibulum (Figs. 24.4 and 24.5). Smith (1) correctly attributed the tufts of hair to re-epithelialization of a cluster of damaged follicular infundibula, such that multiple separate shafts became encased in a single, enlarged infundibulum. A zone of fibrosis eventually separates and surrounds these tufts (Fig. 24.6).

Tufted Folliculitis in Summary

Clinical correlation: "Tufted folliculitis" it is not a specific disease, but an end-stage process shared by several different conditions, most commonly CCCA. The occipital region seems especially prone to tufting. Each tuft consists of a tightly clustered group of hairs surrounded by smooth, shiny skin and a variable amount of erythema and scale.

Histological findings:
- ❖ The infundibular epithelia of several adjacent, inflamed, follicles fuse, forming a large, common infundibulum
- ❖ A zone of fibrosis and variably dense acute and/or chronic inflammation surrounds each tuft
- ❖ Individual follicles surrounding the tufts may demonstrate more disease-specific features
- • Peri-infundibular neutrophilic abscesses may be present

Histological differential diagnosis:
- • All forms of highly inflammatory and destructive alopecias can result in the *tufted folliculitis* pattern
- • Folliculitis decalvans and tufted folliculitis are terms that are sometimes used interchangeably because they both represent nonspecific patterns found in highly inflammatory and destructive alopecias

⚠ **Pitfalls**

A biopsy from the clinically tufted area is less likely to provide useful histopathologic information than one from a peripheral area of "early" disease.

REFERENCES

1. Smith NP. Tufted folliculitis of the scalp. J R Soc Med 1978; 71: 606–8.
2. Elston DM. Tufted folliculitis. J Cutan Pathol 2011; 38: 595–6.
3. Baroni A, Ruocco E, Aiello FS, et al. Tinea capitis mimicking tufted hair folliculitis. Clin Exp Dermatol 2009; 34: e699–701.
4. Jappe U, Schroder K, Zillikens D, Petzoldt D. Tufted hair folliculitis associated with pemphigus vulgaris. J Eur Acad Dermatol Venereol 2003; 17: 223–6.
5. Petronic-Rosic V, Krunic A, Mijuskovic M, Vesic S. Tufted hair folliculitis: a pattern of scarring alopecia? J Am Acad Dermatol 1999; 41: 112–4.
6. Saijyo S, Tagami H. Tufted hair folliculitis developing in a recalcitrant lesion of pemphigus vulgaris. J Am Acad Dermatol 1998; 38(5 Pt 2): 857–9.
7. Luz Ramos M, Munoz-Perez MA, Pons A, Ortega M, Camacho F. Acne keloidalis nuchae and tufted hair folliculitis. Dermatology 1997; 194: 71–3.
8. Rosman IS, Anadkat MJ. Tufted hair folliculitis in a woman treated with trastuzumab. Target Oncol 2010; 5: 295–6.
9. Ena P, Fadda GM, Ena L, Farris A, Santeufemia DA. Tufted hair folliculitis in a woman treated with lapatinib for breast cancer. Clin Exp Dermatol 2008; 33: 790–1.
10. Annessi G. Tufted folliculitis of the scalp: a distinctive clinicohistological variant of folliculitis decalvans. Br J Dermatol 1998; 138: 799–805.
11. Powell J, Dawber R, Gatter K. Folliculitis decalvans including tufted folliculitis: clinical, histological and therapeutic findings. Br J Dermatol 1999; 140: 328–33.

25 Lichen planopilaris

The term lichen planopilaris (LPP) was coined by Pringle in 1905 (1) to describe alopecia with follicular spinous papules in patients with typical cutaneous lesions of lichen planus (2). Today, LPP is regarded as a primary inflammatory cicatricial alopecia characterized by a lymphocyte-mediated lichenoid inflammatory reaction targeting the superficial portions of the folliculosebaceous apparatus. This histopathological pattern has appeared in several distinct clinical scenarios, leading some authors to speculate whether LPP is a single entity or a family of divergent clinical disorders characterized by shared and indistinguishable histological features. The North American Hair Research Society working classification of primary cicatricial alopecias of 2003 (3) proposed a system wherein LPP was subdivided into three main clinical types: (*i*) classic LPP, (*ii*) frontal fibrosing alopecia (FFA) (see chap. 26), and (*iii*) Graham–Little Syndrome. Others have proposed adding fibrosing alopecia in a pattern distribution to this list as well (4) (see chap. 27).

LPP prevalence is not high in the general population. Among patients with a complaint of new hair loss presenting to a tertiary level hair clinic, approximately 1–8% will be diagnosed with LPP (5). LPP is common among the inflammatory cicatricial alopecias, representing as many as 40% of cases in some populations (6,7). Because cicatricial alopecias are chronic and relentlessly progressive (1), an accurate histological diagnosis may be able to guide treatment choices and forestall permanent hair loss.

For many years the cause of LPP was completely unknown. Recently some cases of LPP have been triggered by the use of tumor necrosis factor–alpha (TNF-α) inhibitors (8,9), suggesting the balance between TNF-α and interferon-alpha might be playing a role in disease induction (9). A molecular mechanism linking the permanent loss of the hair follicle, sebaceous gland atrophy, and inflammation via the peroxisome proliferator–activated receptor (PPAR)-γ pathway has recently been identified as playing a crucial role in the early events of LPP (10). In experimental studies, targeted deletion of the PPAR-γ gene in the stem cells of the follicular bulge in mice causes cicatricial alopecia that resembles human disease (10). This critical observation led to a case report documenting the use of a specific PPAR-γ agonist in LPP. In this single report, pioglitazone hydrochloride proved effective in arresting LPP and reducing subjectively reported symptoms (11). Further investigation will determine whether PPAR-γ agonists represent a dependable targeted treatment for LPP.

CLINICAL FINDINGS
LPP typically affects the middle aged, with several studies confirming a mean age of onset of approximately 50 years and an age range from 9 to 79 years (2,7,12,13). Females are more commonly affected by LPP (1,2,7,13,14). Most researchers identify no race predilection, although one study suggested a slight Caucasian predilection over those of African heritage (7,13).

In those with LPP, typical lesions of lichen planus (LP) are seen elsewhere on the body in more than 50% of cases, with alopecia preceding the nonscalp lesions most of the time(1,13). Typical LP lesions on other parts of the body strongly support a diagnosis of LPP, but biopsy is necessary to confirm this impression (15,16). Of those with LP, greater than 40% will have findings of LPP (7). This overlap of LP and LPP argues strongly in favor of the two diseases being closely related although some have pointed out discrepancies, including the fact that LP is more common in males than females (1).

Several clinical presentations of alopecia may result in histopathological findings typical of LPP, prompting some to suggest that LPP may be a heterogeneous collection of diseases characterized by a single histopathological pattern (14).

Graham–Little syndrome (also known as Graham–Little–Piccardi–Lassueur syndrome) consists of: (*i*) LPP of the scalp, (*ii*) noncicatricial pubic/axillary hair loss and follicular keratotic papules resembling keratosis pilaris on the limbs, trunk, and retroauricular areas, and (*iii*) typical cutaneous or mucosal lichen planus (Figs. 25.1–25.4) (13,14,16,17). Graham–Little syndrome is overall quite rare. The authors of this text have encountered only one case fulfilling all of the criteria for diagnosis.

FFA (considered further in chap. 26) typically affects postmenopausal Caucasian women. FFA causes progressive hair loss along the anterior hairline, temples, and eyebrows (14,18,19). Complete loss or reduction of the eyebrows is typical. Despite the completely different clinical characteristics of FFA and LPP patients the histopathological findings for FFA are similar or nearly identical to those seen in LPP (20).

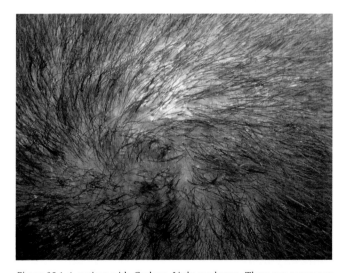

Figure 25.1 A patient with Graham–Little syndrome. There are numerous macules of cicatricial alopecia identified by a loss of follicular ostia. Patchy perifollicular erythema and hyperkeratosis are seen adjacent to emerging hair shafts.

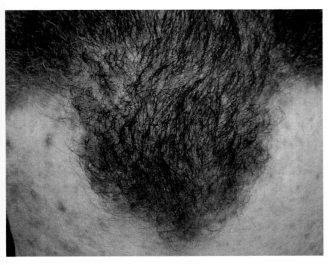

Figure 25.2 A patient with Graham–Little syndrome. Erythema, perifollicular scale, and foci of cicatricial alopecia are present throughout most of the scalp.

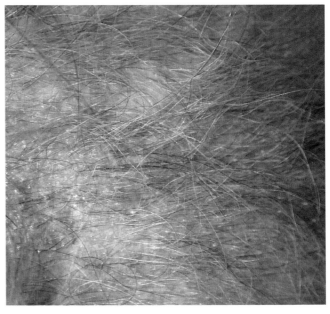

Figure 25.5 Diffusely thinning hair with scalp erythema in a patient with lichen planopilaris.

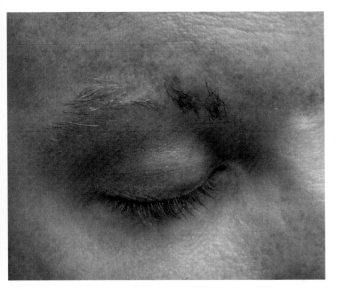

Figure 25.3 This is the same patient pictured in Figs. 25.1 and 25.2. There is irregular loss of eyebrow follicles. Eyelashes are intact.

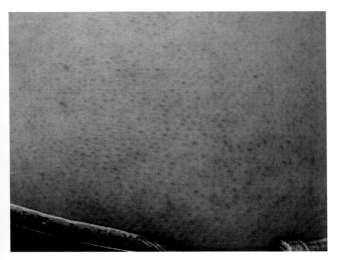

Figure 25.4 This is the same patient pictured in the preceding three images. There are widespread follicular keratotic papules resembling keratosis pilaris over much of the trunk.

Fibrosing alopecia in a patterned distribution (FAPD) (considered further in chap. 27) is another clinically definable pattern with histopathological features sometimes indistinguishable from LPP (4). FAPD has a gradual clinical onset with features typical of androgenetic alopecia, followed by an accelerated inflammatory cicatricial alopecia limited to areas involved by androgenetic alopecia. Histopathologically there are features of typical LPP as well as androgenetic alopecia.

The most common pattern is so-called classic LPP. LPP typically involves the vertex and parietal areas (4,13,14), and least commonly the frontal (12) and occipital (13) areas of the scalp, but can be highly variable. Single, or more commonly, multifocal, patchy areas of alopecia may coalesce to involve nearly the entire scalp (12,14,21). Other commonly involved body sites include the face/beard (sometimes in a linear pattern) (4,22,23), eyebrows, legs (13), arms (13), axillary, and pubic/genital region (24).

Involved areas show irregular white or partially pigmented patches (Figs. 25.5–25.8) of cicatricial alopecia (12). Early changes include violaceous papules and erythema (7). Perifollicular erythema and follicular keratotic spines (Fig. 25.9) are the most common clinical findings (1,2,12–14). These may be most pronounced at the expanding (active) edge of the alopecic patch where a pull test will often extract anagen hairs surrounded by keratin (4,7,21). Perifollicular scale may be pronounced (7,21). In time there will be loss of follicular ostia (21).

The clinical course may be insidious or fulminant. In all cases the course is unpredictable (4). Patients with indolent scalp disease may be asymptomatic. More than half of patients describe pruritus (7,13) and/or pain (13). Patients who also have lesions of LP on the skin or mucosa may have symptoms related to these lesions. Laboratory evaluation is usually unhelpful. Antinuclear antibody testing is negative (7).

By dermoscopy, LPP displays perifollicular scales, diminished follicular ostia, and white dots. Occasionally blue-grey (Fig. 25.10) dots resembling targets are present around the follicles (25).

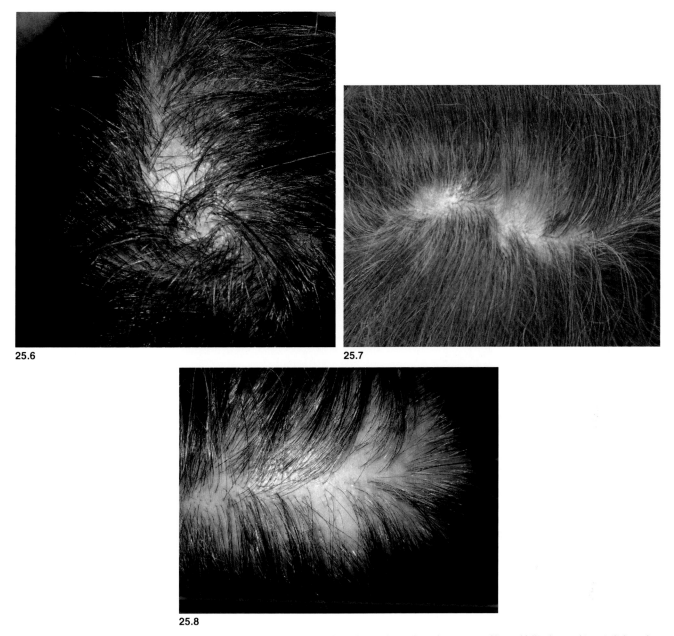

25.6

25.7

25.8

Figures 25.6,25.7,25.8 Irregularly shaped patches of hair loss with variable perifollicular erythema, hyperkeratosis, and loss of follicular markings in lichen planopilaris.

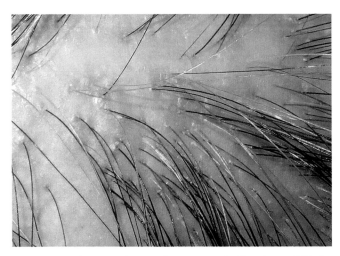

Figure 25.9 Higher magnification of Figure 25.8 detailing the perifollicular hyperkeratosis, subtle perifollicular erythema, and loss of follicular markings.

The clinical differential diagnosis includes alopecia areata, which differs from LPP by having preserved follicular ostia, exclamation point hairs, white hairs, and yellow dots on dermoscopy (4). More challenging is differentiating LPP from chronic cutaneous lupus erythematosus (CCLE), which has inflammation that is less often restricted to perifollicular areas, and frequently causes dyspigmentation, telangiectasia, and scale (4). By dermoscopy, CCLE displays branching capillaries, white patches, and follicular keratin plugs (25). Speckling with blue-grey dots may also be seen (25). A pattern of hair loss suggestive of central, centrifugal cicatricial alopecia (CCCA) can occur. In its final stage (as an end-stage burnt out porcelain scar) LPP can also fall into the catchall group of Brocq's alopecia (see chap. 31). As in all cases of inflammatory cicatricial alopecia, LPP can heal with the formation of polytrichia (tufting). LPP therefore represents one of several causes of so-called tufted folliculitis (see chap. 24).

The treatment of LPP can be challenging and at times will not change the ultimate outcome (16). An in-depth discussion is beyond the scope of this chapter but most experts advocate a tiered approach to therapy based on severity and treatment response. Mid- to high-potency topical corticosteroids are generally considered first-line treatment for LPP, usually in conjunction with intralesional corticosteroids (4,7,16,26). For severe, rapidly progressive disease, initial treatment might consist of oral corticosteroid therapy tapered over at least three months; however, rebound disease and adverse side effects can limit the utility of this therapy alone (16,26). Second-line treatments could include tetracyclines (such as doxycycline) or hydroxychloroquine (26). These should be used in combination with topical corticosteroids. Treatments targeting different pathways may be layered. Others have advocated cyclosporine and the use of mycophenolate mofetil, in particular, is gaining traction (4,7,16,26). A number of additional agents have been used with reported success, including thalidomide and oral retinoids (26). As mentioned in the introduction, there is experimental evidence to advocate on behalf of PPAR-γ agonists, such as pioglitazone hydrochloride, in the treatment of LPP (11).

Meaningful, objective end points are needed to confidently determine the efficacy and safety of current and future treatments. Most LPP studies focus on subjective features, such as symptoms, signs of activity, and progression of hair loss. To address this shortcoming, Price et al. have introduced the LPPAI (lichen planopilaris activity index), a scoring system that endeavors to quantify and objectify disease activity within and across patients (27). This scoring system is a step in the right direction and will hopefully lead to more meaningful comparisons of therapeutic interventions in the future.

HISTOLOGICAL FINDINGS

The typical findings of LPP may be noted in only a few follicles within a single biopsy specimen (1,6). Because of this, vertical sectioning may not capture diagnostic follicles in early/sparse disease (Figs. 25.11–25.12). The inflammatory infiltrate is characterized by a patchy to band-like vacuolar interface dermatitis that specifically affects the infundibulum and isthmus of the follicular epithelium (1,7,12,15,16), sparing the deepest third of the follicle (Figs. 25.13–25.16) (7,14,21). Civatte (cytoid) bodies are sometimes seen (Fig. 25.17) (15,16). There may be an irregular contour or blurring of the basement membrane, but no thickening of it (Fig. 25.18) (6,21,28). Interfollicular epidermal involvement is seen in less than one quarter of cases (1,2,15) and may be associated with prominent pigment incontinence (1). When involved, the epidermis shows either flattening or a saw-tooth configuration of the rete ridges (Figs. 25.19 & 25.20) (7).

A perivascular lymphocytic infiltrate has been described in the reticular dermis in as many as 81% of cases (Fig. 25.21) (16). Perieccrine inflammation, as is commonly encountered in CCLE, does not occur in LPP (Fig. 25.22). Similarly, deep dermal interfollicular mucin is not observed (16) although perifollicular mucinous fibroplasia has been described (16). The infiltrate of LPP is mediated by CD3+ T-lymphocytes with a CD4: CD8 ratio of 1:1–2 (6). A markedly reduced number of CD1a+ Langerhans cells has been described in affected follicles relative to unaffected ones (6).

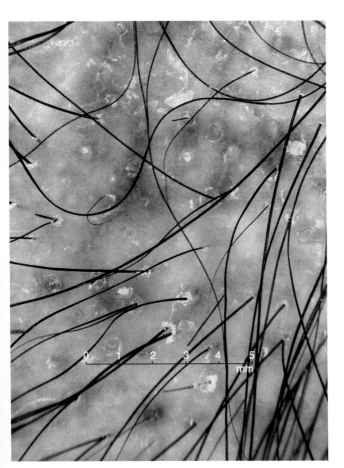

Figure 25.10 Dermoscopic image of lichen planopilaris showing diminished follicular ostia, perifollicular scale, and blue-grey dots that sometimes resemble targets. *Source*: Image courtesy of Antonella Tosti, M.D.

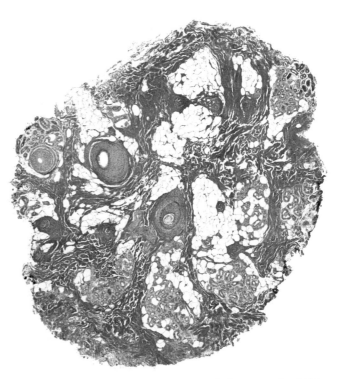

Figure 25.11 This low magnification image reveals three remaining follicles. The one on the left is unaffected by lichen planopilaris.

As in typical lichen planus, the affected follicular epithelium of LPP becomes acanthotic, hypergranulotic, and hyperkeratotic (Figs. 25.23 & 25.24) (7,12,15). In time, follicular ostia become plugged with keratinous debris (1,15). Concentric perifollicular fibrosis ensues (Figs. 25.17,25.25,25.26) (16,21), and with this, the encircling lymphocytic infiltrate

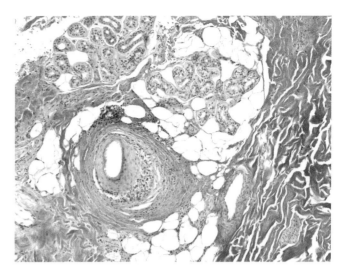

Figure 25.14 Similarly inflamed follicle with changes extending to the deeper isthmus, adjacent to the eccrine glands. In this example, eccentric epithelial thinning is noted. In the inflamed area, concentric perifollicular fibrosis is evident. Lastly, the inner root sheath has desquamated.

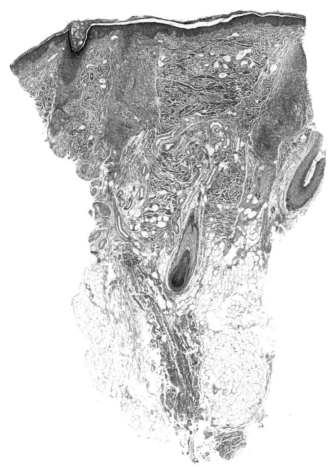

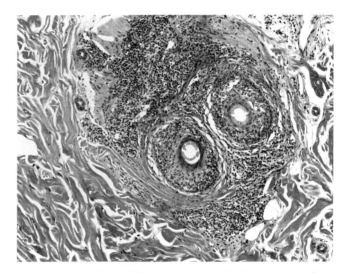

Figure 25.15 Two adjacent follicles demonstrating brisk lymphocytic inflammation in the vicinity of the insertion point of the arrector pili muscle. Inner root sheaths are intact.

Figure 25.12 Because of the patchy nature of the process (revealed in the preceding image) vertical sections may miss affected follicles. In this image, portions of two follicles are uninvolved, whereas two superficially evident follicles are clearly inflamed.

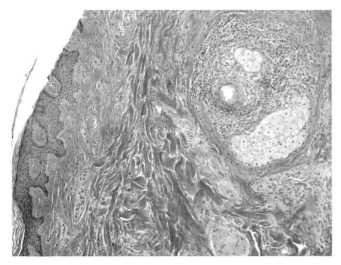

Figure 25.13 The isthmus of a follicle and its sebaceous gland are involved by a brisk infiltrate of small lymphocytes.

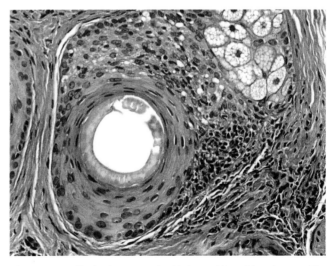

Figure 25.16 Folliculosebaceous unit with intraepidermal lymphocytes. The inner root sheath is intact.

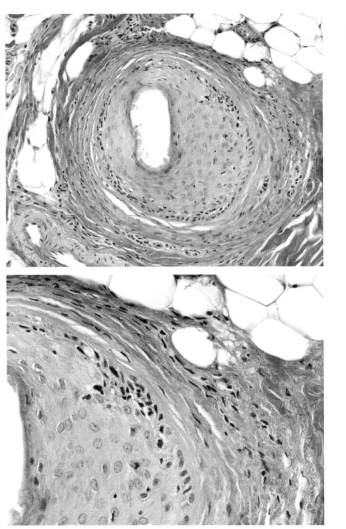

Figure 25.17 Two images demonstrating the deepest extent of involvement of a single follicle. While the inflammatory infiltrate is very mild at this level, involvement is evident by numerous apoptotic (hypereosinophilic) keratinocytes (cytoid bodies) and slight vacuolization of the basalar layer.

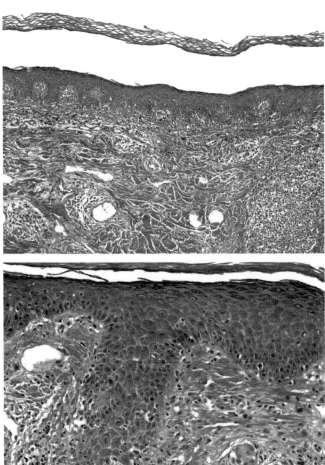

Figure 25.19 Medium-power magnification of a case of lichen planopilaris with interfollicular involvement. There is lymphocyte-mediated necrosis of junctional keratinocytes and pigment incontinence (*top*). On occasion, multinucleated giant cells may develop secondary to follicular destruction and spillage of follicular contents into the dermis (*bottom*).

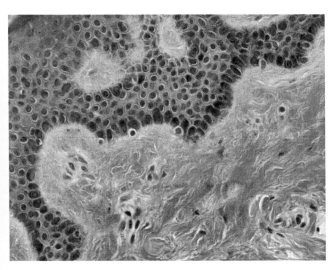

Figure 25.18 The dermal–epidermal junction is not involved between the follicles of this specimen. There is no smudging or thickening of the junction, and no inflammation. Interfollicular epidermal involvement is seen in less than one quarter of lichen planopilaris cases.

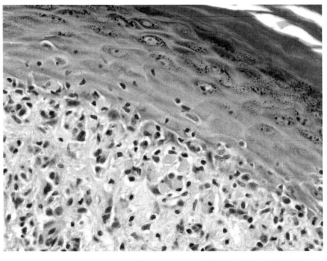

Figure 25.20 Classic high magnification image of lichen planus-like changes (found in this interfollicular zone of lichen planopilaris). There is acanthosis, hyperkeratosis, wedge-shaped hypergranulosis, flattening of the rete ridges, and a band-like lymphocytic infiltrate obscuring the dermal–epidermal junction. Note the numerous dissociated cytoid bodies.

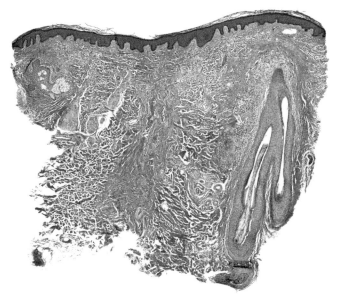

Figure 25.21 Deep inflammation may be seen (*center, base*). This inflammation is in the midst of a scarred follicular tract. Perieccrine lymphocytic inflammation is not a feature of lichen planopilaris.

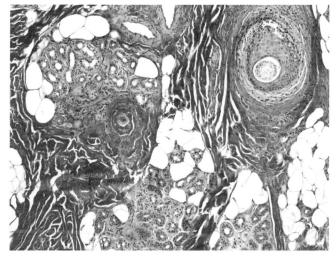

Figure 25.22 The inflammatory infiltrate may extend down the isthmus to the level of the eccrine lobules. Perieccrine lymphocytic inflammation is not a feature of lichen planopilaris.

will appear to "back away" from the follicular epithelium (Figs. 25.27 and 25.28) (15). As with lichen planus, an artifactual cleft (Max–Joseph space (29)) between epithelium and stroma is often found (Fig. 25.29). In horizontally sectioned biopsies the epithelium may seem to "float" within the space formed by this cleft (Fig. 25.30) (15). In perpendicular sections, epithelial atrophy and concentric fibrosis may give rise to an "hourglass" configuration to the follicles (Fig. 25.31) (6,28). The bulge area near the attachment of the arrector pili muscles diminishes, taking with it stem cells necessary for the maintenance of the folliculosebaceous unit (Fig. 25.32). Ki-67+ proliferating bulge cells diminish and may disappear entirely (6). Arrector pili muscles also diminish (16).

Within the isthmus, premature desquamation of the inner root sheath (IRS) may occur, particularly in badly inflamed follicles; this is a feature that may be observed in other cicatricial alopecias, such as CCCA (21). However, clearly inflamed follicles affected by LPP may also have normal desquamation of the IRS, a finding that excludes CCCA from the histological differential diagnosis (Figs. 25.33 & 25.34). Asymmetrical atrophy of the follicular epithelium as viewed in horizontal sections may show eccentricity of the hair shaft placement within the follicle (Figs. 25.35 and 25.36) (21). Residual damaged infundibula may fuse to create compound ostia with polytrichia (tufting) (Figs. 25.37–25.41) (21).

Sebaceous lobules also diminish and disappear (Figs. 25.42–25.44) (6,12,16,21,28,30). In time, the entire folliculosebaceous epithelium vanishes (Fig. 25.45). This sometimes leaves "naked" hair shafts within the dermis (Fig. 25.46), where they can trigger the formation of vertically oriented granulomas (21). Stranded, uninflamed "naked" hair shafts may also be seen. In time, all that remains of the follicle is a tract of connective tissue (28,30). Vellus follicles also disappear (16). Loss of follicles results in a moderate to marked reduction in terminal hair density (16), and in the latest stages will be indistinguishable from the "burnt out" pattern common to most late-stage cicatricial alopecias (see chap. 31).

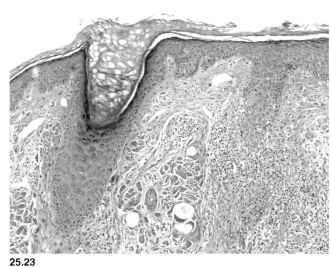

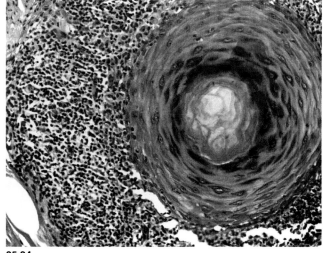

25.23   25.24

Figures 25.23 and 25.24 As in lichen planus, acanthosis, hyperkeratosis, and wedge-shaped hypergranulosis may be seen in the follicular isthmus.

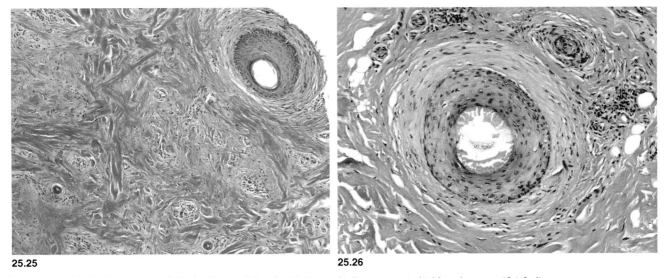

25.25   **25.26**

Figures 25.25 and 25.26 Concentric perifollicular fibrosis of the infundibulum and isthmus are typical (although nonspecific) findings.

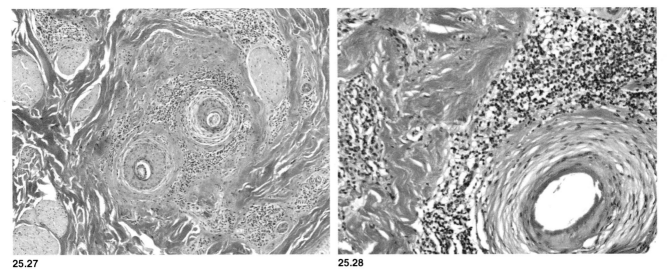

25.27   **25.28**

Figures 25.27 and 25.28 As concentric fibrosis develops in an actively inflamed follicle, the lymphocytic infiltrate will seem to "back away" from the fibrosis.

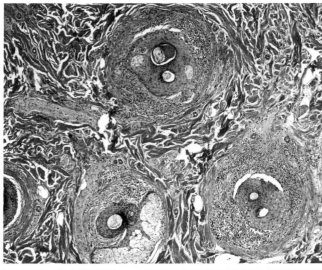

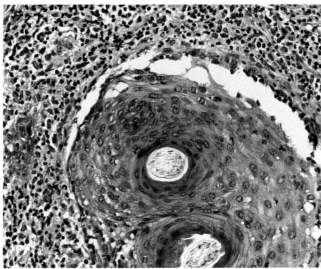

Figures 25.29 As seen at the dermal–epidermal junction in some cases of lichen planus, an artifactual cleft may develop between the follicular epithelium and perifollicular dermis. This cleft is analogous to a so-called Max–Joseph space.

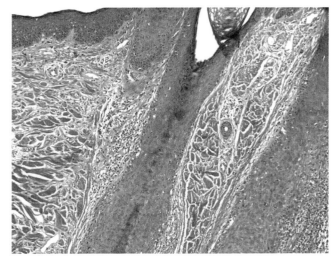

Figure 25.31 Because of fibrosis and loss of follicular volume there may be narrowing of the follicular epithelium resembling an "hourglass."

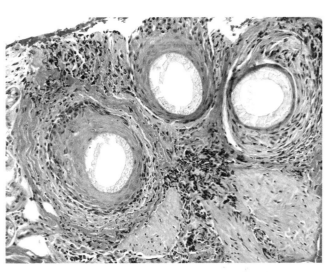

Figure 25.32 The "bulge" area located adjacent to the insertion of the arrector pili muscles is inflamed and eventually destroyed in lichen planopilaris. The loss of this zone results in the loss of follicular stem cells necessary to maintain the folliculosebaceous units. Ultimately this results in the demise of the follicle.

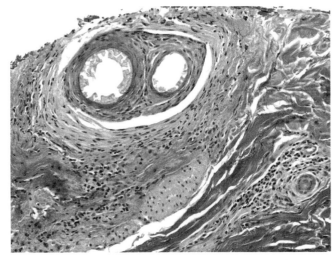

Figure 25.30 Because of the clefting noted in the preceding images, follicles sectioned horizontally may seem to float untethered in the space delineated by fibrosis.

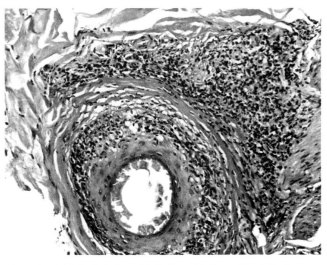

Figures 25.33 Markedly inflamed follicular epithelium with minimal premature desquamation of the inner root sheath.

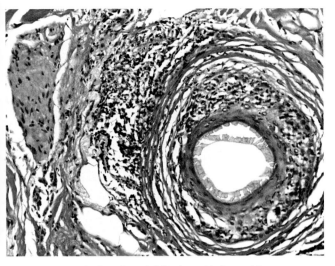

Figures 25.34 Markedly inflamed follicular epithelium without premature desquamation of the inner root sheath. This pattern excludes central, centrifugal cicatricial alopecia as a diagnostic possibility.

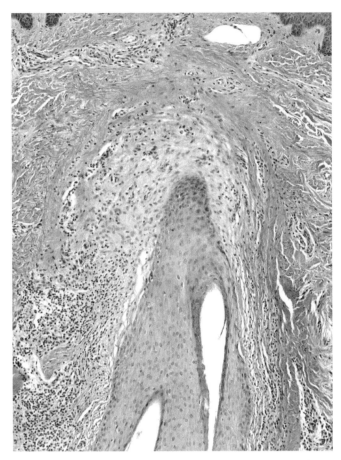

Figure 25.36 Vertical section showing eccentric epithelial atrophy and fusion of adjacent follicular infundibula.

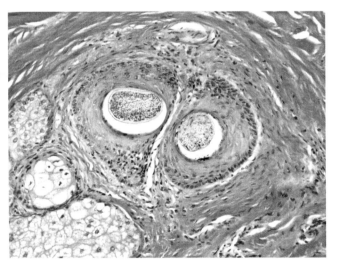

Figure 25.35 Eccentric epithelial atrophy is a feature seen in lichen planopilaris. This may be a precursor to eventual extrusion of the hair shaft or fusion of adjacent follicular infundibula.

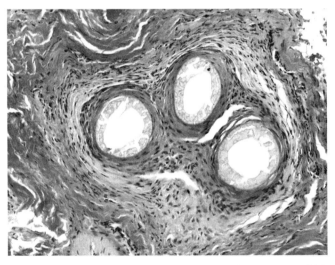

Figure 25.37 Three adjacent involved follicles fusing to form a compound follicle (polytrichia).

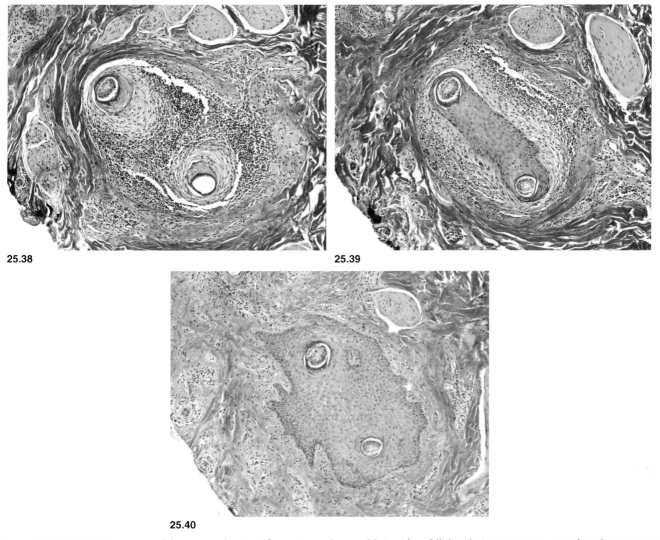

25.38

25.39

25.40

Figures 25.38, 25.39, 25.40 A sequence of three images showing inflammation and eventual fusion of two follicles. The image sequence moves from deeper to more superficial sections.

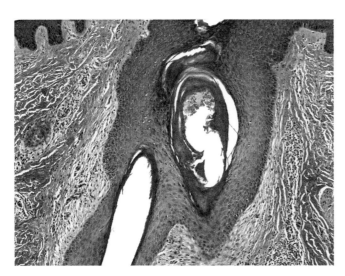

Figure 25.41 Adjacent follicles have fused at the level of the infundibulum.

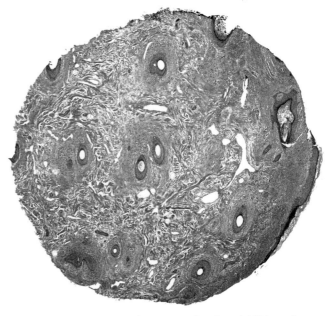

Figure 25.42 Scanning image showing actively inflamed follicles with complete absence of sebaceous lobules.

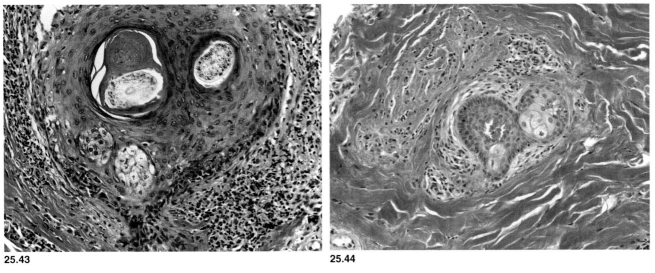

25.43　　　　　　　　　　　　　　**25.44**

Figures 25.43 and 25.44 Two foci of active lichen planopilaris demonstrating nearly involuted sebaceous lobules.

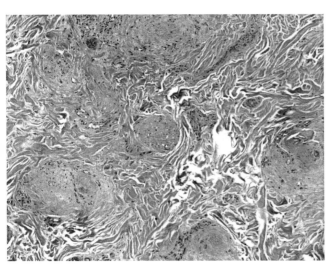

Figures 25.45 An example of end-stage lichen planopilaris showing complete involution of folliculosebaceous structures. Arrector pili muscles are still visible.

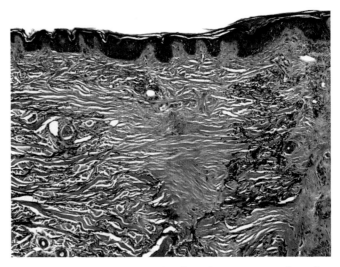

Figure 25.47 Vertical section stained with an elastic stain. Note the wedge-shaped loss of elastic fibers. This is allegedly a pattern specific to lichen planopilaris.

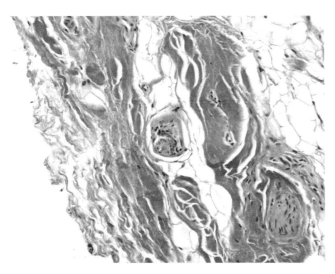

Figure 25.46 After destruction of follicular epithelia, naked hair shafts may become stranded in the dermis. These may or may not induce an inflammatory response.

In the latest stages, cicatricial alopecias are difficult to specifically characterize, although some authors have advocated the use of elastic-Van Gieson (EVG) staining in conjunction with vertically oriented punch biopsy specimens (Fig. 25.47). The perifollicular elastic sheath is destroyed in LPP (6,28) with a marked loss of elastic fibers, (1). These authors contend that the wedge-shaped pattern of superficial perivascular elastic fiber loss (16,31) can be easily and reliably differentiated from elastic loss patterns in other late-stage cicatricial alopecias.

Other authors have advocated the use of direct immunofluorescent microscopy in the evaluation of cicatricial alopecia. Although there is some disagreement in the published studies (32), many authors have found that LPP is associated with globular staining of IgM within junctional and/or follicular Civatte bodies (1,7,15,16,21,33). Linear deposits of immunoreactants (IgG, IgM, and C3) are typical of lupus erythematosus (4).

Lichen Planopilaris in Summary

Clinical correlation: various patterns are seen but most commonly there are scattered foci of partial hair loss. Perifollicular erythema and scaling are common to all cases. Lichen planus lesions elsewhere on the body support the diagnosis of LPP on the scalp.

Histological findings:
❖ Lichenoid interface dermatitis affecting the infundibulum and isthmus
❖ Diminished to absent sebaceous lobules of affected follicles
• Premature desquamation of the inner root sheath in inflamed follicles
• Concentric, lamellar perifollicular fibroplasia with artifactual clefting between the follicular epithelium and the stroma when viewed horizontally, and an hourglass-shaped follicular epithelium when viewed vertically

Histological differential diagnosis:
• **Frontal fibrosing alopecia**: inflammation is often less dense and apoptotic cells more numerous than in LPP. Interfollicular epidermal changes may be present in LPP but are absent in FFA. Vellus hairs are less likely to be affected in LPP
• **Fibrosing alopecia in a pattern distribution**: shows increased vellus:terminal hair ratio, a feature not typical of the involved areas of LPP
• **Chronic cutaneous lupus erythematosus**: differentiating features include perieccrine inflammation, interfollicular dermal mucin deposition, and interfollicular epidermal changes (including follicular plugging and vacuolar alteration with epidermal atrophy). None of these features are seen in LPP. LPP shows globular IgM in Civatte bodies by DIF, whereas CCLE shows linear deposition of IgG, IgM, and C3 at the junction

⚠ **Pitfalls**

Clinical correlation is required to suggest a diagnosis of FFA or fibrosing alopecia in a pattern distribution *versus* LPP as the histological findings of all three entities are too similar to be reliably separated. Unless actively inflamed areas are sampled, histological changes may only show an end-stage cicatricial alopecia.

Abbreviations: LPP, lichen planopilaris; CCLE, chronic cutaneous lupus erythematosus; FFA, frontal fibrosing alopecia.

REFERENCES

1. Mehregan DA, Van Hale HM, Muller SA. Lichen planopilaris: clinical and pathologic study of forty-five patients. J Am Acad Dermatol 1992; 27(6 Pt 1): 935–42.
2. Matta M, Kibbi AG, Khattar J, Salman SM, Zaynoun ST. Lichen planopilaris: a clinicopathologic study. J Am Acad Dermatol 1990; 22: 594–8.
3. Olsen EA, Bergfeld WF, Cotsarelis G, et al. Summary of North American Hair Research Society (NAHRS)-sponsored Workshop on Cicatricial Alopecia, Duke University Medical Center, 2001. J Am Acad Dermatol 2003; 48: 103–10.
4. Assouly P, Reygagne P. Lichen planopilaris: update on diagnosis and treatment. Semin Cutan Med Surg 2009; 28: 3–10.
5. Ochoa BE, King LE Jr, Price VH. Lichen planopilaris: Annual incidence in four hair referral centers in the United States. J Am Acad Dermatol 2008; 58: 352–3.
6. Mobini N, Tam S, Kamino H. Possible role of the bulge region in the pathogenesis of inflammatory scarring alopecia: lichen planopilaris as the prototype. J Cutan Pathol 2005; 32: 675–9.
7. Chieregato C, Zini A, Barba A, Magnanini M, Rosina P. Lichen planopilaris: report of 30 cases and review of the literature. Int J Dermatol 2003; 42: 342–5.
8. Garcovich S, Manco S, Zampetti A, Amerio P, Garcovich A. Onset of lichen planopilaris during treatment with etanercept. Br J Dermatol 2008; 158: 1161–3.
9. Fernandez-Torres R, Paradela S, Valbuena L, Fonseca E. Infliximab-induced lichen planopilaris. Ann Pharmacother 2010; 44: 1501–3.
10. Karnik P, Tekeste Z, McCormick TS, et al. Hair follicle stem cell-specific PPARgamma deletion causes scarring alopecia. J Invest Dermatol 2009; 129: 1243–57.
11. Mirmirani P, Karnik P. Lichen planopilaris treated with a peroxisome proliferator-activated receptor gamma agonist. Arch Dermatol 2009; 145: 1363–6.
12. Annessi G, Lombardo G, Gobello T, Puddu P. A clinicopathologic study of scarring alopecia due to lichen planus: comparison with scarring alopecia in discoid lupus erythematosus and pseudopelade. Am J Dermatopathol 1999; 21: 324–31.
13. Cevasco NC, Bergfeld WF, Remzi BK, de Knott HR. A case-series of 29 patients with lichen planopilaris: the Cleveland Clinic Foundation experience on evaluation, diagnosis, and treatment. J Am Acad Dermatol 2007; 57: 47–53.
14. Sullivan JR, Kossard S. Acquired scalp alopecia. Part I: A review. Australas J Dermatol 1998; 39: 207–19; quiz 220–201.
15. Sperling LC, Cowper SE. The histopathology of primary cicatricial alopecia. Semin Cutan Med Surg 2006; 25: 41–50.
16. Tandon YK, Somani N, Cevasco NC, Bergfeld WF. A histologic review of 27 patients with lichen planopilaris. J Am Acad Dermatol 2008; 59: 91–8.
17. Somani N, Bergfeld WF. Cicatricial alopecia: classification and histopathology. Dermatol Ther 2008; 21: 221–37.
18. Kossard S, Lee MS, Wilkinson B. Postmenopausal frontal fibrosing alopecia: a frontal variant of lichen planopilaris. J Am Acad Dermatol 1997; 36: 59–66.
19. Samrao A, Chew AL, Price V. Frontal fibrosing alopecia: a clinical review of 36 patients. Br J Dermatol 2010; 163: 1296–300.
20. Poblet E, Jimenez F, Pascual A, Pique E. Frontal fibrosing alopecia versus lichen planopilaris: a clinicopathological study. Int J Dermatol 2006; 45: 375–80.
21. Headington JT. Cicatricial alopecia. Dermatol Clin 1996; 14: 773–82.
22. Gerritsen MJ, de Jong EM, van de Kerkhof PC. Linear lichen planopilaris of the face. J Am Acad Dermatol 1998; 38: 633–5.
23. Kuster W, Kind P, Holzle E, Plewig G. Linear lichen planopilaris of the face. J Am Acad Dermatol 1989; 21: 131–2.
24. Grunwald MH, Zvulunov A, Halevy S. Lichen planopilaris of the vulva. Br J Dermatol 1997; 136: 477–8.
25. Duque-Estrada B, Tamler C, Sodre CT, Barcaui CB, Pereira FB. Dermoscopy patterns of cicatricial alopecia resulting from discoid lupus erythematosus and lichen planopilaris. An Bras Dermatol 2010; 85: 179–83.
26. Sperling LC, Nguyen JV. Commentary: treatment of lichen planopilaris: some progress, but a long way to go. J Am Acad Dermatol 2010; 62: 398–401.
27. Chiang C, Sah D, Cho BK, Ochoa BE, Price VH. Hydroxychloroquine and lichen planopilaris: efficacy and introduction of Lichen Planopilaris Activity Index scoring system. J Am Acad Dermatol 2010; 62: 387–92.
28. Moure ER, Romiti R, Machado MC, Valente NY. Primary cicatricial alopecias: a review of histopathologic findings in 38 patients from a clinical university hospital in Sao Paulo, Brazil. Clinics (Sao Paulo) 2008; 63: 747–52.
29. Sperling LC. Scarring alopecia and the dermatopathologist. J Cutan Pathol 2001; 28: 333–42.
30. Nayar M, Schomberg K, Dawber RP, Millard PR. A clinicopathological study of scarring alopecia. Br J Dermatol 1993; 128: 533–6.
31. Elston DM, McCollough ML, Warschaw KE, Bergfeld WF. Elastic tissue in scars and alopecia. J Cutan Pathol 2000; 27: 147–52.
32. Ioannides D, Bystryn JC. Immunofluorescence abnormalities in lichen planopilaris. Arch Dermatol 1992; 128: 214–6.
33. Abell E. Immunofluorescent staining techniques in the diagnosis of alopecia. South Med J 1977; 70: 1407–10.

26 Frontal fibrosing alopecia

Frontal fibrosing alopecia (FFA) was originally described in several Australian, postmenopausal, Caucasian women (1). The disease has since been reported in several countries, including the United States. Although Caucasian women comprise most of the patients, we have seen typical FFA affect African-American women as well.

CLINICAL FINDINGS

Patients are generally postmenopausal women (mean age about 60 years (2)) with pruritus and progressive hair loss along the anterior hairline, temples, and eyebrows (3,4) (Figs. 26.1 and 26.2). There is frequently an atrophic appearance to the alopecic scalp skin left behind the advancing border of the inflammation. Several series of patients have reported premenopausal women (5) and patients with body hair loss (2,6) as well as scalp alopecia. We have also seen several premenopausal women with the condition, and FFA is not uncommon in the African-American population. While the majority of patients do not have lichen planus, (3) a few have been noted to have mucosal lichen planus and even cutaneous lichen planus (5), providing clinical support for the notion that FFA is a variant of lichen planopilaris (LPP) (3,7).

In our experience, treatment is challenging and its efficacy difficult to assess. Some authors have concluded that there is no evidence that the progression of active disease can be halted or slowed by treatment. Others feel that progression of the condition stops in most patients after a variable period on treatment, and resumes upon discontinuation of treatment. This may ultimately lead to a "clown alopecia" appearance (9). Those experienced in treating large numbers of LPP patients generally use hydroxychloroquine as a steroid sparing agent for FFA, finding that the maximal benefits of this drug are evident within the first 6 months of use (4). Mycophenolate mofetil, which can be efficacious in the classic presentation of LPP, may prove to be of use in FFA as well, but adequate studies have not yet been published (10). Oral corticosteroids may be effective to initially "cool-off" rapidly progressing FFA, but long-term therapy with this class of drugs is risky. Topical corticosteroids, intralesional triamcinolone acetonide, oral doxycycline, and 0.1% tacrolimus ointment (5) are relatively safe medications, but their efficacy in FFA has not been critically studied. Finasteride was helpful in limiting disease progression in some patients (11). Topical agents can be combined with systemic agents to maximize the potential for response. Regardless of therapeutic modality, recession of the hair line may progress over many years, and the disease may eventually stabilize in many patients with or without continuing treatment (5).

HISTOLOGICAL FINDINGS

In spite of the completely different clinical characteristics of FFA and LPP patients, the histopathological findings for FFA are similar or nearly identical to those seen in LPP (12). In addition, immunophenotyping fails to reveal any significant differences between the frontal fibrosing and multifocal variants of LPP (3). Common microscopic findings for both FFA and LPP include (12): an inflammatory lymphocytic infiltrate involving the isthmus and infundibulum of the hair follicles (Fig. 26.3); damage to or destruction of the basalar and epibasalar follicular epithelium, with blurring of the epithelial/stromal junction (Fig. 26.4); migration of lymphocytes into the basalar and epibasalar epithelium (Fig. 26.5); apoptotic and/or dyskeratotic cells in the outer root sheath (Fig. 26.6); concentric fibroplasia surrounding the inflamed hair follicles (Fig. 26.7); and subsequent destruction of some follicles (Fig. 26.8). Some authors have found that FFA specimens show less follicular inflammation and contain more apoptotic cells than those from LPP patients (12). In addition, while some cases of LPP show an inflammatory infiltrate involving the interfollicular epidermis, this finding is never present in FFA (12). Direct immunofluorescence was negative

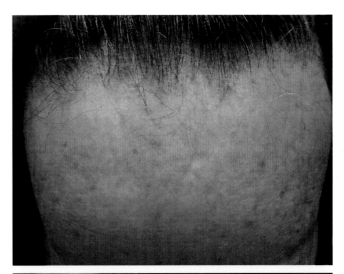

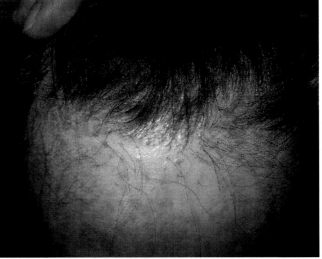

Figure 26.1 Two women with frontal fibrosing alopecia.

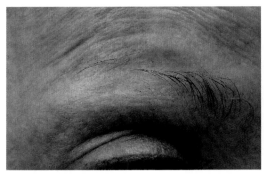 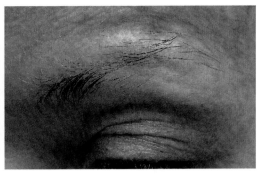

Figure 26.2 Eyebrow loss is commonly found in frontal fibrosing alopecia. As in this case, there is often little visible evidence of inflammation.

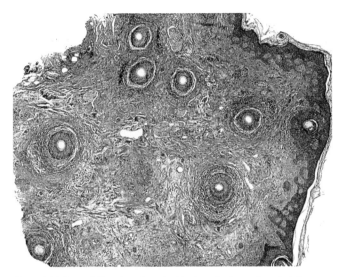

Figure 26.3 Frontal fibrosing alopecia. Moderately dense chronic inflammation surrounds the infundibula of several follicles.

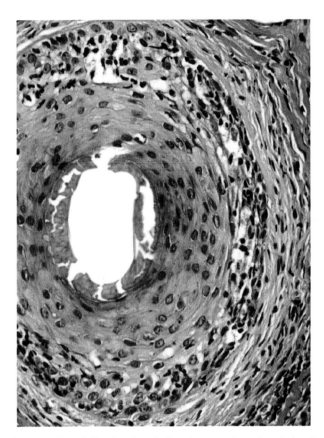

Figure 26.5 Frontal fibrosing alopecia. Lymphocytes migrate into the basalar as well as epibasalar layers.

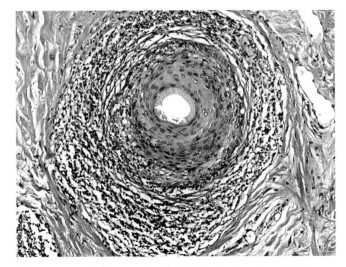

Figure 26.4 Frontal fibrosing alopecia. Moderately dense chronic inflammation surrounds the infundibulum of this follicle, with blurring of the epithelial/stromal junction.

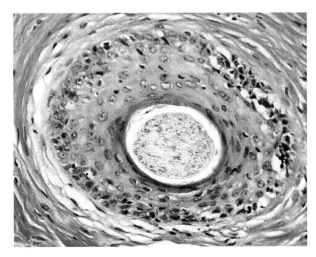

Figure 26.6 Frontal fibrosing alopecia. Dyskeratotic and apoptotic cells are commonly found in the outer root sheaths of affected follicles.

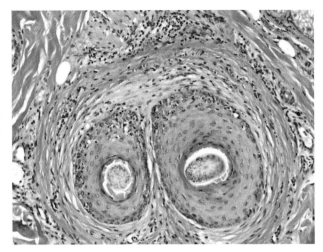

Figure 26.7 Frontal fibrosing alopecia. Concentric, lamellar fibroplasia surrounds two affected follicles, both of which show focal interface alteration and migration of lymphocytes into the outer root sheath.

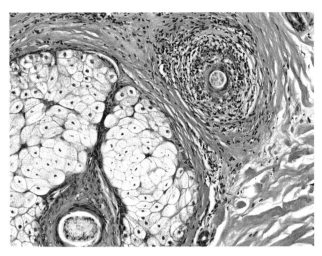

Figure 26.9 In this example of FFA, a small follicle (0.04 mm in diameter) shows prominent inflammatory involvement, while an adjacent terminal follicle is unaffected.

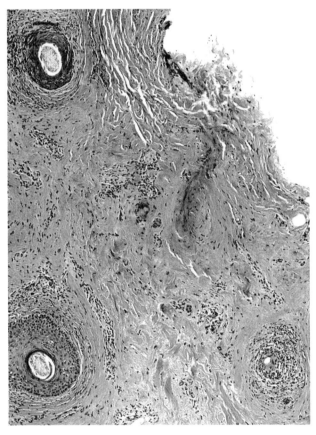

Figure 26.8 Frontal fibrosing alopecia. The follicle on the upper left shows advanced changes with destruction of the basal layer and "squamatization" of the outer root sheath. The follicle on the lower right shows total epithelial destruction with residual chronic and granulomatous inflammation. Between the two is an "empty" zone, the location of follicles long since destroyed.

in two FFA cases studied, but showed deposits of immunoglobulins and/or complement in two of four LPP cases (12).

Most authors, including the authors of this text, stress the similarities between FFA and LPP. However, one group identified a major difference with possible etiologic significance (11). They found that unlike LPP, in FFA the lymphocytic infiltrate and fibrosis selectively affect the indeterminate

(medium-sized) and vellus follicles of the frontal margin and eyebrows (11). They speculated that FFA may represent a variant of LPP with selective involvement of certain androgen-dependent areas (11). Furthermore, they noted that some of the patients treated with finasteride (2.5 mg/day) showed an arrest in the disease progression, indicating that androgens might be involved in disease pathogenesis (11). This also suggests a relationship to "fibrosing alopecia in a pattern distribution," the subject of chapter 27. We have also observed that smaller hairs may be involved in FFA (Fig. 26.9), although in our experience, terminal hairs are frequently involved and ultimately lost as well.

Frontal Fibrosing Alopecia in Summary

Clinical correlation: most often a postmenopausal woman with pruritus and progressive hair loss along the anterior hairline, temples, and eyebrows.

Histological findings:
- ❖ Lichenoid interface dermatitis affecting the infundibulum and isthmus
- ❖ Apoptotic keratinocytes scattered throughout the affected (infundibular and isthmic) follicular epithelium
- Blurring of the epithelial–stromal junction
- Squamatization of the outer root sheath
- Concentric, lamellar perifollicular fibroplasia with artifactual clefting between the follicular epithelium and the stroma

Histological differential diagnosis:
- LPP: the inflammation is often more dense and apoptotic cells less numerous than in FAA. Interfollicular epidermal changes (occasionally seen in LPP) are absent in FFA, and vellus hairs are less likely to be affected in LPP.
- **Fibrosing alopecia in a pattern distribution**: shows increased vellus:terminal hair ratio, a feature not typical of the involved areas of FFA.

- **Discoid lupus erythematosus:** differentiating features include deep perivascular/periadnexal inflammation, mucin deposition, and interfollicular epidermal changes including follicular plugging and vacuolar alteration with epidermal atrophy. None of these features are seen in FAA.

⚠ Pitfalls

Clinical correlation is required to suggest a diagnosis of FFA or fibrosing alopecia in a pattern distribution *vs* LPP, as the histological findings of all three entities are too similar to be reliably separated. Unless actively inflamed areas are sampled, histological changes may only show an end-stage, cicatricial alopecia.

Abbreviations: LPP, lichen planopilaris; FFA, frontal fibrosing alopecia.

REFERENCES

1. Kossard S. Postmenopausal frontal fibrosing alopecia. Scarring alopecia in a pattern distribution. Arch Dermatol 1994; 130: 770–4.
2. Chew AL, Bashir SJ, Wain EM, Fenton DA, Stefanato CM. Expanding the spectrum of frontal fibrosing alopecia: a unifying concept. J Am Acad Dermatol 2010; 63: 653–60.
3. Kossard S, Lee MS, Wilkinson B. Postmenopausal frontal fibrosing alopecia: a frontal variant of lichen planopilaris. J Am Acad Dermatol 1997; 36: 59–66.
4. Samrao A, Chew AL, Price V. Frontal fibrosing alopecia: a clinical review of 36 patients. Br J Dermatol 2010; 163: 1296–300.
5. Tan KT, Messenger AG. Frontal fibrosing alopecia: clinical presentations and prognosis. Br J Dermatol 2009; 160: 75–9.
6. Armenores P, Shirato K, Reid C, Sidhu S. Frontal fibrosing alopecia associated with generalized hair loss. Australas J Dermatol 2010; 51: 183–5.
7. Faulkner CF, Wilson NJ, Jones SK. Frontal fibrosing alopecia associated with cutaneous lichen planus in a premenopausal woman. Australas J Dermatol 2002; 43: 65–7.
8. Rallis E, Gregoriou S, Christofidou E, Rigopoulos D. Frontal fibrosing alopecia: to treat or not to treat? J Cutan Med Surg 2010; 14: 161–6.
9. Moreno-Ramirez D, Camacho Martinez F. Frontal fibrosing alopecia: a survey in 16 patients. J Eur Acad Dermatol Venereol 2005; 19: 700–5.
10. Cho BK, Sah D, Chwalek J, et al. Efficacy and safety of mycophenolate mofetil for lichen planopilaris. J Am Acad Dermatol 2010; 62: 393–7.
11. Tosti A, Piraccini BM, Iorizzo M, Misciali C. Frontal fibrosing alopecia in postmenopausal women. J Am Acad Dermatol 2005; 52: 55–60.
12. Poblet E, Jimenez F, Pascual A, Pique E. Frontal fibrosing alopecia versus lichen planopilaris: a clinicopathological study. Int J Dermatol 2006; 45: 375–80.

27 Fibrosing alopecia in a pattern distribution

Fibrosing alopecia in a pattern distribution (FAPD) was not included in the first edition of this book because it was unclear whether FAPD was a valid entity, distinguishable from other forms of alopecia (1). Since its original description in 2000 (2), only a few journal articles have addressed the condition,(3,4) which seems to have faded into obscurity. We have now seen several alopecia cases that defy easy classification but seem to fit the original description of FAPD. Like frontal fibrosing alopecia (FFA), FAPD may represent a variant of lichen planopilaris (LPP) with distinctive clinical features. Until the condition is better understood, we describe FAPD in a separate chapter to facilitate its recognition.

CLINICAL FINDINGS

FAPD was first described by Zinkernagel and Trüeb (2). They studied 19 patients (15 women and 4 men) who had clinical or histological features supporting a diagnosis of androgenetic alopecia (female pattern or male pattern common balding). Most patients had a biphasic course to their disease, with very gradual thinning over several years followed by an accelerated period of hair loss and scalp inflammation. This accelerated phase had features of an inflammatory, cicatricial alopecia confined to the zone involved by their balding. Perifollicular erythema, loss of follicular ostia, and follicular keratosis, features commonly seen in inflammatory cicatricial alopecia, were present in the majority of patients.

Our own experience has involved male and female patients with erythema, perifollicular scaling and progressive hair loss involving the zone of common balding. The pattern of hair loss in FAPD (Fig. 27.1) closely resembles the symmetrical, centrally accentuated thinning seen in androgenetic alopecia. The clinical impression offered to the pathologist is almost always "androgenetic alopecia *versus* cicatricial alopecia" because features of both seem to be present simultaneously. This provides one clue to the diagnosis. However, this clinical pattern is not unique to FAPD, and histopathological confirmation is required.

HISTOLOGICAL FINDINGS

In their original article on FAPD, Zinkernagel and Trüeb found histological evidence of androgenetic alopecia (increased numbers of miniaturized hairs with underlying fibrous streamers) in 10 of 19 patients. Chronic inflammation was found around the upper portion of some hair follicles in all patients, with a

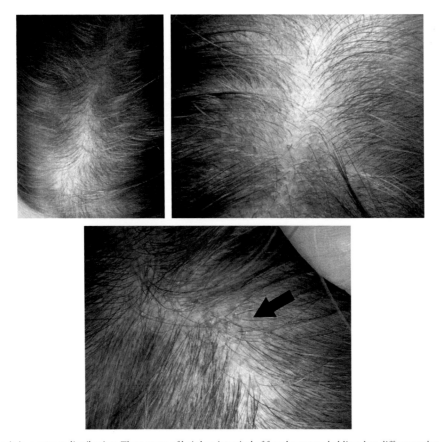

Figure 27.1 Fibrosing alopecia in a pattern distribution. The pattern of hair loss is typical of female pattern balding, but diffuse erythema and perifollicular scaling (arrow) are present.

vacuolar interface dermatitis pattern in about half the cases. Both terminal and vellus hairs could be affected. A combination of focal liquefaction degeneration of the follicular basal layer in concert with prominent apoptosis of follicular keratinocytes was seen in about 30% of cases. Concentric perifollicular lamellar fibrosis was seen in over 90% of cases. The authors concluded that follicular interface dermatitis targeting the upper follicle represented early disease, and the perifollicular lamellar fibroplasia indicated late lesions.

Our histological diagnoses of FAPD were based on the features described by Zinkernagel and Trüeb. There is clear-cut evidence of cicatricial alopecia in all specimens (Fig. 27.2). The number of vellus hairs is disproportionately large, and hair shaft size variability is marked, as would be expected in common balding (Fig. 27.3).

Inflammation is restricted to the upper half of affected follicles. It may vary in intensity between specimens and often within the same specimen. There is vacuolar interface alteration of the follicular epithelium, with some spongiosis and exocytosis of lymphocytes (Fig. 27.4). Civatte bodies (colloid bodies) are occasionally seen, but are not a prominent feature.

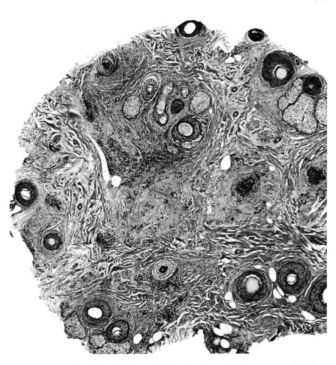

Figure 27.3 Hair miniaturization in fibrosing alopecia in a pattern distribution. In this field, 10 of 18 follicles are miniaturized/vellus hairs; additional vellus hairs are found in more superficial levels. There is also a column of connective tissue scar centrally within the specimen.

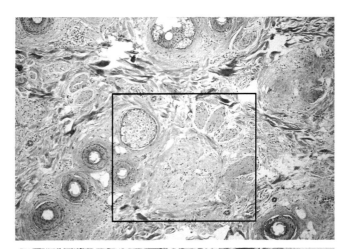

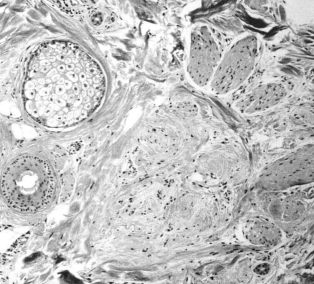

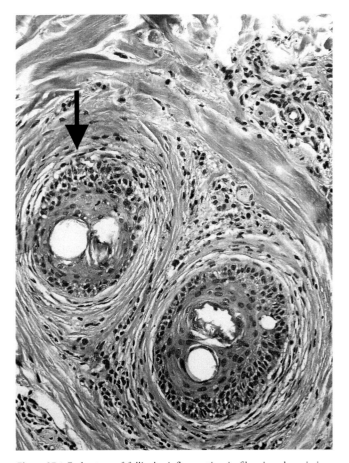

Figure 27.2 Fibrosing alopecia in a pattern distribution. The upper panel shows a reduction in the number of follicles. The boxed area surrounds a follicular unit (magnified in the lower panel) in which all follicles have been destroyed and replaced by connective tissue (true follicular scars).

Figure 27.4 Early stage of follicular inflammation in fibrosing alopecia in a pattern distribution. The arrow indicates vacuolar interface alteration of the follicular epithelium.

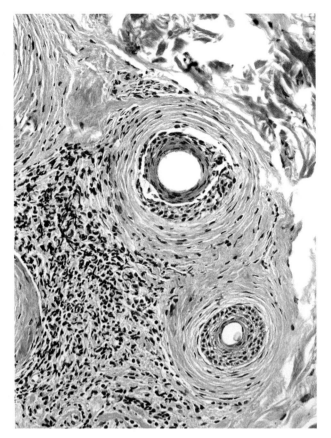

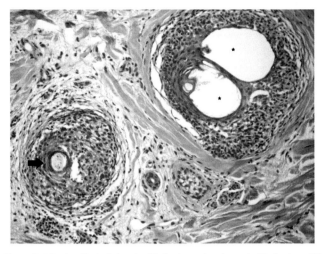

Figure 27.7 Both vellus/miniaturized hairs (*arrow*) and terminal hairs (*asterisk*) are involved in the inflammatory process of fibrosing alopecia in a pattern distribution.

Figure 27.5 Damage to the follicular basal layer in fibrosing alopecia in a pattern distribution sometimes results in an artifactual cleft between the epithelium and stroma.

As in LPP, artifactual clefting between the epithelium and stroma may be seen (Fig. 27.5). There is a variably dense accumulation of lymphocytes surrounding affected follicles; often a perifollicular zone of fibrosis separates the lymphocytes from the epithelium (Fig. 27.6). Both terminal hairs and vellus hairs are affected (Fig. 27.7). This differs from the typical case of LPP, in which terminal hairs are the usual target of inflammation and destruction. The validity of this observation has never been critically studied.

Without a good clinical history, the histological findings of FAPD are indistinguishable from LPP. Common balding is so prevalent in the population that it would not be surprising for an otherwise typical LPP patient to have manifestations of both diseases in a single biopsy specimen. This would be especially true if the sample were taken from the crown/vertex region. We suspect that FAPD represents a variant of LPP, analogous to the situation with FFA. Clear-cut cases of LPP can sometimes affect the crown of the scalp in a symmetrical, "patterned" fashion. While FAPD patients lack cutaneous lesions of lichen planus or interfollicular epidermal inflammation, this does not necessarily exclude a diagnosis of LPP. The absence of these findings is more the rule than the exception in many cases of LPP. The question remains whether androgenetic alopecia and the lichenoid inflammation of FAPD are pathogenically related. In other words, does the cicatricial process specifically target hairs that are undergoing or will undergo miniaturization during the course of androgenetic alopecia?

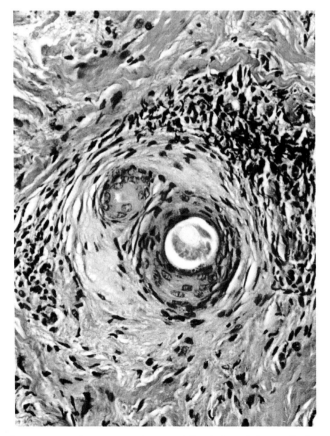

Figure 27.6 Lymphocytes around a zone of fibroplasia encircling a vellus hair. This more intense inflammation likely represents a later stage of fibrosing alopecia in a pattern distribution than the changes seen in Figure 27.4.

Fibrosing Alopecia in a Pattern Distribution in Summary

Clinical correlation: the pattern of hair loss is typical of common balding, but diffuse erythema and perifollicular scaling are present in the zone of thinning.

Histological findings:

❖ Increased percentage of vellus hairs (evidence of miniaturization)

❖ Vacuolar interface alteration of the upper portion of the follicular epithelium
❖ Variably dense, perifollicular, lymphocytic inflammation
• Both vellus and terminal hairs may be inflamed or destroyed
• A zone of fibroplasia may separate the follicular epithelium and the inflammatory infiltrate
• Interfollicular epidermis is spared

Histological differential diagnosis:
• **Lichen planopilaris:** few vellus hairs are affected, but otherwise the follicular changes are indistinguishable from FAPD
• **Chronic cutaneous lupus erythematosus:** increased deep dermal mucin, dense foci of deep inflammation, eccrine and arrector pili inflammation, and increased plasma cells may be seen
• **Androgenetic alopecia:** does not show interface dermatitis, lichenoid inflammation, significant superficial perifollicular fibrosis, or true follicular scars. Mild spongiosis can occasionally be seen superficially, especially if there is concurrent seborrheic dermatitis

⚠ **Pitfalls**
When both vellus and terminal hairs have been destroyed in large numbers, it will be impossible to reliably document the presence of hair miniaturization.

Abbreviation: FAPD, fibrosing alopecia in a pattern distribution

REFERENCES

1. Sperling LC, Solomon AR, Whiting DA. A new look at scarring alopecia. Arch Dermatol 2000; 136: 235–42.
2. Zinkernagel MS, Trueb RM. Fibrosing alopecia in a pattern distribution: patterned lichen planopilaris or androgenetic alopecia with a lichenoid tissue reaction pattern? Arch Dermatol 2000; 136: 205–11.
3. Amato L, Chiarini C, Berti S, Bruscino P, Fabbri P. Case study: fibrosing alopecia in a pattern distribution localized on alopecia androgenetica areas and unaffected scalp. Skinmed 2004; 3: 353–5.
4. Chiu HY, Lin SJ. Fibrosing alopecia in a pattern distribution. J Eur Acad Dermatol Venereol 2010; 24: 1113–4.

28 Chronic cutaneous lupus erythematosus

Chronic cutaneous lupus erythematosus (CCLE) is the preferred term for a variety of chronic cutaneous expressions of lupus erythematosus, including tumid lupus, discoid lupus erythematosus (DLE), and lupus panniculitis. DLE, the dominant subtype of CCLE (1,2), enjoys such common usage that the two terms are often used interchangeably. DLE is classically localized to the head and neck, but may occur on other parts of the body; scalp involvement occurs in 60% of patients with discoid lesions, and is the sole area of involvement in 10% (3). Overall, the discoid lesions of CCLE are a common cause of primary cicatricial alopecia (3,4). The average age of onset is 41.6 years, with fewer than 2% of cases reported in children (5,6). Women are 2–3 times more likely than men to develop the discoid lesions of CCLE (5,7). Fewer than 5–10% of patients with CCLE ultimately progress to systemic lupus erythematosus (SLE) (3,8). Although the precise cause is not known, the fundamental pathology leading to cicatricial alopecia is the likely destruction of follicular stem cells located in the bulge region of the hair follicle (9,10).

CLINICAL FINDINGS

Patients with CCLE may be asymptomatic or may describe burning, pruritus, or tenderness in involved areas (11). Discoid lesions begin as scaly, indurated papules (1) that gradually expand to form ill-defined, irregular, or round plaques (Figs. 28.1 and 28.2) with variable atrophy, follicular plugging, telangiectasia, and depigmentation (Figs. 28.3–28.5) (8,11). The

plaques commonly exhibit central erythema (Fig. 28.6) (12). An uncommon but distinctive pattern of alopecia is the solitary, elongated patch of hair loss in the crown, aligned along the longitudinal (mid-sagittal) plane (Figs. 28.5 and 28.7). In dark-skinned individuals, central hypopigmentation and peripheral hyperpigmentation are characteristic. In well-established lesions there is frequently adherent scale, which upon retraction may have keratotic spikes on its underside, the so-called "carpet-tack" sign (13). Although follicular ostia may be present in early disease, they gradually disappear as hair follicles are irreversibly destroyed (14). In late lesions, a depressed, smooth, depigmented hairless area will remain (12,13). Dermoscopy will reveal the above-described findings as well as the loss of acrosyringia (15), the presence of arborizing vessels, and a "follicular red dot" pattern thought to be due to dilated infundibula surrounded by ectatic vessels with red blood cell extravasation (16). A history of Raynaud's phenomenon may be elicited in up to 15% of patients (17). In general, abnormal laboratory findings are uncommon in CCLE, although some researchers have reported positive antinuclear antibody (ANA) tests in up to 53% of those with CCLE (2,5). One study associated the presence of antiribosomal protein P with alopecia (18).

The clinical differential of CCLE in its inflammatory stage may include alopecia areata and bacterial and/or fungal infection (6). In some cases discoid plaques of CCLE may merge to form large, irregularly shaped zones of cicatricial alopecia. If centered on the crown or vertex this pattern may resemble

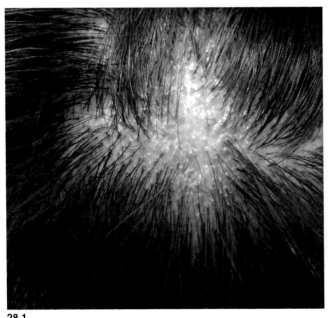
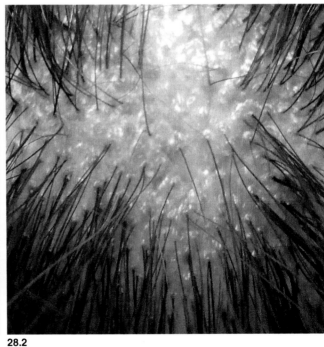

28.1   **28.2**

Figures 28.1 and 28.2 Two different magnifications showing slightly scaly confluent erythematous papules forming an irregular zone of alopecia in a patient with chronic cutaneous lupus erythematosus.

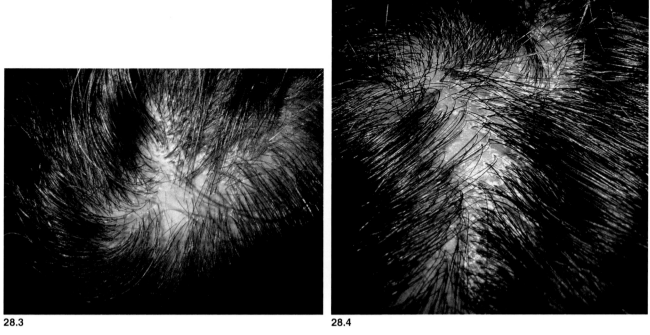

28.3   **28.4**

Figures 28.3 and 28.4 Two patients with chronic cutaneous lupus erythematosus manifesting erythematous papules, scaling, and focal loss of follicular markings.

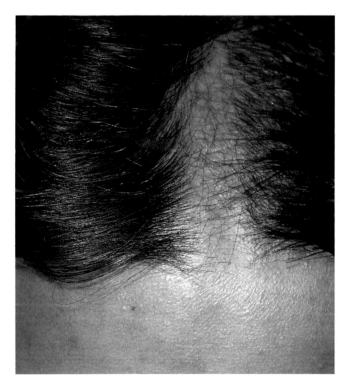

Figure 28.5 A patient with chronic cutaneous lupus erythematosus demonstrating an atrophic linear focus of alopecia with loss of follicular markings. The pattern can resemble linear morphea (*en coup de sabre*) clinically.

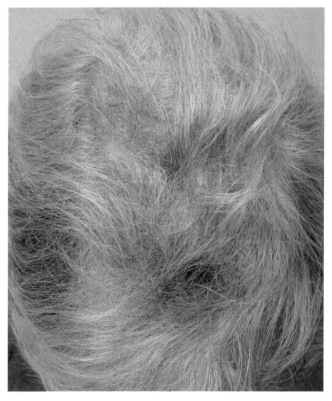

Figure 28.6 A patient with chronic cutaneous lupus erythematosus with erythema, scaling, and irregular borders.

central, centrifugal cicatricial alopecia (CCCA). Late stages of CCLE become clinically indistinguishable from other primary cicatricial alopecias, including lichen planopilaris, CCCA, and Brocq's alopecia (pseudopelade). Because CCLE of the scalp can have many clinical patterns, the diagnosis cannot be based on clinical findings alone, and therefore a biopsy is indicated.

Those at risk for CCLE are encouraged to photoprotect, as ultraviolet light is a known trigger for CCLE (6). Patients in the early inflammatory stages of CCLE are treated with a variety of agents, including hydroxychloroquine, and topical, intralesional, and sometimes systemic corticosteroids. Common second-line agents include oral retinoids, methotrexate, thalidomide, and immunomodulatory drugs, such as cyclosporine (4).

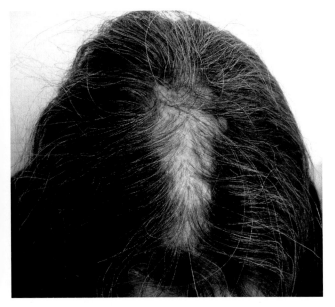

Figure 28.7 A patient with chronic cutaneous lupus erythematosus with an elongated patch of hair loss on the crown oriented in the mid-sagittal plane. *Source*: Image courtesy of Dr. Brett Krasner.

HISTOLOGICAL FINDINGS

The quality of histopathological findings depends on biopsy site selection. A symptomatic site with residual follicles is ideal. Active disease can be identified by anagen hairs that are easily extractable by a hair pull test (10,19). The most characteristic finding in CCLE, seen in 74% of cases in one large study (20), is vacuolar interface change with apoptotic keratinocytes along the hair follicular basal layer and frequently at the dermal–epidermal junction between follicles (Figs. 28.8–28.11) (3,6,8,21,22). Typically, the infiltrate is lymphoplasmacytic, and characteristically involves the superficial and deep dermis along blood vessels, eccrine ducts, and eccrine glands (Figs. 28.12–28.20) (6,8,22). The density of the infiltrate and the degree of keratinocyte apoptosis are highly variable. On occasion the infiltrate extends into the fat with the formation of lymphoid follicles (19). The infiltrate may involve the length of the entire follicle. Some authors have noted an accentuation of the infiltrate in the bulge region of the follicle (23). Sebaceous lobules within the affected follicular units are frequently reduced in

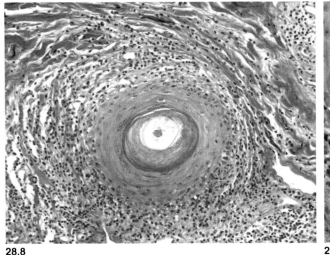

28.8

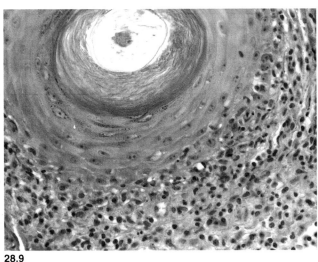

28.9

Figures 28.8 and 28.9 Two magnifications of an involved follicle with a dense surrounding vacuolar interface dermatitis mediated by lymphocytes. There is evidence of dermal pigment incontinence in the interfollicular zone.

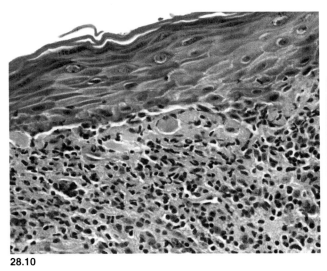

28.10

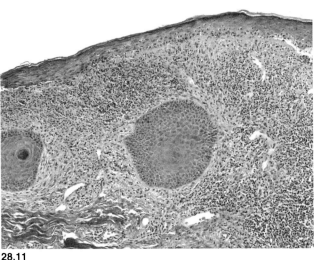

28.11

Figures 28.10 and 28.11 High and low magnification showing interfollicular involvement of the dermal–epidermal junction by a dense infiltrate of lymphocytes. The hypergranulosis typical of lichen planopilaris is not seen. Necrotic keratinocytes are evident as dull pink globules, deep to which is a lymphoplasmacytic infiltrate.

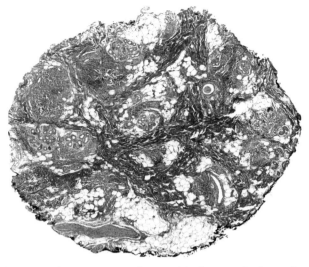

Figure 28.12 This scanning magnification of the deep reticular dermis identifies no viable follicles. There is a dense inflammatory infiltrate that involves the perivascular and perieccrine areas.

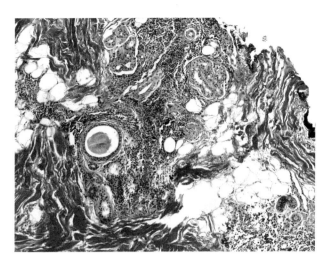

Figure 28.15 Perieccrine inflammation with dilation of an eccrine duct.

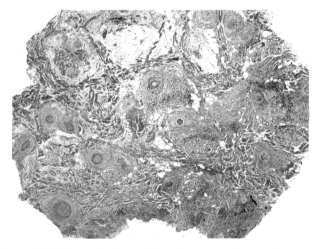

Figure 28.13 This scanning image of chronic cutaneous lupus erythematosus sectioned in the deep dermis demonstrates active vacuolar inflammation of the deep follicles, with additional periadnexal and perivascular inflammation. A marked shift to catagen:telogen is noted among most of the follicular epithelia. This shift, along with deep inflammation, can sometimes create the impression of alopecia areata.

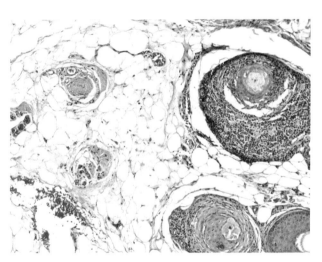

Figure 28.16 Markedly inflamed follicles seated in the fat, with adjacent stele. Complete inflammatory destruction of the follicle may strand the hair shaft in the dermis.

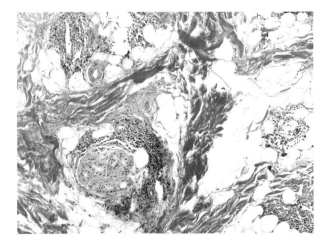

Figure 28.14 Loss of follicular epithelia with deep perivascular and perieccrine inflammation is a clue to CCLE. Deep mucin is not seen in this image, and is not always present in CCLE. *Abbreviation*: CCLE, chronic cutaneous lupus erythematosus.

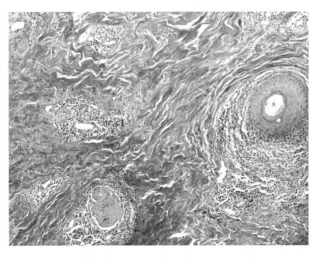

Figure 28.17 Deep follicular, perivascular, and perieccrine inflammation in a patient with chronic cutaneous lupus erythematosus.

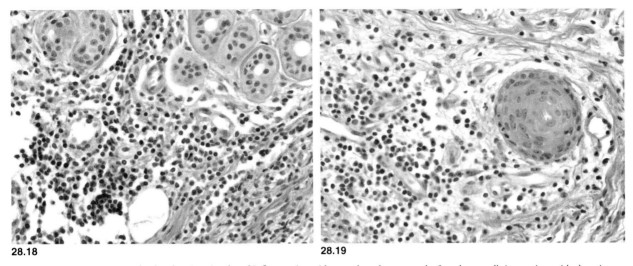

28.18   **28.19**

Figures 28.18 and 28.19 Perieccrine gland and perieccrine ductal inflammation with many lymphocytes and a few plasma cells in a patient with chronic cutaneous lupus erythematosus.

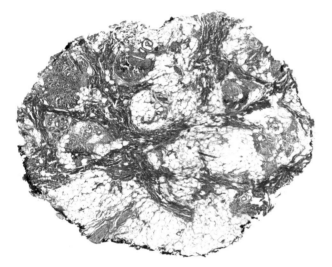

Figure 28.20 Scanning magnification of a nearly end-stage case of CCLE. There are no preserved follicles at this level, although scarred tracts can be seen. A perieccrine and perivascular infiltrate, along with aggregates of lymphocytes at the dermal–subcutaneous junction, favor CCLE as the cause. *Abbreviation*: CCLE, chronic cutaneous lupus erythematosus

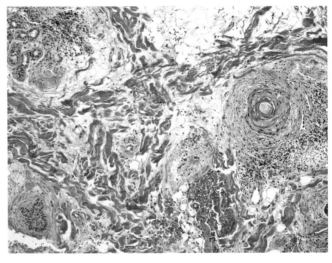

Figure 28.22 Deep follicular vacuolar inflammation with perieccrine and perivascular lymphocytes and dermal mucin deposits identify this as a case of chronic cutaneous lupus erythematosus sectioned in the deep dermis.

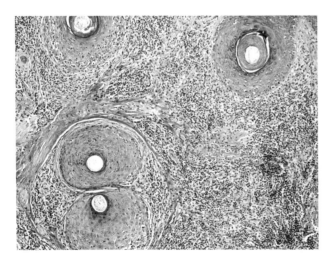

Figure 28.21 CCLE. There is dense, active, predominantly lymphocytic inflammation in the peri-infundibular area. Sebaceous lobules are absent. The perifollicular fibrosis typical of lichen planopilaris is not developed in this case of CCLE. There is incipient fusion of the two follicular epithelia in the bottom left corner. *Abbreviation*: CCLE, chronic cutaneous lupus erythematosus.

number early in the disease process, and eventually are lost entirely (Fig. 28.21) (19,24). Follicular hyperkeratosis with ostial plugging is seen in 91% of the cases (6,20).

Apoptotic loss of keratinocytes (Fig. 28.22) eventually results in epidermal and follicular atrophy (88%) with thickening of the basement membrane (Fig. 28.23) (77%) (20). A periodic acid–Schiff stain may be useful in highlighting the latter finding (8). Dermal edema and pigment incontinence (8) (Fig. 28.24) may be noted early, followed sometimes by dermal sclerosis and vascular ectasia (21). Deep dermal mucin deposition is a common finding in CCLE (Figs. 28.25 and 28.26). This can be highlighted with an Alcian blue or colloidal iron stain for acid mucopolysaccharides (Fig. 28.27) (6,8,22). Widespread alteration and loss of elastic fibers identified by Verhoeff–van Gieson staining may be noted in the perifollicular and interfollicular dermis (8,25). Destruction of anagen follicular epithelium may result in the formation of granulomas surrounding residual hair shaft fragments (Figs. 28.28 and 28.29) (10,13).

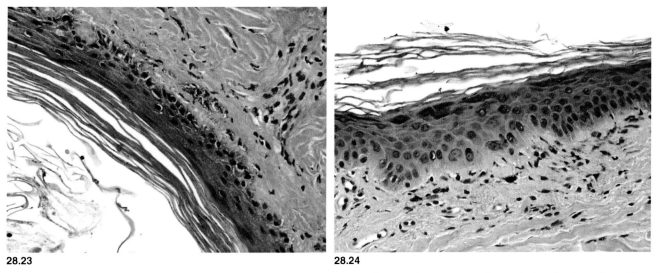

28.23 **28.24**

Figures 28.23 and 28.24 The dermal–epidermal junction in this case of chronic cutaneous lupus erythematosus reveals vacuolar interface dermatitis, epidermal atrophy, thickening of the basement membrane and underlying pigment incontinence.

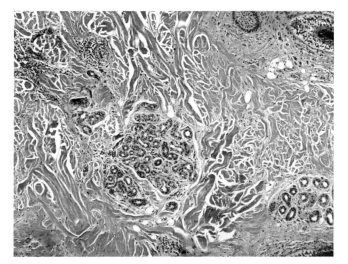

Figure 28.25 Deep dermal mucin is identified as hematoxyphilic web-like strands between collagen bundles. This mucin can be highlighted with special stains, such as Alcian blue and colloidal iron stains, although it is quite evident in this H&E-stained section.

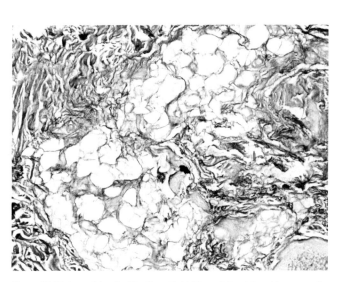

Figure 28.27 A special stain, like the colloidal iron stain pictured here, may be useful to highlight mucin.

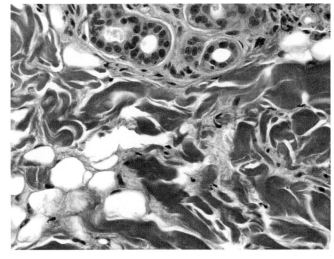

Figure 28.26 Higher magnification showing increased deep dermal mucin.

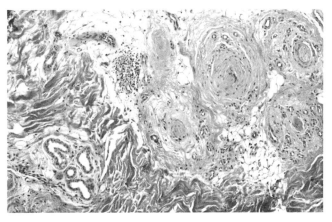

Figure 28.28 Complete destruction of follicles in CCLE may result in stranded "naked" hair shafts, as seen in the top right corner of this image.

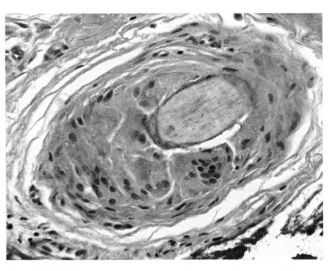

Figure 28.29 High magnification of a stranded hair shaft surrounded by multinucleated giant cells forming a hair "granuloma."

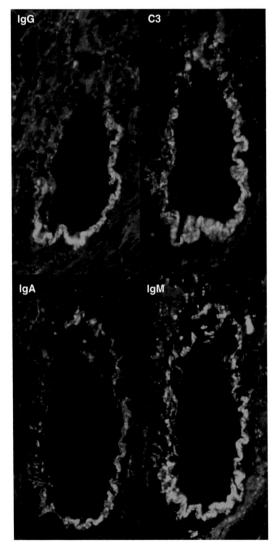

Figure 28.30 A composite direct immunofluorescence image of a patient with chronic cutaneous lupus erythematosus demonstrating a bright band of immunoreactant deposition along the basement membrane of a follicular epithelium.

Direct immunofluorescence (DIF) studies may be useful in certain cases. One study suggests that 31.5% of CCLE cases were *only* diagnosable when DIF techniques were used (20). The best DIF results are obtained by sampling a lesion that is 2–3 months old and has not been treated for 3 weeks (19). A site with active disease should be chosen, as the center of scarred plaques may not yield characteristic findings (26). A positive DIF is seen in 70–95% of cases of CCLE and is characterized by dense linear granular deposition of IgG and C3 along the dermal–epidermal and follicular basement membrane (Fig. 28.30) (6,8,12,27). IgM and IgA staining may also be seen (3,6,27). In CCLE, only lesional skin will reveal DIF findings, whereas in SLE even normal skin may show the pattern outlined above (26).

The final common pathway for all types of primary cicatricial alopecia is hair follicular stem cell failure leading to loss of the folliculosebaceous apparatus (10). Consequently, the appearance of end-stage cicatricial alopecias of many types may be histopathologically identical. In such cases, there may be no other diagnosis to offer than "end-stage cicatricial alopecia," although the presence of small amounts of residual inflammation, dermal mucin, elastic changes, and DIF findings may enable the diagnostician to favor one diagnostic possibility over another. Because of the loss of follicles, hair regrowth is impossible.

Chronic Cutaneous Lupus Erythematosus in Summary

Clinical correlation: Indurated papules that become variably atrophic irregular alopecic plaques with follicular plugging, telangiectasia, central erythema, depigmentation, and adherent scale. Follicular markings disappear as follicles are destroyed. Central hypopigmentation and peripheral hyperpigmentation are commonly seen in dark-skinned individuals.

Histological findings:

❖ Vacuolar interface change with apoptotic keratinocytes along the hair follicular basal layer (infundibulum > isthmus) and frequently at the dermal–epidermal junction between follicles
❖ A variably dense lymphoplasmacytic infiltrate that involves the superficial and deep dermis along blood vessels and adnexal structures
• Deep dermal mucin may be seen
• Diminished numbers of sebaceous lobules
• Follicular hyperkeratosis with ostial plugging
• Follicular epithelial and/or epidermal thinning
• Thickening of the basement membrane
• Widespread loss of elastic fibers in perifollicular and interfollicular areas by Verhoeff–Van Gieson staining
• Direct immunofluorescence: IgG and C3 along the dermal epidermal junction in 70–95% of cases

Histological differential diagnosis:
- **Lichen planopilaris:** differs from CCLE by the presence of follicular hypergranulosis, diminished elastic fibers in a wedge shape around follicular infundibula, more frequent colloid bodies, absence of deep dermal mucin and deep periadnexal and perivascular inflammation

⚠ **Pitfalls**

Late stages of all cicatricial alopecias are commonly indistinguishable

Abbreviation: CCLE, Chronic cutaneous lupus erythematosus.

REFERENCES

1. Klein R, Moghadam-Kia S, Taylor L, et al. Quality of life in cutaneous lupus erythematosus. J Am Acad Dermatol 2011; 64: 849–58.
2. Vera-Recabarren MA, Garcia-Carrasco M, Ramos-Casals M, Herrero C. Comparative analysis of subacute cutaneous lupus erythematosus and chronic cutaneous lupus erythematosus: clinical and immunological study of 270 patients. Br J Dermatol 2010; 162: 91–101.
3. Trueb RM. Involvement of scalp and nails in lupus erythematosus. Lupus 2010; 19: 1078–86.
4. Hamilton T, Otberg N, Wu WY, Martinka M, Shapiro J. Successful hair re-growth with multimodal treatment of early cicatricial alopecia in discoid lupus erythematosus. Acta Derm Venereol 2009; 89: 417–8.
5. Bae YI, Yun SJ, Lee JB, et al. A clinical and epidemiological study of lupus erythematosus at a tertiary referral dermatology clinic in Korea. Lupus 2009; 18: 1320–6.
6. Miettunen PM, Bruecks A, Remington T. Dramatic response of scarring scalp discoid lupus erythematosus (DLE) to intravenous methylprednisolone, oral corticosteroids, and hydroxychloroquine in a 5-year-old child. Pediatr Dermatol 2009; 26: 338–41.
7. Feng JB, Ni JD, Yao X, et al. Gender and age influence on clinical and laboratory features in Chinese patients with systemic lupus erythematosus: 1,790 cases. Rheumatol Int 2010; 30: 1017–23.
8. Stefanato CM. Histopathology of alopecia: a clinicopathological approach to diagnosis. Histopathology 2010; 56: 24–38.
9. Harries MJ, Meyer KC, Paus R. Hair loss as a result of cutaneous autoimmunity: frontiers in the immunopathogenesis of primary cicatricial alopecia. Autoimmun Rev 2009; 8: 478–83.
10. Headington JT. Cicatricial alopecia. Dermatol Clin 1996; 14: 773–82.
11. Harries MJ, Sinclair RD, Macdonald-Hull S, et al. Management of primary cicatricial alopecias: options for treatment. Br J Dermatol. 2008; 159: 1–22.
12. Berlin JM, Wang AL, McDuffie BC, Leeman DR. JAAD Grand rounds quiz. Cicatricial alopecia. J Am Acad Dermatol 2010; 63: 547–8.
13. Hordinsky M. Cicatricial alopecia: discoid lupus erythematosus. Dermatol Ther 2008; 21: 245–8.
14. Hemmati I, Otberg N, Martinka M, et al. Discoid lupus erythematosus presenting with cysts, comedones, and cicatricial alopecia on the scalp. J Am Acad Dermatol 2009; 60: 1070–2.
15. Abraham LS, Pineiro-Maceira J, Duque-Estrada B, Barcaui CB, Sodre CT. Pinpoint white dots in the scalp: dermoscopic and histopathologic correlation. J Am Acad Dermatol 2010; 63: 721–2.
16. Tosti A, Torres F, Misciali C, et al. Follicular red dots: a novel dermoscopic pattern observed in scalp discoid lupus erythematosus. Arch Dermatol 2009; 145: 1406–9.
17. Patel P, Werth V. Cutaneous lupus erythematosus: a review. Dermatol Clin 2002; 20: 373–85, v.
18. Hoffman IE, Peene I, Meheus L, et al. Specific antinuclear antibodies are associated with clinical features in systemic lupus erythematosus. Ann Rheum Dis 2004; 63: 1155–8.
19. Somani N, Bergfeld WF. Cicatricial alopecia: classification and histopathology. Dermatol Ther 2008; 21: 221–37.
20. Fabbri P, Amato L, Chiarini C, Moretti S, Massi D. Scarring alopecia in discoid lupus erythematosus: a clinical, histopathologic and immunopathologic study. Lupus 2004; 13: 455–62.
21. Annessi G, Lombardo G, Gobello T, Puddu P. A clinicopathologic study of scarring alopecia due to lichen planus: comparison with scarring alopecia in discoid lupus erythematosus and pseudopelade. Am J Dermatopathol 1999; 21: 324–31.
22. Sperling LC. Scarring alopecia and the dermatopathologist. J Cutan Pathol 2001; 28: 333–42.
23. Al-Refu K, Edward S, Ingham E, Goodfield M. Expression of hair follicle stem cells detected by cytokeratin 15 stain: implications for pathogenesis of the scarring process in cutaneous lupus erythematosus. Br J Dermatol 2009; 160: 1188–96.
24. Wilson CL, Burge SM, Dean D, Dawber RP. Scarring alopecia in discoid lupus erythematosus. Br J Dermatol 1992; 126: 307–14.
25. Elston DM, McCollough ML, Warschaw KE, Bergfeld WF. Elastic tissue in scars and alopecia. J Cutan Pathol 2000; 27: 147–52.
26. Jordon RE. Subtle clues to diagnosis by immunopathology. Scarring alopecia. Am J Dermatopathol Summer 1980; 2: 157–9.
27. Abell E. Immunofluorescent staining technics in the diagnosis of alopecia. South Med J 1977; 70: 1407–10.

29 Dissecting cellulitis of the scalp (perifolliculitis capitis abscedens et suffodiens)

Dissecting cellulitis is an uncommon but distinctive disease. It most commonly affects young adult men, especially African-American men, but it can also occur in Caucasians (1,2) and the pediatric population (3,4). While dissecting cellulitis is part of the "follicular occlusion tetrad" that also includes hidradenitis suppurativa, acne conglobata, and pilonidal sinus, scalp disease often occurs alone.

CLINICAL FINDINGS
Lesions begin as multiple, firm scalp nodules, most commonly on the crown, vertex, and upper occiput (Fig. 29.1). The nodules rapidly progress, forming boggy, fluctuant, oval and linear ridges that eventually discharge purulent material. Lesions often interconnect, so that pressure on one fluctuant area may result in a purulent discharge from perforations several centimeters away (Fig. 29.2). Despite massive, deep inflammation, there can be surprisingly little pain, and patients often present with a chief complaint of hair loss or a foul-smelling discharge.

The disease typically waxes and wanes for years, but eventually leads to dense dermal fibrosis, sinus tract formation, hypertrophic scarring, and permanent alopecia. Squamous cell carcinoma has rarely been reported to arise in the setting of longstanding disease.

Treatment is difficult, and the literature on the subject consists of case reports and small case series. Intralesional corticosteroids are useful for short-term improvement. Several patients have responded to oral isotretinoin (2,5,6) and adalimumab (7,8). Other modalities that have been tried with success (in at least 1 patient) include infliximab, (9) a combination of dapsone and isotretinoin, (10) and even therapeutic scalping (11). For severe, intractable disease, X-ray epilation (12) can be very successful although it exposes the patient to the long-term risks of radiotherapy.

HISTOLOGICAL FINDINGS
The earliest findings have seldom been described, probably because patients typically consult physicians after the disease is firmly established. Also, clinicians are more likely to obtain biopsy specimens from nodular or cystic lesions that represent more advanced, longstanding disease. If an appropriate site is selected (Fig. 29.3), the earliest change is moderately dense, perifollicular lymphocytic inflammation affecting the lower half of the dermis and extending into the fat (Figs. 29.4 and 29.5). At this stage, numerous intact and seemingly undamaged terminal follicles are bathed in a sea of acute and chronic inflammation (Fig. 29.6). Terminal anagen hairs are reduced in number because many have converted to the catagen/telogen phase (Fig. 29.7).

Initially, lymphocytes dominate the infiltrate, but eventually neutrophils become more numerous, especially in longstanding,

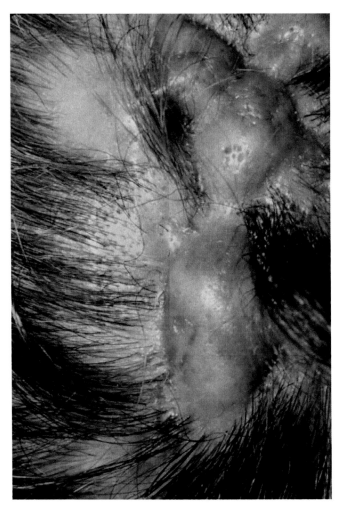

Figure 29.2 Interconnecting, fluctuant nodules of dissecting cellulitis in a Caucasian man. Photograph courtesy of Jeffrey Miller, M.D.

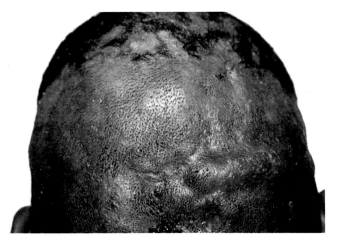

Figure 29.1 Dissecting cellulitis in an African-American man.

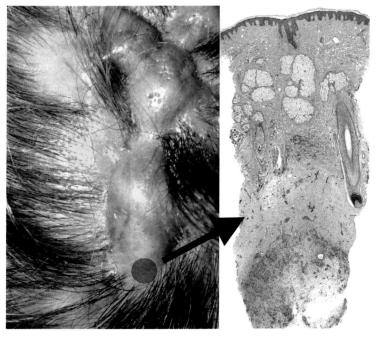

Figure 29.3 The center of a fluctuant or fibrotic nodule usually represents end-stage disease showing only nonspecific histological changes. A more productive biopsy site, indicated by a circle (*left panel*), can result in a biopsy specimen similar to that shown in the *right panel*, and magnified in Figure 29.4.

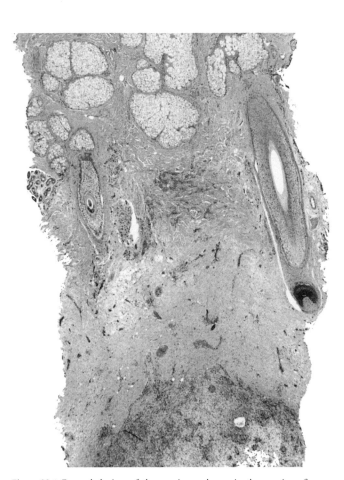

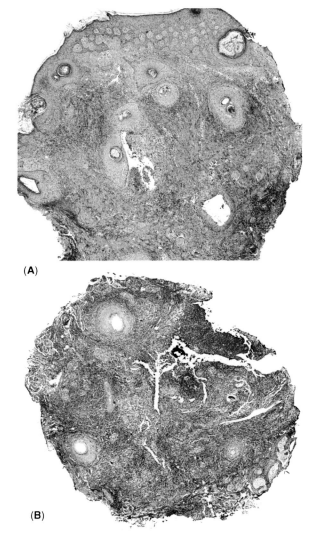

(A)

(B)

Figure 29.4 Expanded view of the specimen shown in the previous figure. Note that the upper half of the specimen appears relatively normal, with intact follicles and sebaceous glands. Inflammation is concentrated at the level of the deep dermis/superficial fat, corresponding to the level of the terminal hair bulbs.

Figure 29.5 A horizontally sectioned specimen from a different patient with dissecting cellulitis shows that the inflammation in the upper dermis (A) is much less intense than that at the deep dermal level (B).

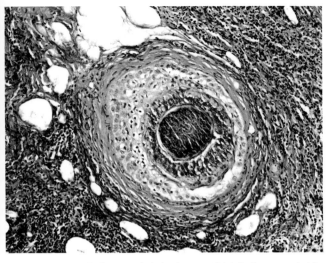

Figure 29.6 A terminal anagen hair in the superficial fat is surrounded by intense chronic inflammation but remains (as of yet) uninjured.

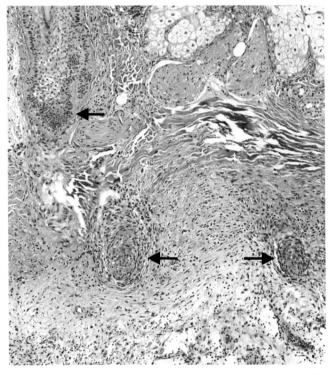

Figure 29.7 Terminal catagen/telogen hairs (*arrows*) are greatly increased in number.

fluctuant lesions. Still later, plasma cells increase in number. Repetitive injury to the follicles results in acneiform dilation of the infundibula, with perifollicular neutrophilic inflammation. Infundibular distention can be found at any stage of the disease (Figs. 29.8 and 29.9). As the disease evolves, a vascular proliferation accompanies the infiltrate and the deep dermis and subcutaneous fat begin to resemble granulation tissue (Fig. 29.10).

In most other forms of inflammatory, cicatricial alopecia, sebaceous glands are the first structures to disappear. In dissecting cellulitis, sebaceous glands remain intact well into the course of the disease (Fig. 29.11). This relative sparing of sebaceous glands (at least initially) may be related to the depth of the infiltrate in the earlier stages of disease.

The intense inflammation of dissecting cellulitis triggers the conversion of anagen hairs into catagen/telogen hairs, whose shafts are ultimately shed. Therefore, the hair loss seen in the early stages of dissecting cellulitis is temporary. With the passage of time, however, inflammation extends throughout the dermis, causing epithelial injury and follicular destruction. The result is a permanent, cicatricial alopecia. If fluctuant nodules and sinuses are sampled, large perifollicular and mid-to-deep dermal abscesses composed of neutrophils, lymphocytes, and often numerous plasma cells are seen. Eventually, chronic abscesses become lined with squamous epithelium derived from the overlying epidermis, and true sinus tracts are formed. As follicles are completely destroyed, inflammation subsides and is replaced by dense fibrosis of the dermis and the superficial fat.

Dissecting Cellulitis of the Scalp in Summary

Clinical correlation: young adult, usually male and often African-American, with boggy nodules and a purulent discharge on the scalp. Lesions are scattered, but most concentrated on the crown, vertex, and upper occiput.

Histological findings:
- ❖ Early lesions show moderately dense, lymphocytic, perifollicular inflammation surrounding the lower half of the follicle
- ❖ Fully developed, fluctuant lesions show perifollicular and mid-to-deep dermal abscesses composed of neutrophils, lymphocytes, and often abundant plasma cells
- ❖ Sebaceous glands may persist well into the course of the disease
- • Eventually, granulation tissue, epithelial-lined lined sinus tracts, and fibrosis are seen
- • Increased numbers of catagen/telogen hairs

⚠ Pitfalls

Rare instances of tinea capitis may mimic dissecting cellulitis both clinically and histologically. Fungi may be difficult to locate even with special stains; therefore, culture data may be necessary to rule out fungal infection (13).

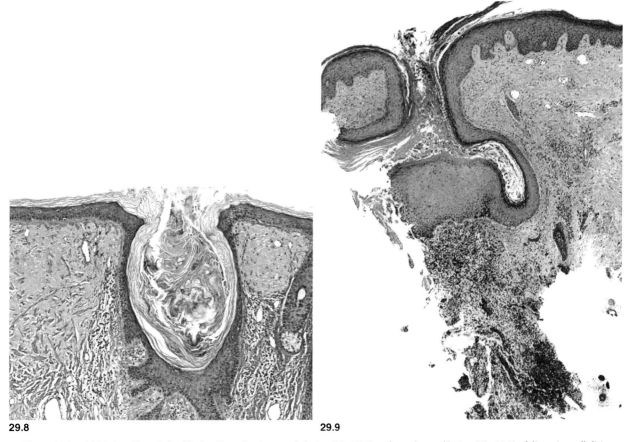

29.8   **29.9**

Figures 29.8 and 29.9 Acneiform infundibular distension in an early lesion (Fig. 29.8) and an advanced lesion (Fig. 29.9) of dissecting cellulitis.

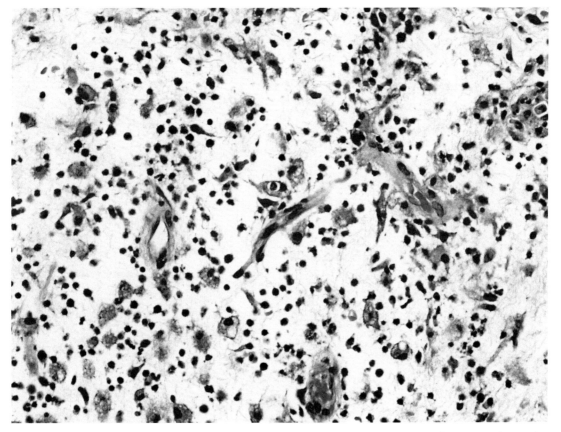

Figure 29.10 In well-established dissecting cellulitis, the deep dermis and superficial fat are replaced by a dense, mixed inflammatory infiltrate, edema, and vascular proliferation, resembling granulation tissue.

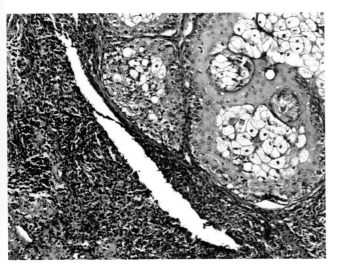

Figure 29.11 Despite the presence of dense inflammation, sebaceous glands persist well into the course of the disease (see also Figure 29.4).

REFERENCES

1. Stites PC, Boyd AS. Dissecting cellulitis in a white male: a case report and review of the literature. Cutis 2001; 67: 37–40.
2. Koca R, Altinyazar HC, Ozen OI, Tekin NS. Dissecting cellulitis in a white male: response to isotretinoin. Int J Dermatol 2002; 41: 509–13.
3. Ramesh V. Dissecting cellulitis of the scalp in 2 girls. Dermatologica 1990; 180: 48–50.
4. Arneja JS, Vashi CN, Gursel E, Lelli JL. Management of fulminant dissecting cellulitis of the scalp in the pediatric population: Case report and literature review. Can J Plast Surg 2007; 15: 211–4.
5. Khaled A, Zeglaoui F, Zoghlami A, Fazaa B, Kamoun MR. Dissecting cellulitis of the scalp: response to isotretinoin. J Eur Acad Dermatol Venereol 2007; 21: 1430–1.
6. Scerri L, Williams HC, Allen BR. Dissecting cellulitis of the scalp: response to isotretinoin. Br J Dermatol 1996; 134: 1105–8.
7. Navarini AA, Trueb RM. 3 cases of dissecting cellulitis of the scalp treated with adalimumab: control of inflammation within residual structural disease. Arch Dermatol 2010; 146: 517–20.
8. Sukhatme SV, Lenzy YM, Gottlieb AB. Refractory dissecting cellulitis of the scalp treated with adalimumab. J Drugs Dermatol 2008; 7: 981–3.
9. Brandt HR, Malheiros AP, Teixeira MG, Machado MC. Perifolliculitis capitis abscedens et suffodiens successfully controlled with infliximab. Br J Dermatol 2008; 159: 506–7.
10. Bolz S, Jappe U, Hartschuh W. Successful treatment of perifolliculitis capitis abscedens et suffodiens with combined isotretinoin and dapsone. J Dtsch Dermatol Ges 2008; 6: 44–7.
11. Moschella SL, Klein MH, Miller RJ. Perifolliculitis capitis abscedens et suffodiens. Report of a successful therapeutic scalping. Arch Dermatol 1967; 96: 195–7.
12. McMullan FH, Zeligman I. Perifolliculitis capitis abscedens et suffodiens; its successful treatment with x-ray epilation. AMA Arch Derm 1956; 73: 256–63.
13. Twersky JM, Sheth AP. Tinea capitis mimicking dissecting cellulitis: a distinct variant. Int J Dermatol 2005; 44: 412–4.

30 Erosive pustular dermatosis

Named by Pye in 1979 (1), erosive pustular dermatosis (EPD) is an uncommon condition of uncertain nosology, but the medical literature suggests that it is a distinct disease (2). Laboratory data is noncontributory, bacteriological and mycological studies are usually negative, and histopathological findings are nonspecific (3). Nevertheless, the clinical picture is sufficiently distinctive to evoke the diagnosis, and in the proper clinical setting, the histological findings are supportive.

CLINICAL FINDINGS
The condition almost always occurs in elderly patients, most often in women (1,2,4,5). The presence of pre-existing balding (3,6,7) and chronic sun damage (7,8) seems to be a common denominator. The condition is frequently reported in association with injury to the skin, such as herpes zoster (6), CO_2 laser vaporization to treat multiple actinic keratoses (8), scalp surgery (4,9), cryosurgery (10), radiation therapy (11), photodynamic therapy with methyl 5-aminolevulinic acid (5), and 5-fluorouracil treatment (8). Lesions are described or illustrated as persistent, large, moist, eroded plaques with variable degrees of pustule formation and crusting (Figs. 30.1 and 30.2).

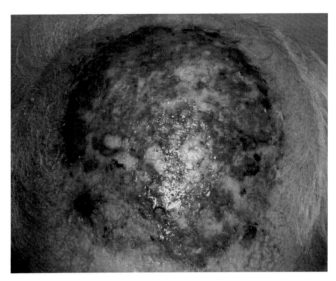

Figure 30.1 Typical clinical appearance of erosive pustular dermatosis. *Source:* Image courtesy of Dr. Almut Böer-Auer.

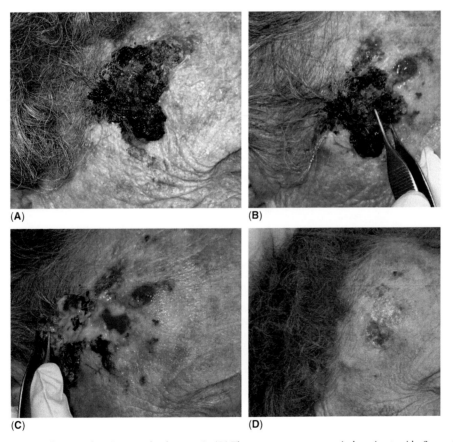

(A) (B)

(C) (D)

Figure 30.2 (**A–C**) Typical clinical features of erosive pustular dermatosis. (**D**) The response to potent topical corticosteroids. *Source:* Images courtesy of Dr. Mary Maloney.

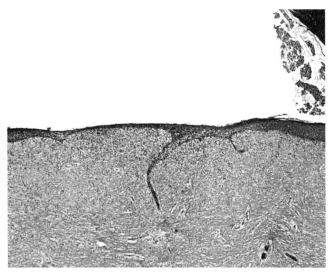

Figure 30.3 A typical case of erosive pustular dermatosis showing marked epidermal atrophy and non-specific upper dermal fibroplasia, inflammation, and loss of follicular structures. (Case contributed by Dr. Almut Böer-Auer)

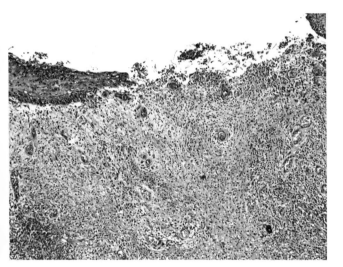

Figure 30.4 Same case as shown in Figure 30.3, showing a zone of epidermal erosion and a dense, dermal, polymorphous inflammation with vascular proliferation, suggestive of granulation tissue. (Case contributed by Dr. Almut Böer-Auer)

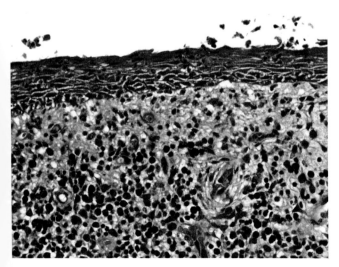

Figure 30.5 The epidermal atrophy and plasma cell-rich infiltrate in this case of erosive pustular dermatosis are very reminiscent of Zoon's mucositis. (Case contributed by Dr. Almut Böer-Auer)

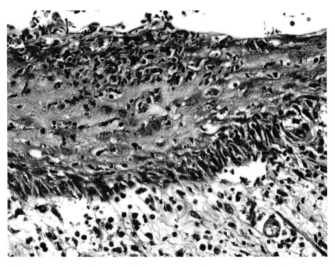

Figure 30.6 Spongiform pustule in a patient with erosive pustular dermatosis.

Several treatments have been suggested in anecdotal reports or small case series, including potent topical corticosteroids (1), oral isotretinoin (3), and topical tacrolimus (6,8,12).

HISTOLOGICAL FINDINGS

Other authors have reported that the histological features of EPD are nonspecific, showing an atrophic epidermis and a diffuse, dermal, mixed infiltrate of chronic inflammatory cells, including plasma cells (1–3,6,12). Our experience is similar (Figs. 30.3–30.5). There is also a variable degree of intraepidermal micro- or macropustulation, reminiscent of that seen in psoriasis (Fig. 30.6).

Erosive Pustular Dermatosis in Summary

Clinical correlation: persistent erosions and pustule formation on the balding, sun-damaged scalp of an elderly person. Lesions often have a thick crust, which when removed reveals pus within an ulcer.

Histological findings:
- ❖ Marked epidermal atrophy with focal erosions
- ❖ Upper dermal mixed inflammatory infiltrate
- • Intraepidermal accumulations of neutrophils (often)
- • Dermal infiltrate rich in plasma cells (often)

⚠ **Pitfalls**
Histological findings are not specific, and good clinical correlation is required to establish the diagnosis.

REFERENCES
1. Pye RJ, Peachey RD, Burton JL. Erosive pustular dermatosis of the scalp. Br J Dermatol 1979; 100: 559–66.
2. Caputo R, Veraldi S. Erosive pustular dermatosis of the scalp. J Am Acad Dermatol 1993; 28: 96–8.
3. Mastroianni A, Cota C, Ardigò M, Minutilli E, Berardesca E. Erosive pustular dermatosis of the scalp: a case report and review of the literature. Dermatology 2005; 211: 273–6.

4. Ena P, Lissia M, Doneddu GM, Campus GV. Erosive pustular dermatosis of the scalp in skin grafts: report of three cases. Dermatology 1997; 194: 80–4.

5. Guarneri C, Vaccaro M. Erosive pustular dermatosis of the scalp following topical methylaminolaevulinate photodynamic therapy. J Am Acad Dermatol 2009; 60: 521–2.

6. Kim KR, Lee JY, Kim MK, Yoon TY. Erosive pustular dermatosis of the scalp following herpes zoster: successful treatment with topical tacrolimus. Ann Dermatol 2010; 22: 232–4.

7. Petersen BO, Bygum A. Erosive pustular dermatosis of the scalp: a case treated successfully with isotretinoin. Acta Derm Venereol 2008; 88: 300–1.

8. Tavares-Bello R. Erosive pustular dermatosis of the scalp. A chronic recalcitrant dermatosis developed upon CO2 laser treatment. Dermatology 2009; 219: 71–2.

9. Layton AM, Cunliffe WJ. Erosive pustular dermatosis of the scalp following surgery. Br J Dermatol 1995; 132: 472–3.

10. Rongioletti F, Delmonte S, Rossi ME, Strani GF, Rebora A. Erosive pustular dermatosis of the scalp following cryotherapy and topical tretinoin for actinic keratoses. Clin Exp Dermatol 1999; 24: 499–500.

11. Trueb RM, Krasovec M. Erosive pustular dermatosis of the scalp following radiation therapy for solar keratoses. Br J Dermatol 1999; 141: 763–5.

12. Cenkowski MJ, Silver S. Topical tacrolimus in the treatment of erosive pustular dermatosis of the scalp. J Cutan Med Surg 2007; 11: 222–5.

31 Brocq's alopecia (pseudopelade of Brocq) and end-stage cicatricial alopecia

The term "pseudopelade of Brocq" is a source of much confusion and fruitless debate, and should be abandoned. Weedon recommends using the term "idiopathic scarring alopecia" as an alternative designation (1). In recent decades, *pseudopelade* has been used to describe some patients with central, centrifugal cicatricial alopecia (CCCA), a very different condition than that described by Louis–Anne–Jean Brocq in 1905. To avoid confusion, we will refer to the entity described by Brocq (2) as *Brocq's alopecia* (BA). We propose that Brocq's alopecia is not a distinct disease (1) but a clinical *pattern* of cicatricial alopecia. BA represents an end-stage or clinical variant of various other forms of cicatricial alopecia, and is a diagnosis of exclusion.

The pattern of hair loss observed in Brocq's alopecia can be seen in "burnt-out" lichen planopilaris (LPP), discoid lupus erythematosus (DLE), and other forms of cicatricial hair loss (3). If a definitive diagnosis of DLE, LPP, CCCA, or another form of cicatricial alopecia can be made based on clinical, histological, or immunofluorescence features, then the term Brocq's alopecia cannot be used. If a "primary" form of Brocq's alopecia exists, it has yet to be convincingly defined with a clinical-histopathological correlate. The frequently cited manuscript by Braun-Falco (4) (see section Histological Findings below) does little to dispel this notion. An attempt to prove that Brocq's alopecia and LPP are distinct diseases using gene expression patterns (5) also fails to shed light on the matter; the study only shows that an active inflammatory disease and an end-stage pauci-inflammatory state express different genes, a foregone conclusion.

CLINICAL FINDINGS

Patients meeting the clinical characteristics of Brocq's original observations are very uncommon. An example of such a patient would be a Caucasian adult who is surprised to discover discrete, asymptomatic areas of scalp hair loss. As would be expected in an entity that likely includes a number of distinct and different diseases, more than one pattern of progression has been described. It has been reported as slowly progressive in some patients, with new areas of alopecia developing over a period of months-to-years; in others, the condition worsens in spurts, with periods of activity followed by dormancy. It is important to recognize that the slow but steady centrifugal expansion of cicatricial alopecia originating on the vertex is a distinct clinical pattern of CCCA, even when seen in Caucasians, and should not fall into the pseudopelade nosological wastebasket. Reported cases of BA with exclusive crown or vertex involvement may actually represent examples of "burnt-out" CCCA. In contradistinction, descriptions of Brocq's alopecia are of irregularly shaped and often widely distributed or grouped bald patches on the scalp.

The individual lesion of BA is hypopigmented ("porcelain white" is a classic description) and slightly depressed (atrophic). Lesions are often irregularly shaped (Fig. 31.1), as opposed to the round or oval patches usually seen in alopecia areata and most cases of CCCA. The classic description of "footprints in the snow" refers to both the hypopigmentation and the dermal atrophy causing a slight depression below the surrounding normal scalp. However, many purported cases of Brocq's alopecia do not demonstrate this depression. Usually only mild erythema and slight perifollicular scaling are present, and often there is no clinical evidence of inflammation. Just as in other forms of cicatricial alopecia, a few isolated hairs may remain within an otherwise smooth, shiny, bald patch.

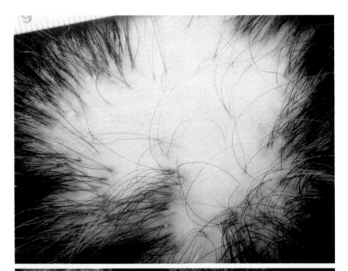
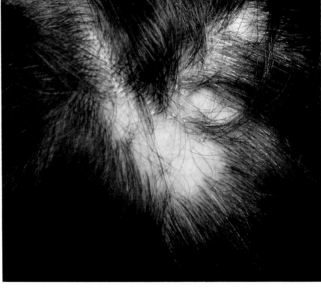

Figure 31.1 Typical lesions of Brocq's alopecia in two women whose hairdressers discovered the bald spots. There was no clinical evidence of active inflammation in either patient, and the histological findings were those of an end-stage or "burnt-out" cicatricial alopecia.

HISTOLOGICAL FINDINGS

The histopathological findings of Brocq's alopecia have yet to be clearly defined. The criteria established by Pinkus (6) in 1978 are *not* correlated in any way with clinical features. Instead, "patterns of elastic fibers in the perifollicular and interfollicular dermis" were utilized in a retrospective fashion to differentiate "pseudopelade of Brocq from pseudopelade-like states secondary to lupus erythematosus and other disease processes." The retrospective review by Braun-Falco (4) lists the following features as being characteristic of Brocq's alopecia: little or only moderate lymphocytic infiltrate; absence of significant follicular plugging; absent or diminished sebaceous glands; and negative direct immunofluorescence studies. These features are all nonspecific in that they are found in many different cicatricial processes.

A more recent retrospective study (7) also depended on histological features alone to define Brocq's alopecia as a condition showing "an absence of criteria seen in CCLE and LPP and preservation of the elastic sheet around the follicles." Thus "pseudopelade of Brocq" as described by these authors is a histological and not a clinical entity. Elastic tissue stains may be useful (8), but their precise role in the classification of cicatricial alopecia has yet to be critically studied. In most cases of Brocq's alopecia, the "active" lesion is elusive, and the typical histological findings are those of an end-stage cicatricial alopecia (see the following section).

In summary, we believe that Brocq's alopecia represents the end-stage of several different forms of cicatricial alopecia. A prospective study of Brocq's alopecia with sound clinical correlation has yet to be performed.

END-STAGE OR "BURNT-OUT" CICATRICIAL ALOPECIA

All too often, pathologists must render the diagnosis of a "burnt-out" or "end-stage" cicatricial alopecia. The histological term *end-stage cicatricial alopecia*, similar to the clinical term *Brocq's alopecia*, does not indicate a specific disease but a pattern common to several entities. There are two possible reasons for the existence of this pattern. First, the patient's disease may, in fact, have truly "burnt-out" like an extinguished forest fire, with no further follicular destruction. More commonly, however, the end-stage pattern is the result of an unfortunate choice of biopsy site. Frequently, bald or nearly bald areas are sampled, instead of foci where numerous hairs are still present. The advancing border of a zone of cicatricial alopecia is usually a more productive site for histopathological examination than a bald zone. Areas with subtle findings such as perifollicular erythema or scaling prove more fruitful than those showing the advanced findings of pustules, papules, extensive hair loss, or obliteration of follicular ostia. Just a few millimeters may separate fruitful from suboptimal biopsy sites, but even experienced clinicians cannot see below the surface of the skin. For clinicians evaluating patients with progressive hair loss, the histological diagnosis of "end-stage cicatricial alopecia" should serve as an invitation for additional biopsy specimens.

End-stage cicatricial alopecia is characterized by the following: markedly decreased total number of hairs, especially terminal hairs (Fig. 31.2); loss of the sebaceous glands; residual, "naked" hair shafts surrounded by mild, granulomatous inflammation (Fig. 31.3); follicular stelae without overlying follicles (Fig. 31.4); and cylindrical columns of connective tissue representing the sites of former follicles or entire follicular units (Figs. 31.5 and 31.6).

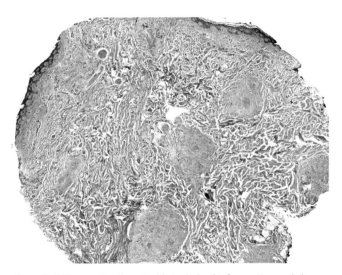

Figure 31.2 The paucity of terminal hairs, lack of inflammation, and absence of sebaceous glands are typical of end-stage or "burnt-out" cicatricial alopecia. This particular example was taken from a patient who proved to have central, centrifugal cicatricial alopecia (based on additional specimens and a typical clinical presentation).

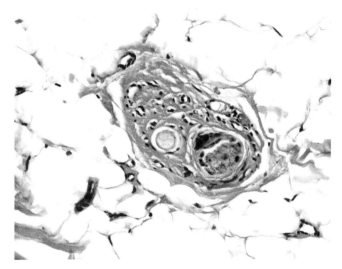

Figure 31.3 A "naked" hair shaft surrounded by granulomatous inflammation and fibrosis. Deeply seated hair shaft fragments can incite surprisingly little inflammation.

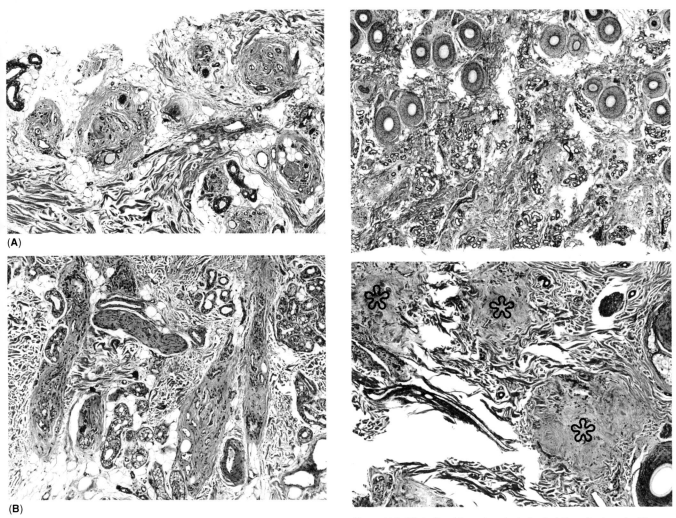

Figure 31.4 In this example of end-stage cicatricial alopecia, numerous follicular stele can be found in transverse (**A**) and vertical (**B**) sections.

Figure 31.5 Clinically, this patient had classical Brocq's alopecia. The *top panel* shows a clear demarcation between normal and diseased scalp. The *bottom panel* shows three follicular scars (*) that probably replaced entire follicular units.

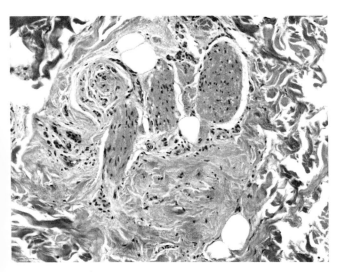

Figure 31.6 Transverse section of a typical follicular scar (probably representing an entire follicular unit) with loss of sebaceous glands but retention of arrector pili.

Brocq's Alopecia (Pseudopelade of Brocq) and End-stage Cicatricial Alopecia in Summary

Clinical correlation: the term Brocq's alopecia can apply to a Caucasian adult who discovers discrete, asymptomatic, hypopigmented or depigmented, slightly depressed (atrophic) and irregularly shaped bald patches affecting any portion of the scalp. This represents a clinical subset of end-stage, cicatricial alopecia. It includes patients with various forms of inflammatory, cicatricial alopecia that are no longer active and classifiable at the time of presentation.

Histological findings:
* ❖ Markedly decreased total number of hairs, especially terminal hairs
* ❖ Loss of the sebaceous glands
* ❖ Cylindrical columns of connective tissue at the sites of former follicles
* • Residual, "naked" hair shafts surrounded by mild, granulomatous inflammation
* • Follicular stelae without overlying follicles

Histological differential diagnosis:

- **End-stage traction alopecia:** shows retention of sebaceous glands and vellus hairs in follicular units that have lost terminal hairs
- **Aplasia cutis congenita:** lacks all follicular structures, including arrector pili

⚠ **Pitfalls**

Routine vertical sections cannot be used to assess the extent of follicular loss in end-stage cicatricial alopecia. Transverse sections must be viewed at multiple levels to document the permanent loss of follicular epithelium.

REFERENCES

1. Weedon D. Skin Pathology. Vol 1. 3rd ed. London: Churchill Livingstone Elsevier, 2010.
2. Brocq L, Lenglet E, Ayrignac J. Recherches sur l'alopecie atrophiante, variete pseudopelade. Ann Dermatol Syphilol (France) 1905; 6: 1–32; P 97–127 P 209–237.
3. Amato L, Mei S, Massi D, Gallerani I, Fabbri P. Cicatricial alopecia; a dermatopathologic and immunopathologic study of 33 patients (pseudopelade of Brocq is not a specific clinico-pathologic entity). Int J Dermatol 2002; 41: 8–15.
4. Braun-Falco O, Imai S, Schmoeckel C, Steger O, Bergner T. Pseudopelade of Brocq. Dermatologica 1986; 172: 18–23.
5. Yu M, Bell RH, Ross EK, et al. Lichen planopilaris and pseudopelade of Brocq involve distinct disease associated gene expression patterns by microarray. J Dermatol Sci 2010; 57: 27–36.
6. Pinkus H. Differential patterns of elastic fibers in scarring and non-scarring alopecias. J Cutan Pathol 1978; 5: 93–104.
7. Moure ER, Romiti R, Machado MC, Valente NY. Primary cicatricial alopecias: a review of histopathologic findings in 38 patients from a clinical university hospital in Sao Paulo, Brazil. Clinics (Sao Paulo) 2008; 63: 747–52.
8. Elston DM, McCollough ML, Warschaw KE, Bergfeld WF. Elastic tissue in scars and alopecia. J Cutan Pathol 2000; 27: 147–52.

32 Aplasia cutis congenita of the scalp

Aplasia cutis congenita (ACC) refers to the congenital absence of skin. An exhaustive review of the subject was performed by Demmel in 1975 (1) and Frieden in 1986 (2), and a variety of classification schemes have been proposed since that time. This chapter will focuses on ACC of the scalp without associated anomalies (Frieden's Group I), which is by far the most common subtype of ACC.

CLINICAL FINDINGS

Solitary lesions of ACC are the most common presentation. However, occasionally two or even three foci may occur together on the scalp. Involved areas are often located near the hair whorl on the vertex of the scalp and can be various shapes and sizes (0.5–10 cm). At the time of birth, the defects may be deeply ulcerated, superficially eroded, or completely healed with scarring (Fig. 32.1). Occasionally, lesions are bullous (3). Familial cases have been reported (4). We have seen a lesion of ACC in a patient with temporal triangular alopecia (5), an association that we believe is purely coincidental. Most lesions heal spontaneously (before or after birth) and seldom result in significant morbidity (6).

A hair collar sign may be present either in simple cases or in those with underlying structural defects; in the presence of a hair collar, radiological imaging is warranted prior to further intervention. Large foci are more likely to be associated with involvement of the skull or defects extending to the meninges. Parents of affected infants or non-dermatologist clinicians may mistakenly attribute ACC to trauma inflicted from forceps or scalp electrodes used for intrauterine fetal monitoring.

HISTOLOGICAL FINDINGS

Biopsy specimens from patients with ACC are often obtained long after birth when involved areas are excised for cosmetic reasons. The epidermis often demonstrates flattening of the rete ridges, particularly in the central portion of the lesion. A few residual hair follicles may remain stranded in a dermis that is otherwise devoid of follicles and sweat glands. When the central portion of the lesion is compared with the surrounding normal scalp skin, the dermis usually appears thickened because the superficial subcutaneous fat has been replaced by collagenous tissue (Figs. 32.2–32.4). However, in some instances, the dermis is relatively thinned.

In the majority of cases of ACC, collagen is thickened and sclerotic, often oriented in bundles parallel to the skin surface as would be expected in a well-healed scar (7) (Figs. 32.4 and 32.5).

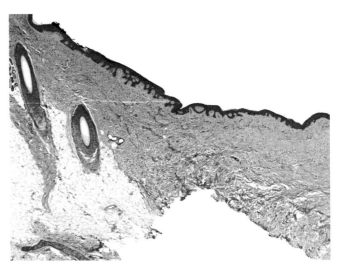

Figure 32.2 Dermal thickening and loss of follicles is evident in the central portion (*right side*) of this focus of aplasia cutis congenita as compared with the border (*left side*).

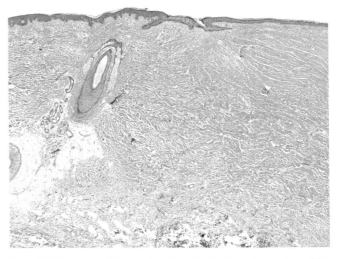

Figure 32.3 Flattening of the rete ridges is evident in the central portion of this lesion of aplasia cutis congenita (*right side*) as compared with the border (*left side*). Loss of adnexal structures and thickening of the dermis are also noted.

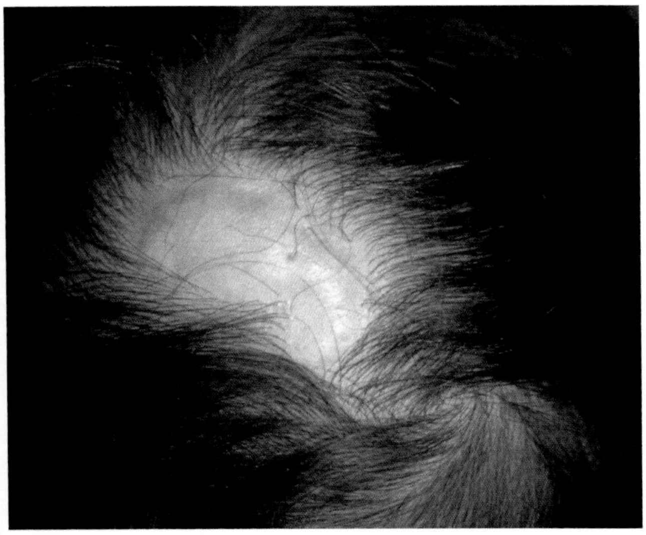

Figure 32.1 Scar-like lesion of aplasia cutis congenita located near the scalp whorl.

178

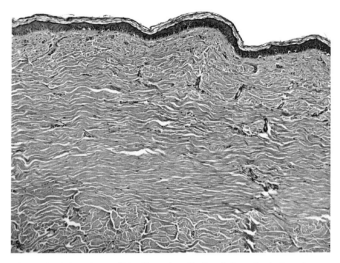

Figure 32.4 Sclerotic, parallel collagen bundles in a lesion of aplasia cutis congenita.

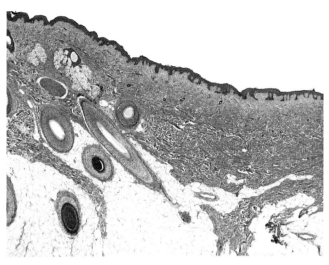

Figure 32.7 In this lesion of aplasia cutis congenita (*right side of image*), the dermis appears relatively normal. However, when compared with perilesional skin (*left side of image*), it is clear that adnexal structures are missing.

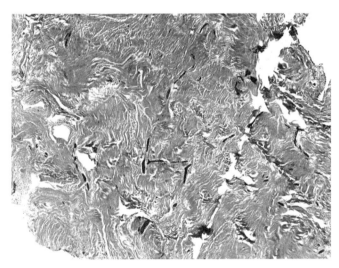

Figure 32.5 Transverse section at the level of the mid-dermis showing sclerotic, parallel collagen bundles in a lesion of aplasia cutis congenita.

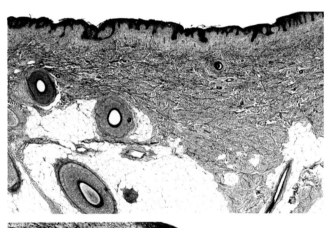

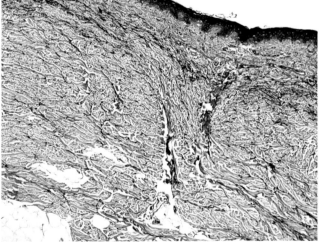

Figure 32.8 Elastic stain of a lesion of aplasia cutis congenita. The upper panel demonstrates that the elastic fiber distribution within the lesional skin (*right side*) appears relatively normal as compared to the normal scalp (*left side*). The *lower panel* magnifies a view within the abnormal (bald) zone.

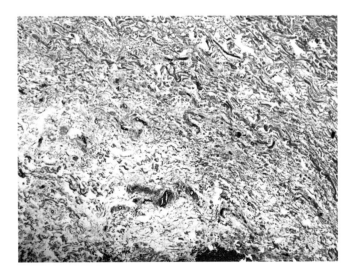

Figure 32.6 In this example of aplasia cutis congenita, the deeper portion of the specimen shows a loose, edematous stroma.

Some authors have described a fibrovascular and edematous stroma (Fig. 32.6) (3) which we have also observed in the deeper portions of some samples (Fig. 32.7) Occasionally, the thickened dermal collagen appears deceptively normal due to the random orientation of collagen bundles. However, even in these cases, adnexal structures are absent or rare (Fig. 32.8). Inflammation is not seen in completely healed lesions of ACC. Elastic tissue staining may vary greatly from case to case. We have seen examples with a thickened dermis devoid of adnexal structures but with a relatively normal elastic tissue distribution (Fig. 32.8). In other cases, however, elastic fibers are greatly diminished. The elastic tissue staining pattern is not a dependable diagnostic feature.

Aplasia Cutis Congenita in Summary

Clinical correlation: a single (rarely multiple) hairless plaque, most often located near the hair whorl on the vertex of the scalp. ACC is present at birth and can be of various shapes and sizes. At birth, the defects may be deeply ulcerated, superficially eroded, or completely healed with scarring. Most lesions are excised long after birth when they are completely healed.

Histological findings:
❖ Relative flattening of the epidermal rete ridges
❖ Absence of most or all adnexal structures, including follicles and sweat glands
❖ Thickening, sclerosis, and parallel orientation of dermal collagen fibers
• Thickening of the dermis with replacement of fat by connective tissue
• Loose, edematous stroma in the deeper aspects of some lesions
• Elastic fibers may be normal or decreased

Histological differential diagnosis:
• **End-stage cicatricial alopecia:** arrector pili and sweat glands should be present
• **Scar secondary to thermal injury:** (see Pitfalls)

⚠ **Pitfalls**

Without a clinical history, ACC may be impossible to differentiate from a traumatic scar, especially from a well-healed burn injury.

Abbreviation: ACC, aplasia cutis congenita.

REFERENCES
1. Demmel U. Clinical aspects of congenital skin defects. I. Congenital skin defects on the head of the newborn. Eur J Pediatr 1975; 121: 21–50.
2. Frieden IJ. Aplasia cutis congenita: a clinical review and proposal for classification. J Am Acad Dermatol 1986; 14: 646–60.
3. Colon-Fontanez F, Fallon Friedlander S, Newbury R, Eichenfield LF. Bullous aplasia cutis congenita. J Am Acad Dermatol 2003; 48(5 Suppl): S95–8.
4. Itin P, Pletscher M. Familial aplasia cutis congenita of the scalp without other defects in 6 members of three successive generations. Dermatologica 1988; 177: 123–5.
5. Kenner JR, Sperling LC. Pathological case of the month. Temporal triangular alopecia and aplasia cutis congenita. Arch Pediatr Adolesc Med 1998; 152: 1241–2.
6. Santos de Oliveira R, Barros Juca CE, Lopes Lins-Neto A, et al. Aplasia cutis congenita of the scalp: is there a better treatment strategy? Childs Nerv Syst 2006; 22: 1072–9.
7. Kruk-Jeromin J, Janik J, Rykala J. Aplasia cutis congenita of the scalp. Report of 16 cases. Dermatol Surg 1998; 24: 549–53.

33 Tinea capitis

Tinea capitis (fungal infection of scalp hair) most commonly affects children (1), and African-American children are especially prone to this infection (2–4). Any inflamed or scaly alopecic area on the scalp of a child of African descent should be considered to be tinea capitis until proven otherwise. Hispanic children are also at increased risk (4). Less commonly, adults can be affected. Among adults, African-American women have a higher rate of infection than other racial groups, likely due in part to their primary role in the care of affected children (5,6). If treated early, tinea capitis heals without scarring or hair loss. Highly inflammatory lesions or untreated lesions may eventuate in permanent hair loss (7). Inflammatory tinea capitis is one of several causes of the end-stage clinical pattern of "tufted folliculitis" (polytrichia; see also chap. 24).

The vast majority of cases of tinea capitis seen in North America are caused by *Trichophyton tonsurans*, a large-spore endothrix infection (8). Disease caused by *Microsporum canis*, an ectothrix infection, is much less commonly seen. Predominant species differ worldwide by geographic area, and immigration patterns can increase the local prevalence of otherwise rare species (9).

CLINICAL FINDINGS
As an endothrix fungus, *T. tonsurans* invades and multiplies within the hair shaft below the surface of the skin, causing hair fragility and breakage. Classically, this results in bald patches with follicular ostia filled with keratinous debris or "black dots," the residua of infected, pigmented hair shafts (Figs. 33.1 and 33.2). Using the dermatoscope, these broken hairs characteristically show a corkscrew or comma-shape (Fig. 33.3) (10,11). Many different clinical presentations are possible, however, depending both on the causative fungus and the host inflammatory response (12). These range from a normal-appearing scalp in the carrier state, to an alopecic area with minimal-to-no scale, to a mild seborrheic dermatitis-like presentation, to a cicatricial pattern, to the highly inflamed, purulent, edematous, and crusted plaques known as kerions (Fig. 33.4) (1,12,13). Rarely, tinea capitis may present with an inflammatory pattern that resembles dissecting cellulitis, both clinically and histologically (Figs. 33.5 and 33.6).

Pustular lesions on the scalp should always raise suspicion for and evaluation of tinea capitis. Lymphadenopathy is often present and can help to distinguish tinea capitis from other forms of patchy noninfectious alopecia, such as alopecia areata or the alopecia of lupus erythematosus. Culture via scalp brushings, swab, or collection of hair stubs (scraped from the follicular ostia) is important to document infection and guide therapy. Examining long, plucked hair shafts is fruitless—these hairs are not infected.

The affected individual should be treated with a systemic antifungal agent to ensure adequate drug delivery to the infected hair shafts. Micronized griseofulvin and terbinafine (which comes in granules for ease of use in children) are the two most commonly used agents, and the ones approved by the FDA for use in tinea capitis. Screening and treatment of household carriers with an antifungal shampoo, and regular bleach disinfection of combs and other hair-care instruments can prevent repeat infections in susceptible individuals.

HISTOLOGICAL FINDINGS
The common denominator and pathognomonic finding in all cases of endothrix tinea capitis is the presence of spores (and sometimes hyphae) within the hair shaft (Figs. 33.7–33.11).

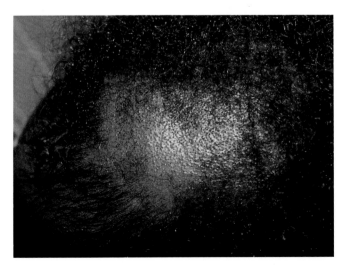

Figure 33.1 This image portrays a nine-month-old African-American baby with "black dot" tinea capitis caused by *Trichophyton tonsurans*. Although there is extensive hair loss, clinical inflammation (erythema, scaling) is not present.

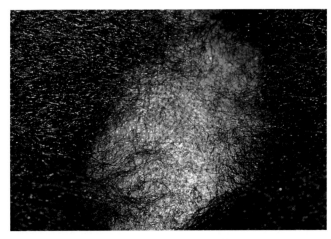

Figure 33.2 "Black dot" tinea capitis in another African-American patient; again, clinical signs of inflammation are not present.

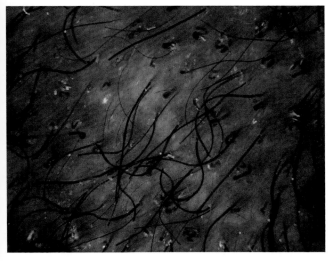

Figure 33.3 Corkscrew and comma shaped broken-off hairs are visible in this dermoscopic image from a patient with "black dot" tinea capitis. The infected hairs are weakened, fragile, and easily broken. *Source*: Image courtesy of Antonella Tosti, M.D.

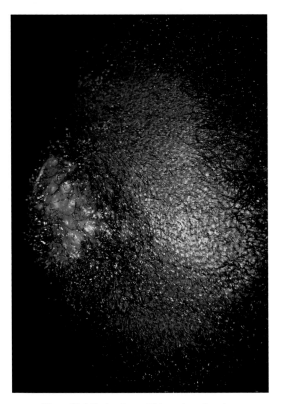

Figure 33.4 Kerion in an African-American boy.

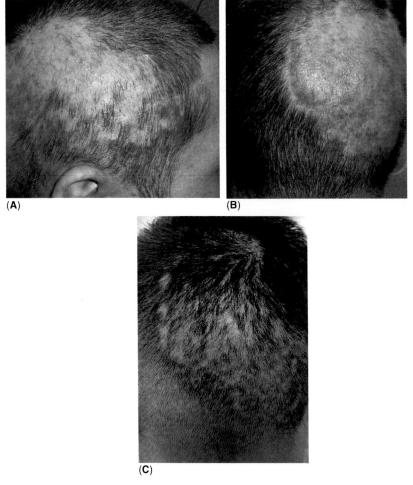

Figure 33.5 Highly inflammatory tinea capitis caused by *Trichophyton tonsurans* and mimicking dissecting cellulitis in a Caucasian patient, shown before (**A** and **B**) and during treatment (**C**).

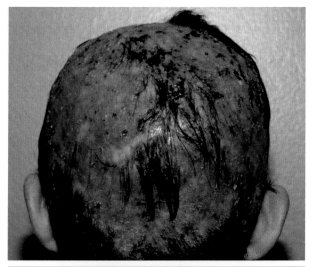

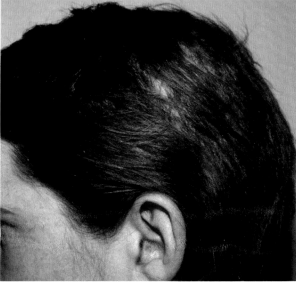

Figure 33.6 Another case of severe, inflammatory tinea capitis in a 13-year-old Caucasian patient, shown before (*upper panel*) and 5 months after (*lower panel*) systemic treatment. Complete regrowth was ultimately achieved in this patient.

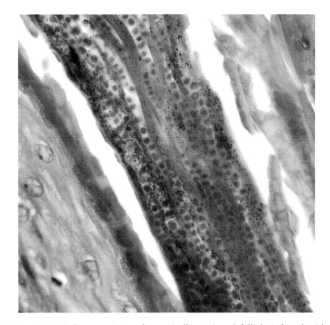

Figure 33.7 High-power view of a vertically sectioned follicle infected with endothrix fungal spores.

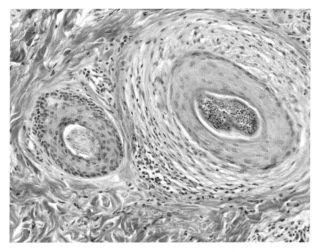

Figure 33.8 Transverse section of follicle infected with fungal spores (endothrix). The affected shaft (*right side*) is adjacent to another that is spared.

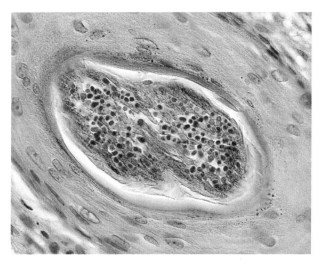

Figure 33.9 Transverse section of follicle infected with fungal spores (endothrix). This is a higher power view of the same follicle seen in Figure 33.8. The fungal spores are clearly visible, even with this hematoxylin and eosin stain.

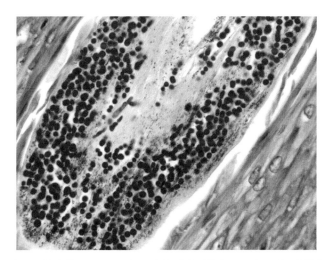

Figure 33.10 Transverse section of the infundibular portion of a follicle infected with fungal spores (endothrix), PAS stain. The fungal spores are further highlighted with a PAS stain. *Abbreviations*: PAS, periodic acid–Schiff.

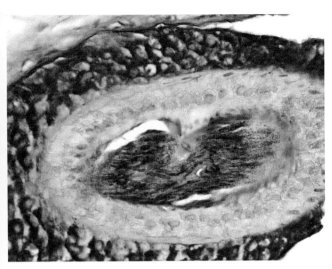

Figure 33.11 Transverse section of the suprabulbar portion of a follicle infected with fungal hyphae (endothrix), PAS stain. The PAS stain is helpful in visualizing the hyphae at this level. The stain also highlights glycogen within the outer root sheath. *Abbreviations*: PAS, periodic acid–Schiff.

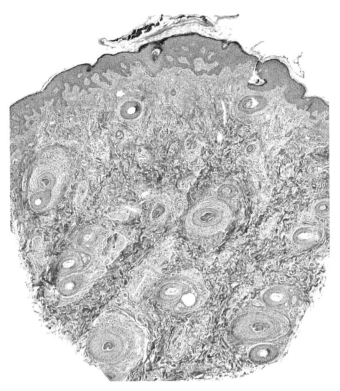

Figure 33.13 There is a mix of affected and unaffected follicles within this specimen. There is relatively mild perifollicular fibrosis and inflammation surrounding affected follicles. The overlying scale-crust also serves as a clue to the diagnosis.

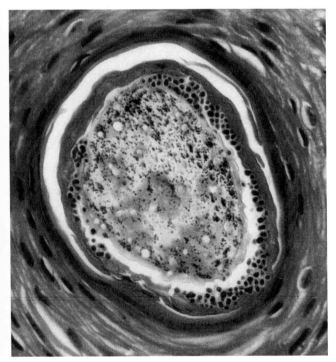

Figure 33.12 Transverse section of a follicle infected with ectothrix fungal spores. The spores are surrounding the hair shaft, but not invading the shaft itself.

In ectothrix infections, such as *M. canis*, the organisms will surround the hair shaft (Fig. 33.12). Only a few follicles within a specimen may demonstrate the finding, and therefore, transverse sectioning is the most reliable way to establish the diagnosis. The degree of inflammation seen on histopathology is highly variable. In some cases, hairs packed with spores incite surprisingly little inflammation (Figs. 33.13 and 33.14).

A superficial and/or deep perifollicular infiltrate rich in neutrophils, eosinophils, and lymphocytes may be present (Figs. 33.15–33.17). Such cases are often associated with pustules or a purulent discharge and crusting. Prolonged brisk inflammation can result in follicular destruction with granulomatous inflammation. Biopsy of a kerion reveals dense suppurative and mixed inflammation with follicular destruction and a granulomatous response (Fig. 33.18).

Exceptional cases of inflammatory tinea capitis resembling dissecting cellulitis (Figs. 33.19–33.28) have a deep, dense lymphocytic infiltrate that surrounds hair bulbs and extends into the fat (14) (Fig. 33.19). Hairs adjacent to the zone of inflammation may be converted to the catagen/telogen phase (Figs. 33.26 and 33.27), although this is not always the case (Fig. 33.28). Ironically, although clinical findings and degree of histological inflammation are quite dramatic, infected follicles may be difficult to find. In these cases, fungal cultures may be required to establish the diagnosis.

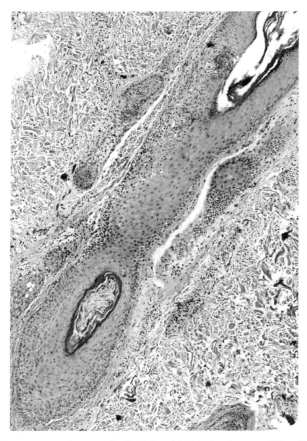

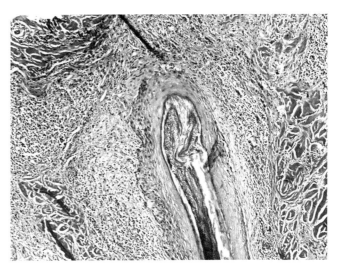

Figure 33.16 Fungal spores disrupt the hair shaft superiorly. There is exocytosis of lymphocytes into the outermost aspect of the follicular epithelium.

Figure 33.14 Another example of an infected follicle showing very mild perifollicular inflammation despite the densely packed fungal spores within the shaft.

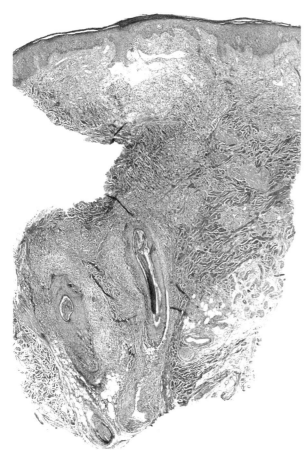

Figure 33.15 The inflammatory response is much more brisk in this specimen as compared with the previous figure.

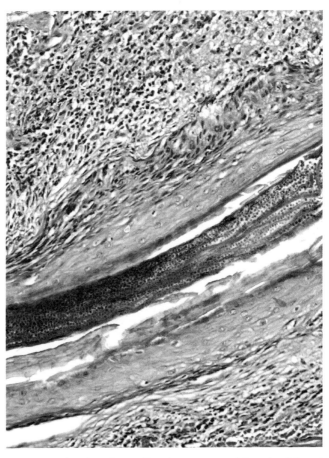

Figure 33.17 There is a mixture of lymphocytes, neutrophils, eosinophils, and plasma cells surrounding the infected follicle.

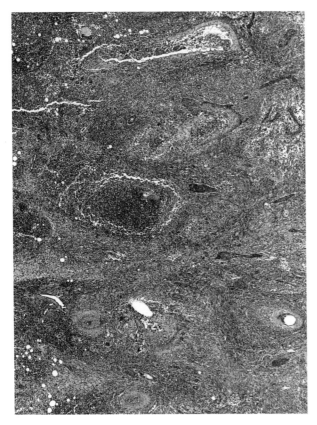

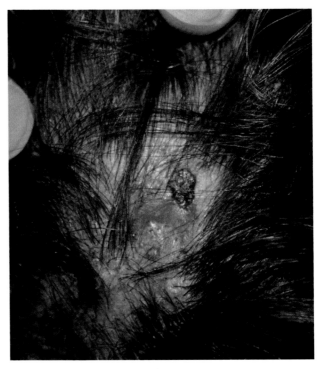

Figure 33.20 Tinea capitis resembling dissecting cellulitis in a 20-year-old wrestler who also had Majocchi's granuloma on the abdomen (Figs. 33.21, 33.22). There were multiple foci of involvement within the scalp.

Figure 33.18 This biopsy of a kerion shows dense suppurative and mixed inflammation with destruction of the follicles leading to a granulomatous response.

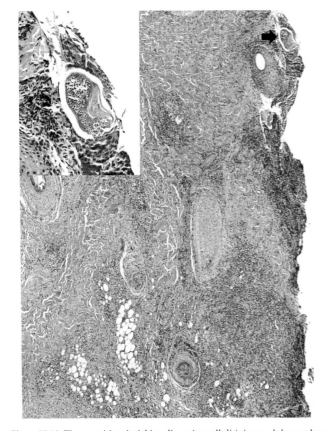

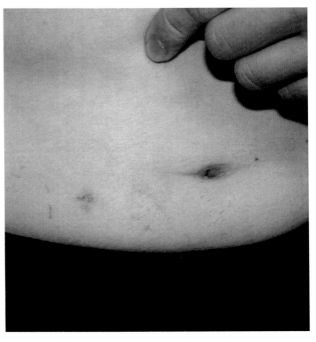

Figure 33.21 Majocchi's granuloma on the abdomen of the wrestler pictured in Figure 33.20.

Figure 33.19 Tinea capitis mimicking dissecting cellulitis in an adolescent boy. The dense inflammation preferentially involves the deep dermis and superficial panniculus. After multiple sections, only one shaft demonstrated the fungal organism (arrow indicates the affected shaft, which is shown at higher power in the inset image). A culture identified the causative organism as *Trichophyton tonsurans*.

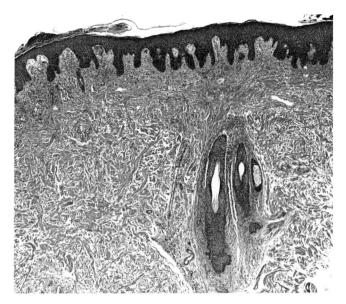

Figure 33.22 Low power view of Majocchi's granuloma on the abdomen of the wrestler pictured in Figures 33.20 and 33.21.

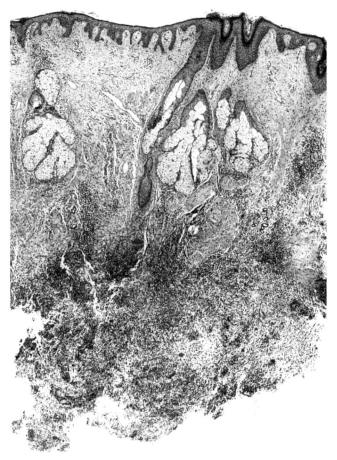

Figure 33.24 Tinea capitis resembling dissecting cellulitis (same patient as in Figs. 33.20–33.23). Infected follicles were not identified in the scalp biopsy despite numerous sections and periodic acid–Schiff stains. The sample from the abdomen helped to solidify the diagnosis. The patient responded to treatment with systemic antifungals with clearance of the plaque and regrowth of >50% of the hair in the affected scalp after two months.

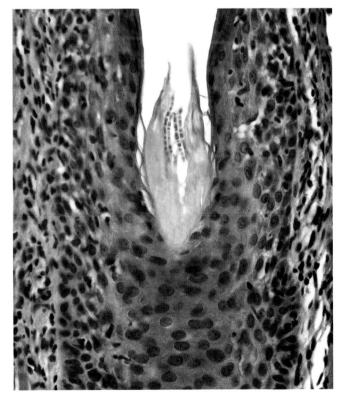

Figure 33.23 High-power view of the Majocchi's granuloma pictured in Figure 33.22, with visible fungal hyphae within the follicle.

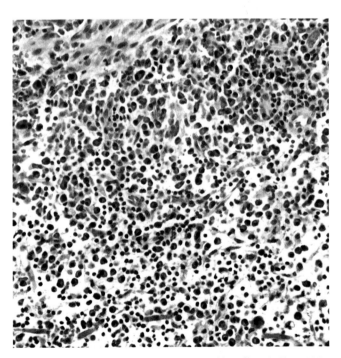

Figure 33.25 High-power view of the deep portion of the infiltrate in Figure 33.24. The infiltrate is composed predominantly of plasma cells and lymphocytes.

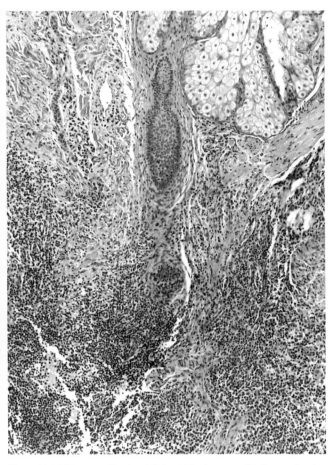

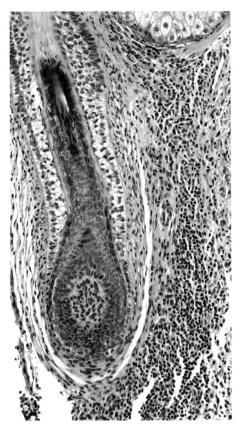

Figure 33.28 Occasionally anagen hairs may remain seemingly unaffected despite being surrounded by dense inflammation.

Figure 33.26 The centrally placed hair within the zone of inflammation has shifted into the catagen/telogen phase. Its bulb is nearly obscured by the dense lymphoplasmacytic infiltrate.

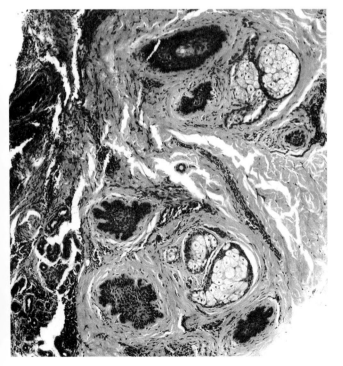

Figure 33.27 Several hairs adjacent to the zone of inflammation have shifted into the catagen/telogen phase.

Tinea Capitis in Summary

Clinical correlation: patients are most often children with alopecic, scaly alopecic patches on the scalp. In children with darkly pigmented hair widened follicular ostia containing the broken pigmented shafts ("black dots") may be visible. The clinical manifestations of inflammation are highly variable and range from mild scaling without erythema to intense redness, induration, pustules, and a purulent discharge.

Histological findings:
❖ Spores (and sometimes hyphae) within (or surrounding) hair shafts are diagnostic
• The amount of perifollicular inflammation is highly variable
• A superficial and/or deep perifollicular infiltrate rich in neutrophils, eosinophils, and lymphocytes may be present

Histological differential diagnosis:
• None, when spores or hyphae are identified
• In the absence of obvious fungal elements, the histopathological findings can be those of an inflammatory cicatricial alopecia without a specific pattern suggestive of another disease; rarely it can mimic the deep inflammatory pattern of dissecting cellulitis

⚠ **Pitfalls**

- Infected follicles may be few; therefore, vertical sections can lead to a false-negative evaluation if an affected follicle is not sectioned
- Infected follicles may be difficult to find in cases of dissecting cellulitis-like tinea capitis; therefore, fungal culture may be a more reliable way to establish the diagnosis

REFERENCES

1. Elewski BE. Tinea capitis: a current perspective. J Am Acad Dermatol 2000; 42(1 Pt 1): 1–20; quiz 21–24.
2. Tack DA, Fleishcer A Jr, McMichael A, Feldman S. The epidemic of tinea capitis disproportionately affects school-aged African Americans. Pediatr Dermatol 1999; 16: 75.
3. Lobato MN, Vugia DJ, Frieden IJ. Tinea capitis in California children: a population-based study of a growing epidemic. Pediatrics 1997; 99: 551–4.
4. Coley MK, Bhanusali DG, Silverberg JI, Alexis AF, Silverberg NB. Scalp hyperkeratosis and alopecia in children of color. J Drugs Dermatol 2011; 10: 511–6.
5. Silverberg NB, Weinberg JM, DeLeo VA. Tinea capitis: focus on African American women. J Am Acad Dermatol 2002; 46(2 Suppl Understanding): S120–4.
6. Aly R. Ecology, epidemiology and diagnosis of tinea capitis. Pediatr Infect Dis J 1999; 18: 180–5.
7. Kralund H, Paulsen E. [Protracted case of kerion Celsi in otherwise healthy seven year-old girl]. Ugeskr Laeger 20 2011; 173: 1805–6.
8. Kemna ME, Elewski BE. A U.S. epidemiologic survey of superficial fungal diseases. J Am Acad Dermatol 1996; 35: 539–42.
9. Coloe JR, Diab M, Moennich J, et al. Tinea capitis among children in the Columbus area, Ohio, USA. Mycoses 2010; 53: 158–62.
10. Hughes R, Chiaverini C, Bahadoran P, Lacour JP. Corkscrew hair: a new dermoscopic sign for diagnosis of tinea capitis in black children. Arch Dermatol 2011; 147: 355–6.
11. Slowinska M, Rudnicka L, Schwartz RA, et al. Comma hairs: a dermatoscopic marker for tinea capitis: a rapid diagnostic method. J Am Acad Dermatol 2008; 59(5 Suppl): S77–9.
12. Mirmirani P, Willey A, Chamlin S, Frieden IJ, Price VH. Tinea capitis mimicking cicatricial alopecia: what host and dermatophyte factors lead to this unusual clinical presentation? J Am Acad Dermatol 2009; 60: 490–5.
13. Tangjaturonrusamee C, Piraccini BM, Vincenzi C, Starace M, Tosti A. Tinea capitis mimicking folliculitis decalvans. Mycoses 2011; 54: 87–8.
14. Sperling LC. Inflammatory tinea capitis (kerion) mimicking dissecting cellulitis. Occurrence in two adolescents. Int J Dermatol 1991; 30: 190–2.

34 Trichodysplasia of immunosuppression

Trichodysplasia of immunosuppression (TI; also known as trichodysplasia spinulosa (1), viral-associated trichodysplasia in patients who are immunocompromised (2), and pilomatrix dysplasia (3)) was first described by Haycox in 1999 (1). Most reports describe patients who are undergoing drug-induced immunosuppression to prevent organ transplant rejection, but involvement in patients with other states of immunosuppression, such as lymphoma (4) or leukemia (5), has been described. One patient with chronic lymphocytic leukemia (in remission) developed trichodysplasia spinulosa 2 months after ceasing chemotherapy (5). At least 20 patients with TI have been reported (6), and the majority of them were kidney or heart transplant recipients on a variety of multidrug, immunosuppressive "cocktails." Patients of all ages have been described, several of them in the pediatric age group (7–9).

CLINICAL FINDINGS
Patients have numerous erythematous papules concentrated in the central portion of the face. There is a variable degree of

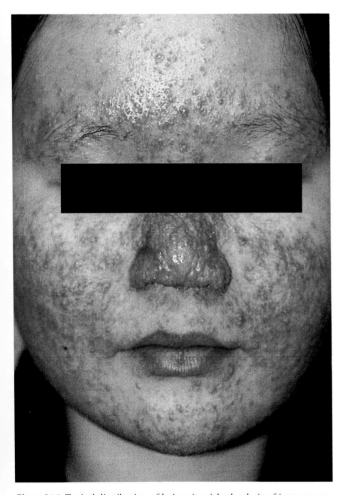

Figure 34.1 Typical distribution of lesions in trichodysplasia of immunosuppression. Note loss of eyebrow hair. The patient's scalp hair was normal. *Source:* Image courtesy of Dr. Douglas Thomas.

hair loss, most severely affecting facial hair (Fig. 34.1). Eyebrow hairs are often prominently affected. Many patients have friable follicular spines (hence the term *spinulosa* (1)) emerging from follicular ostia, particularly on the nose (Fig. 34.2).

The first reported successful treatment for TI was cidofovir 3% cream (2), and this has been used with success in other patients (10). More recently, oral valganciclovir therapy has been used with success in some patients (7,11), but failed to work in another (8). In one patient with acute lymphocytic leukemia, the TI resolved once the patient's immune function returned to normal (total disease duration of 2 years) (12).

HISTOLOGICAL FINDINGS
The histological picture of these facial papules is so distinctive that it is unlikely to be confused with any other condition (1–4). Hair follicles stain brilliantly on hematoxylin and eosin, are markedly distended, and have a bulbous appearance (Fig. 34.3). The infundibula are shaftless, dilated, and plugged with hyperkeratotic material (Fig. 34.4). Hair bulbs lack an obvious hair papilla (Fig. 34.5). A thin rim of basaloid, germinative-type cells surrounds a proliferation of inner root sheath (IRS)-type cells containing abnormally large trichohyaline granules (Fig. 34.6). These cells abruptly cornify without the presence of a granular layer into a pale pink acellular material consistent with IRS. In the suprabulbar zone, and persisting throughout the lower segment of the follicle, are nucleated cells with enlarged trichohyaline granules. These occupy most of the follicular epithelium, and are surrounded with only a thin outer root sheath (Fig. 34.7). The overall histological picture suggests that the entire machinery of the follicular bulb is devoted to the manufacture of IRS-type keratin (Fig. 34.8) (4). The infundibular plugs, seen clinically as "spiny" projections, are not hair shafts. They are cornified IRS cells. IRS-type cornification can be identified by intense staining with toluidine blue (Fig. 34.9).

ELECTRON MICROSCOPY FINDINGS
When Haycox et al. first used electron microscopy (EM) to study tissue from a patient with TI, they found intracellular viral particles with a size and appearance consistent with those in the Papovaviridae family (1). EM of negatively stained extract from a homogenized lesion also demonstrated icosahedral viruses with papovavirus morphology (1). Similar intranuclear viral particles were found in the second reported case of TI (Fig. 34.10) (2). Recently, through the use of a newly designed quantitative, viral-specific polymerase chain reaction, the "trichodysplasia spinulosa-associated polyomavirus (TSV)" has been identified as a close relative of Bornean orangutan polyomavirus, and a distant relative of the Merkel cell polyomavirus (10). TSV has been found in other patients by other investigators (6).

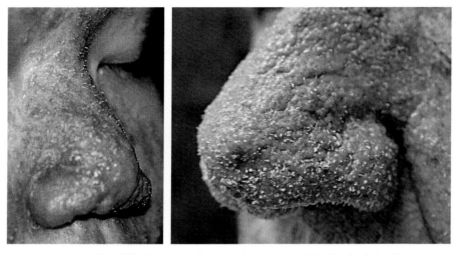

Figure 34.2 Minute, spiny projections emerging from follicular ostia on the noses of two patients with trichodysplasia of immunosuppression. *Source*: The image on the left is courtesy of Dr. Douglas Thomas and the image on the right is courtesy of Dr. Jeff Heller.

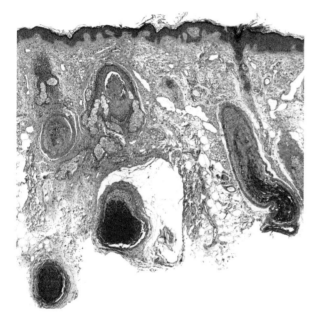

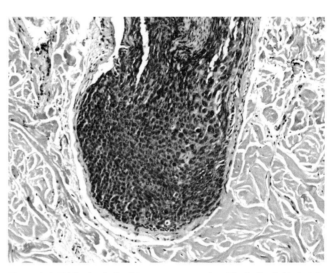

Figure 34.5 Trichodysplasia of immunosuppression. The bulb of this hair is enlarged and has no apparent hair papilla.

Figure 34.3 In trichodysplasia of immunosuppression, the follicular bulbs are bulbous and the lumina are distended with eosinophilic, cornified material.

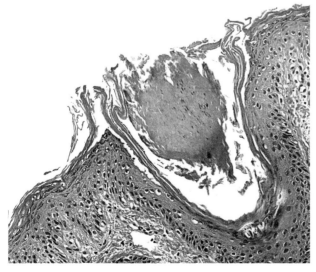

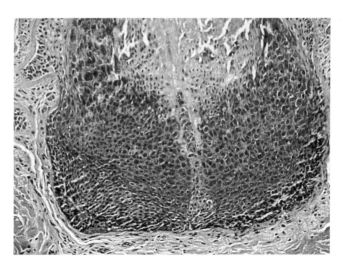

Figure 34.4 The infundibulum is distended with a cornified plug. No hair shaft is present.

Figure 34.6 Trichodysplasia of immunosuppression, showing an abnormally broad hair bulb with a relatively thin rim of basophilic, germinative cells and a wide, central zone of more eosinophilic cells.

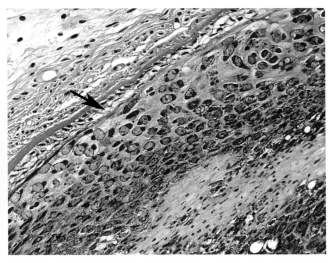

Figure 34.7 Trichodysplasia of immunosuppression. The suprabulbar zone consists of a central zone of homogenous, eosinophilic material surrounded by a broad zone of inner root sheath-type cells containing enlarged trichohyaline granules (stained magenta in this image). The outer root sheath (*arrow*) is abnormally thin.

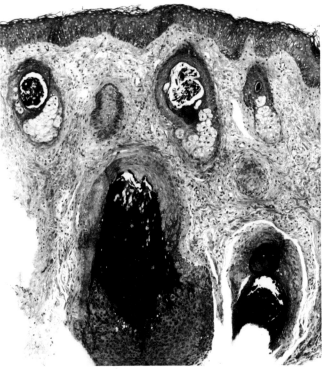

Figure 34.9 Toluidine blue highlights the inner root sheath material filling the lumen of these trichodysplasia of immunosuppression follicles.

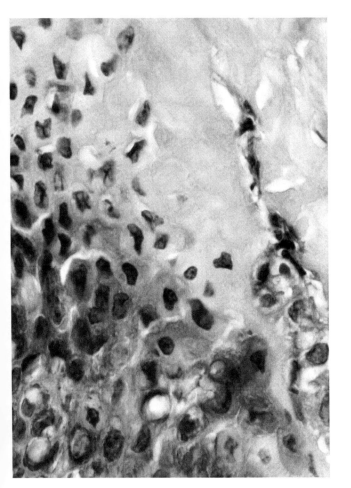

Figure 34.8 Trichodysplasia of immunosuppression. The zone above the central portion of the hair bulb, normally the site of a newly forming hair shaft, is instead filled with cornified inner root sheath material.

Trichodysplasia of Immunosuppression in Summary

Clinical correlation: an immunosuppressed patient, such as an organ transplant recipient, or a patient with a hematopoietic malignancy (lymphoma or leukemia), who develops numerous central facial papules and alopecia of the eyebrows.

Histological findings:
❖ Bulbous and markedly distended hair follicles
❖ Absence of hair shafts, with follicular lumina instead filled by inner root sheath-like cornified debris
❖ Enlarged bulbs with an abnormally thin germinative layer and inconspicuous hair papilla
• Clusters of intranuclear viral particles can be found with electron microscopy

Histological differential diagnosis:
• Unlikely to be confused with any other entity

⚠ Pitfalls
Despite the distinctive clinical and histological features the condition is rare, and therefore unfamiliar to many dermatologists and dermatopathologists.

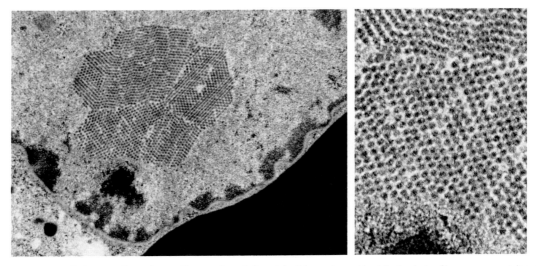

Figure 34.10 Electron micrograph showing a large cluster of intranuclear viral particles from patient with trichodysplasia of immunosuppression; on the *left panel*, the nuclear membrane is highlighted in pink; on the right side, viral particles are seen magnified further, and are the size and shape of polyomavirus capsids.

REFERENCES

1. Haycox CL, Kim S, Fleckman P, et al. Trichodysplasia spinulosa–a newly described folliculocentric viral infection in an immunocompromised host. J Investig Dermatol Symp Proc 1999; 4: 268–71.
2. Sperling LC, Tomaszewski MM, Thomas DA. Viral-associated trichodysplasia in patients who are immunocompromised. J Am Acad Dermatol 2004; 50: 318–22.
3. Chastain MA, Millikan LE. Pilomatrix dysplasia in an immunosuppressed patient. J Am Acad Dermatol 2000; 43(1 Pt 1): 118–22.
4. Osswald SS, Kulick KB, Tomaszewski MM, Sperling LC. Viral-associated trichodysplasia in a patient with lymphoma: a case report and review. J Cutan Pathol 2007; 34: 721–5.
5. Lee JS, Frederiksen P, Kossard S. Progressive trichodysplasia spinulosa in a patient with chronic lymphocytic leukaemia in remission. Australas J Dermatol 2008; 49: 57–60.
6. Matthews MR, Wang RC, Reddick RL, Saldivar VA, Browning JC. Viral-associated trichodysplasia spinulosa: a case with electron microscopic and molecular detection of the trichodysplasia spinulosa-associated human polyomavirus. J Cutan Pathol.
7. Benoit T, Bacelieri R, Morrell DS, Metcalf J. Viral-associated trichodysplasia of immunosuppression: report of a pediatric patient with response to oral valganciclovir. Arch Dermatol 146: 871–4.
8. Schwieger-Briel A, Balma-Mena A, Ngan B, Dipchand A, Pope E. Trichodysplasia spinulosa–a rare complication in immunosuppressed patients. Pediatr Dermatol 27: 509–13.
9. Wyatt AJ, Sachs DL, Shia J, Delgado R, Busam KJ. Virus-associated trichodysplasia spinulosa. Am J Surg Pathol 2005; 29: 241–6.
10. van der Meijden E, Janssens RW, Lauber C, et al. Discovery of a new human polyomavirus associated with trichodysplasia spinulosa in an immunocompromized patient. PLoS Pathog 6: e1001024.
11. Holzer AM, Hughey LC. Trichodysplasia of immunosuppression treated with oral valganciclovir. J Am Acad Dermatol 2009; 60: 169–72.
12. Sadler GM, Halbert AR, Smith N, Rogers M. Trichodysplasia spinulosa associated with chemotherapy for acute lymphocytic leukaemia. Australas J Dermatol 2007; 48:110–4.

35 Chemotherapy-induced alopecia

Hair loss due to systemic chemotherapy has traditionally been viewed as an anagen effluvium or anagen arrest (as opposed to telogen effluvium or cicatricial alopecia). The reasonable hypothesis is that the follicular machinery is suppressed by the chemotherapeutic agent, resulting in the formation of hair shafts of diminished thickness. The shafts taper down to a point, and are then shed as "pencil point" or tapered hairs, as described in chapter 36. This hypothesis presupposes that most hairs remain in the anagen phase while shaft production is greatly diminished. Prompt hair regrowth at the end of a chemotherapy session would seem to support the concept of anagen effluvium.

The mechanism of hair loss is partly dependent on the chemotherapeutic agent. Certain medications, such as methotrexate, 5-fluorouracil, and the retinoids often result in a telogen effluvium (1). In contrast, cyclophosphamide, etoposide, topotecan, and paclitaxel typically result in an anagen effluvium. Mouse models have been used to explore the underlying pathophysiology of hair loss during chemotherapy. In one study examining mice exposed to cyclophosphamide (2), the authors demonstrated that p53 is essential for the process because in contrast to wild-type mice, p53-deficient mice show neither hair loss nor apoptosis of the follicular keratinocytes.

One revealing study (3) examined shed and plucked hairs in breast cancer patients who were about to receive cycles of chemotherapy with cyclophosphamide, methotrexate, and 5-fluorouracil. The authors did not perform biopsies. During chemotherapy, shed hairs were predominantly telogen hairs, although fractured shafts were fairly common. The major anatomic change noted was proximal hair shaft tapering. Many of the abnormal, tapered telogen hairs had diminutive bulbs. Fracturing of hairs with diminutive bulbs produced typical "exclamation mark" hairs. The authors concluded that the major effect of cytotoxic drugs used in this study were tapering of the proximal hair shaft and premature entry of the follicle into telogen. This conflicts with the conventional view that affected hair follicles continue in anagen. Given the tapering of hair shafts, the authors proposed the term "atrophic telogen effluvium" to describe the pattern of hair loss. We feel that the findings described are strikingly reminiscent of those seen in rapidly progressive alopecia areata, a concept that is discussed later in this chapter.

CLINICAL FINDINGS

Most patients treated with systemic chemotherapy have some degree of diffuse alopecia, the severity determined by the medication, the dosage, and probably patient-specific predispositions. Although most hair loss is temporary, it is possible that a majority of patients permanently lose at least a fraction of their hair, but only permanent alopecia that is clinically obvious has been evaluated histologically. The following findings must be regarded as tentative, pending good prospective studies with adequate histological correlation.

HISTOLOGICAL FINDINGS

There are several articles that address some of the histopathological features occurring in patients with permanent hair loss due to chemotherapy (1,4–9). This information pertains to an unusual situation (permanent hair loss) and describes the end result of damage that occurred long before the time of biopsy. Although hair loss is very common with the use of systemic chemotherapy, there are no prospective (or even good retrospective) studies of the histopathology of hair loss *during* treatment. In part this is because hair loss is usually temporary and regrowth is predictable. Also, any research study involving elective biopsies in an emotionally vulnerable population is an unappealing prospect for patients, physicians, and institutional review boards alike. Nevertheless, certain studies do shed light on the effects of chemotherapy on hair. One group of authors (9) described an unusual case of permanent alopecia in a patient who received adjuvant chemotherapy for breast carcinoma. They found a "unique histologic finding" of replacement of anagen hair follicles by linear columns of basaloid epithelium (Fig. 35.1).

One intriguing data set that may shed some light on the subject has been collected by Dr. David Whiting in Dallas, Texas (personal communication). He studied biopsy specimens from a group of patients who had received docetaxal (a taxane) in combination with other chemotherapeutic agents. These patients lost the expected amount of hair during treatment, but hair regrowth was incomplete with a variable degree of persistent alopecia. In most cases the pattern of hair loss was diffuse or resembled the pattern of common balding, and most biopsies were performed a few years after termination of chemotherapy. The histological findings are remarkably similar between specimens and may prove to be a paradigm for the changes that occur during or after chemotherapy. The common denominators in Dr. Whiting's collection of specimens include the following: (*i*) a normal or nearly normal total number of follicles (Fig. 35.2); (*ii*) a marked increase in the percentage of miniaturized hairs (Figs. 35.3 and 35.4); (*iii*) a marked increase in the percentage of telogen follicles, especially when miniaturized follicles are included in the counts (Figs. 35.5 and 35.6); (*iv*) preservation of sebaceous glands (Fig. 35.7); and (*v*) no significant deep or destructive inflammation.

This set of histological features is consistent with severe androgenetic alopecia, but also resembles the findings seen in alopecia areata, with the exception of the peribulbar inflammation found in alopecia areata. In fact, these post-docetaxal/chemotherapy specimens are an exact mimic of the "noninflammatory" pattern of alopecia areata, replete with nanogen follicles. Perhaps chemotherapy-induced hair loss and alopecia areata share pathogenic features, at least for portions of the physiological cascade resulting in hair loss. Alternatively, chemotherapy-induced alopecia may uncover, exacerbate, or accelerate androgenetic alopecia, at least in a subset of patients. These possibilities provide avenues for future research and treatment.

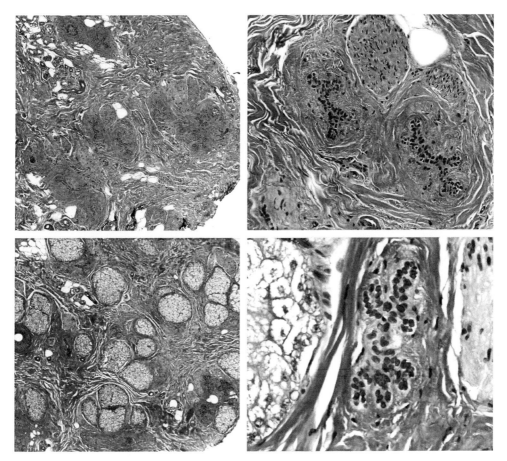

Figure 35.1 Biopsy from a patient with permanent alopecia following chemotherapy for breast carcinoma. Anagen hair follicles are replaced by linear columns of basaloid epithelium. *Source*: Images courtesy of Dr. Lynne Goldberg.

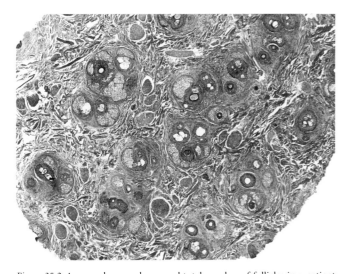

Figure 35.2 A normal or nearly normal total number of follicles in a patient treated with docetaxal. Slide contributed by Dr. David Whiting.

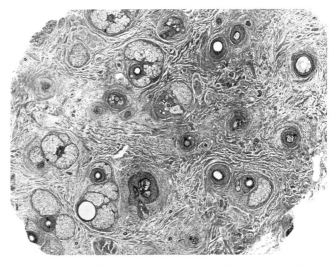

Figure 35.3 A marked increase in the percentage of miniaturized hairs in a patient treated with docetaxal. Slide contributed by Dr. David Whiting.

Several published reports document permanent hair loss in a small number of patients who receive chemotherapy (4–7,9,10). The pathological features described in permanent alopecia from busulfan (10) include reduced follicular density in the absence of fibrosis, suggesting that alopecia resulted either from hair follicle stem cell destruction or from acute damage to the keratinocytes of the lower portion of some follicles. In a report of 10 cases of permanent alopecia from chemotherapy (4), taxanes were implicated in 6 and busulfan in 3.

Biopsy samples were obtained at least 12–24 months after completion of chemotherapy. The characteristic findings were a decrease in hair density and percentage of anagen hairs, and an increase in the percentage of telogen hairs, miniaturized hairs, and follicular streamers. Many follicular units contained two or more telogen hairs. These findings are very similar to those seen in androgenetic alopecia, although the clinical setting is inconsistent with common balding. In cases with very high catagen/telogen counts and numerous nanogen hairs producing little if any hair shaft, the noninflammatory form of alopecia areata would have to be added to the histological differential diagnosis. The increased percentage of miniaturized hairs suggests the possibility of clinical improvement with the use of topical minoxidil solution (11).

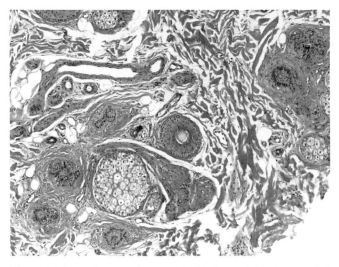

Figure 35.6 Biopsy from a patient treated with docetaxal showing a marked increase in the percentage of telogen follicles, especially when miniaturized follicles are included in the counts. Slide contributed by Dr. David Whiting.

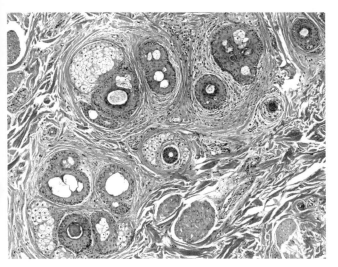

Figure 35.4 A marked increase in the percentage of miniaturized hairs in a patient treated with docetaxal. Slide contributed by Dr. David Whiting.

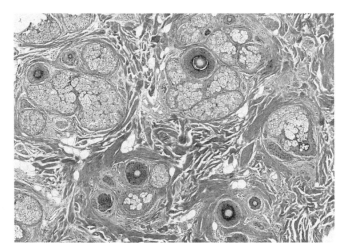

Figure 35.7 Preservation of sebaceous glands in a patient treated with docetaxal. Slide contributed by Dr. David Whiting.

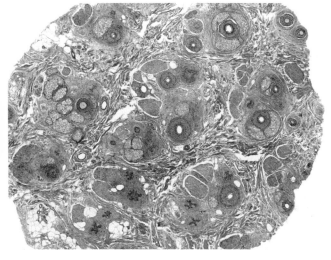

Figure 35.5 Biopsy from a patient treated with docetaxal showing a marked increase in the percentage of telogen follicles, especially when miniaturized follicles are included in the counts. Slide contributed by Dr. David Whiting.

Chemotherapy-induced Alopecia in Summary

Clinical correlation: diffuse alopecia, with severity determined by medication, dosage, and probably patient-specific predispositions. Most hair loss is temporary. It is possible that most patients permanently lose a fraction of their hair. The following findings must be regarded as tentative, pending good prospective studies with adequate histological correlation.

Histological findings (following chemotherapy):
❖ Normal or nearly normal total number of follicles
❖ Marked increase in the percentage of miniaturized hairs
❖ Marked increase in the percentage of telogen follicles, especially when miniaturized follicles are included in the counts
❖ No significant deep or destructive inflammation
• Preservation of sebaceous glands

Histological differential diagnosis:

- **Alopecia areata:** reveals at least a few follicles with peribulbar inflammation
- **Androgenetic alopecia:** the percentage of telogen terminal hairs is usually much less than with chemotherapy
- **Psoriatic alopecia:** shares the catagen/telogen shift and miniaturization but shows diminished sebaceous glands

Histological findings (permanent alopecia secondary to chemotherapy):

- ❖ Decreased total number of follicles
- ❖ Marked increase in the percentage of miniaturized hairs
- ❖ Increase in the percentage of telogen follicles, especially when miniaturized follicles are included in the counts
- Preservation of sebaceous glands
- No significant deep or destructive inflammation

Histological differential diagnosis:

- **Androgenetic alopecia:** total number of hairs usually not reduced; historical information should allow for differentiation

⚠ **Pitfalls**

Separating components of telogen effluvium, androgenetic alopecia, and chemotherapy effect may be impossible. All three processes may be simultaneously present.

REFERENCES

1. Yeager CE, Olsen EA. Treatment of chemotherapy-induced alopecia. Dermatol Ther 2011; 24: 432–42.
2. Botchkarev VA, Komarova EA, Siebenhaar F, et al. p53 is essential for chemotherapy-induced hair loss. Cancer Res 2000; 60: 5002–6.
3. Bleiker TO, Nicolaou N, Traulsen J, Hutchinson PE. 'Atrophic telogen effluvium' from cytotoxic drugs and a randomized controlled trial to investigate the possible protective effect of pretreatment with a topical vitamin D analogue in humans. Br J Dermatol 2005; 153: 103–12.
4. Miteva M, Misciali C, Fanti PA, et al. Permanent alopecia after systemic chemotherapy: a clinicopathological study of 10 cases. Am J Dermatopathol 2011; 33: 345–50.
5. Tran D, Sinclair RD, Schwarer AP, Chow CW. Permanent alopecia following chemotherapy and bone marrow transplantation. Australas J Dermatol 2000; 41: 106–8.
6. de Jonge ME, Mathot RA, Dalesio O, et al. Relationship between irreversible alopecia and exposure to cyclophosphamide, thiotepa and carboplatin (CTC) in high-dose chemotherapy. Bone Marrow Transplant 2002; 30: 593–7.
7. Masidonski P, Mahon SM. Permanent alopecia in women being treated for breast cancer. Clin J Oncol Nurs 2009; 13: 13–4.
8. Al-Mohanna H, Al-Khenaizan S. Permanent alopecia following cranial irradiation in a child. J cutan Med Surg 2010; 14: 141–3.
9. Tallon B, Blanchard E, Goldberg LJ. Permanent chemotherapy-induced alopecia: case report and review of the literature. J Am Acad Dermatol 2010; 63: 333–6.
10. Tosti A, Piraccini BM, Vincenzi C, Misciali C. Permanent alopecia after busulfan chemotherapy. Br J Dermatol 2005; 152: 1056–8.
11. Prevezas C, Matard B, Pinquier L, Reygagne P. Irreversible and severe alopecia following docetaxel or paclitaxel cytotoxic therapy for breast cancer. Br J Dermatol 2009; 160: 883–5.

36 Overview of hair shaft disorders

Pathologists, dermatopathologists, and dermatologists are sometimes called upon to identify a hair shaft disorder based on a submitted sample of hair. This section will focus on describing the morphologic features of shaft disorders as seen by light microscopy. Several excellent general reviews of hair shaft disorders are available and are listed in the reference section (1–6). The genetic basis of many of these disorders has also been reviewed (7,8).

TRICHORRHEXIS NODOSA

The basic cause of trichorrhexis nodosa is trauma to the hair shafts, but any inherent weakness of the shaft may result in this defect. All of the various forms of weathering (grooming, washing, styling, and so on) can cause or worsen the disorder. Examples of physical trauma include excessive brushing, the application of heat (9), hair pulling or twisting (10), and scratching due to pruritic scalp disorders (11,12). Examples of chemical trauma include permanent straightening (13)

("relaxing"), permanent waving, dyeing, and shampooing. Clinically, trichorrhexis nodosa may appear as small, white or gray specks on the hair shafts. Affected hairs are susceptible to fracture, which can result in patchy or diffuse alopecia, depending on the extent of involvement (Fig. 36.1). Although scalp hair is usually affected, trichorrhexis nodosa can be found on pubic hair and other hairy areas of the body (12).

Trichorrhexis nodosa is often found in association with other types of hair shaft abnormalities caused by weathering or inherited hair fragility disorders, such as trichothiodystrophy (TTD) (14) and argininosuccinicaciduria (5,15). Therefore, *trichoclasis* ("greenstick fractures"), *trichoptilosis* ("split ends"; Fig. 36.2) and *trichoschisis* (see below) are often found in hairs from the same patient or even the same shaft (Fig. 36.3).

The "nodes" of trichorrhexis nodosa represent foci of frayed cortical fibers that bulge out through a ruptured cuticle. Scanning electron microscopy has shown that the earliest change is a focal loss of cuticular cells, which eventually results in hair

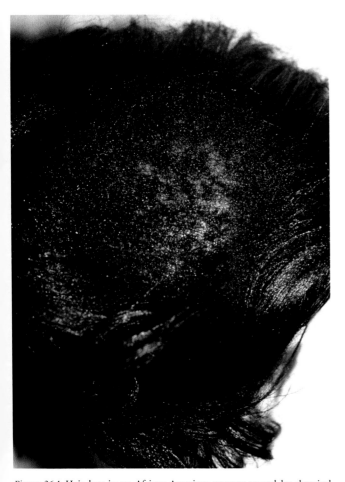

Figure 36.1 Hair loss in an African-American woman caused by chemical relaxers. Longer hairs along the margins of the "bald spot" showed dramatic trichorrhexis nodosa of the proximal shafts. Hair loss was due to fractures of the damaged shafts.

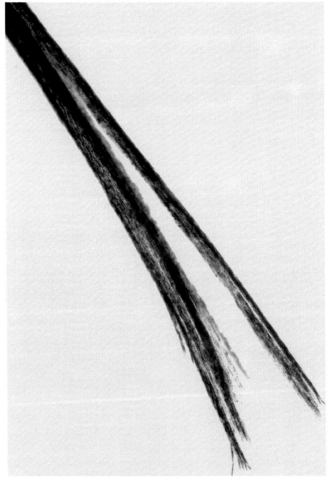

Figure 36.2 Trichoptilosis (split ends)

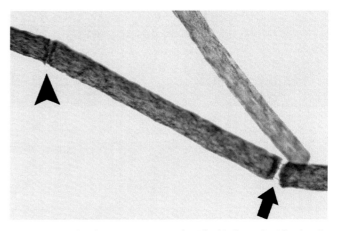

Figure 36.6 Trichoschisis in a patient with trichothiodystrophy. The sharply defined transverse fracture results in marked hair fragility. The arrowhead points to an incipient fracture, and the arrow shows a nearly complete fracture.

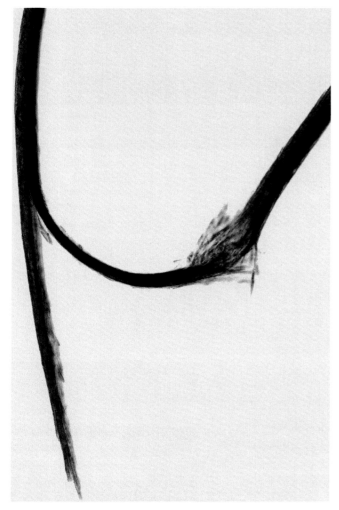

Figure 36.3 Trichoclasis ("greenstick fracture" of hair) and trichorrhexis nodosa are often found in the same weathered shaft.

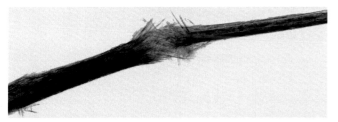

Figure 36.4 Focal loss of the hair cuticle results in cortical fiber separation and the fragile "nodes" of trichorrhexis nodosa.

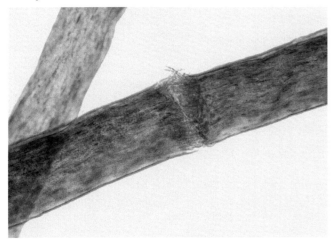

Figure 36.5 Trichoschisis in a patient with trichothiodystrophy. A localized absence of cuticle cells can be found at the site of the fracture.

fiber separation and fracture. By light microscopy, each node then takes on the appearance of two paintbrushes whose bristles have been pushed together (Fig. 36.4). Each "bristle" represents a cornified cortical cell, which can separate from adjacent cells once the binding function of the cuticle is impaired.

TRICHOSCHISIS

The term *trichoschisis* describes a narrow, transverse fracture across the hair shaft through cuticle and cortex (Fig. 36.5). Although trichoschisis is occasionally found in normal hair, it usually occurs in the setting of TTD (see the following section).

TRICHOTHIODYSTROPHY

Patients with TTD have congenitally brittle hair with low sulfur content (16). This hair defect serves as the common denominator for patients with neuroectodermal abnormalities and mutations in the xeroderma pigmentosum-B, xeroderma pigmentosum-D, and p8/TTDA helicase/ATPase subunits of the dual functional DNA repair/basal transcription factor TFIIH (17).

Depending on the precise mutation, patients may have some or all of the following clinical manifestations: developmental delay/intellectual impairment, short stature, ichthyosis, ocular abnormalities, infections, photosensitivity, and a wide variety of less common abnormalities. The 2008 review by Faghri and colleagues (18) is particularly useful.

Hair from patients with TTD demonstrates several abnormalities that are visible with light microscopy. The first is trichoschisis, as described above, which accounts for the brittleness of the hair (Figs. 36.6 and 36.7). Hair shafts may be focally flattened and ribbon-like (Figs. 36.8 and 36.9). One prominent and consistent finding is alternating light and dark banding seen with polarized light (Figs. 36.10 and 36.11). The hair is placed between polarizing filters, and the banding is most evident when the filters are rotated into the "crossed" or "extinguished" position (background is dark). Banding can be transverse or diagonal, and can be reversed (i.e., light becomes dark) by rotating one of the filters about 45°. This banding is due to the undulating nature of cortical fibers found in TTD (Fig. 36.12) (19).

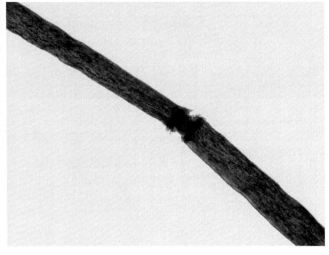

Figure 36.7 Partial hair fracture in a trichothiodystrophy patient with tricho-schisis.

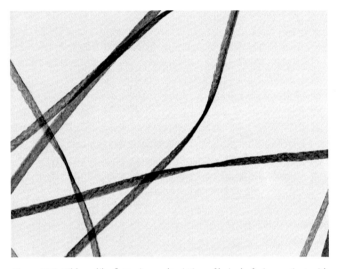

Figure 36.8 Ribbon-like flattening and twisting of hair shafts in a patient with trichothiodystrophy.

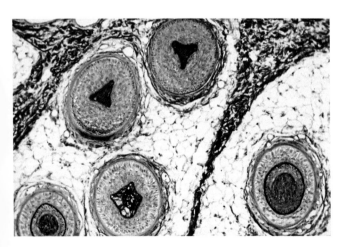

Figure 36.9 Transverse sections demonstrating the dramatic flattening and grooving of trichothiodystrophy hairs, first apparent just above the hair bulb.

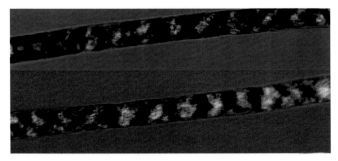

Figure 36.10 Alternating light and dark banding ("tiger tail phenomenon") in a patient with trichothiodystrophy. The image on top shows a polarized hair with the filters in the "crossed" position. The bottom shows the same shaft with filters rotated about 45°.

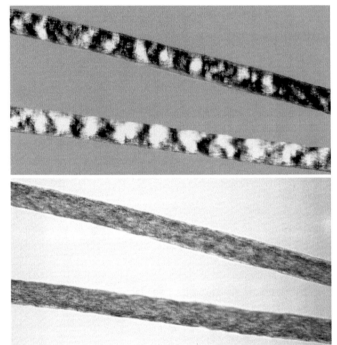

Figure 36.11 Two trichothiodystrophy hair shafts shown with polarization (top) and without (bottom).

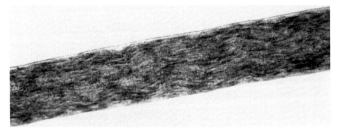

Figure 36.12 Trichothiodystrophy cortical fibers undulate in a closely set, regular pattern.

TRICHORRHEXIS INVAGINATA AND NETHERTON SYNDROME

Trichorrhexis invaginata is a rare congenital hair shaft abnormality seen in Netherton syndrome (20), which manifests with a combination of short, brittle hair and ichthyosiform erythroderma (especially ichthyosis linearis circumflexa). Atopic dermatitis is also found in the majority of patients. The defective gene in Netherton syndrome is SPINK5, which

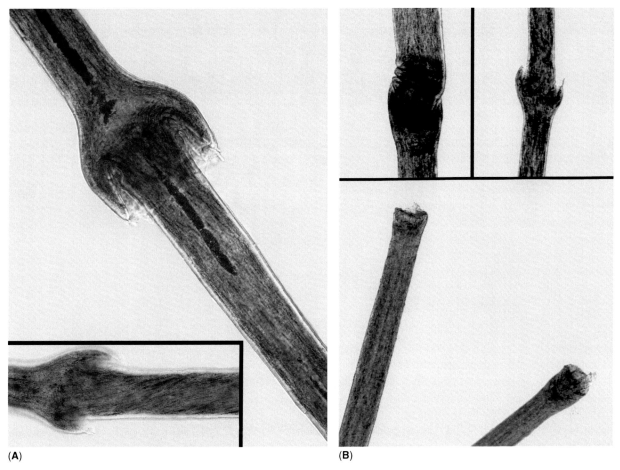

(A)   **(B)**

Figure 36.13 (**A**) Netherton syndrome. The distal portion of this hair shaft (*upper left*) has sunken into the proximal portion (*lower right*) to create a node of trichorrhexis invaginata. Inset: the cortical fibers of the distal portion twist as they intussuscept into the "socket."; (**B**) Netherton syndrome. The *upper left panel* shows an incipient node undergoing torsion. The *upper right panel* shows a fully formed trichorrhexis invaginata node, and the lower panel shows two shafts after nodal fractures.

encodes a serine protease inhibitor called LEKTI (21). Also called "bamboo hair," trichorrhexis invaginata appears as multiple small swellings spaced along the shaft at irregular intervals. Each swelling consists of a cup-like expansion of the proximal hair cortex that surrounds a rounded distal fragment, giving the defect the appearance of a ball-and-socket joint (Fig. 36.13). It appears as if the distal segment has intussuscepted down into the proximal segment. These nodes are extremely fragile and susceptible to fracture, and consequently the hair of affected persons is short, thin, and friable. The likelihood of finding the hair shaft defect may be increased by also examining eyebrow hairs (22).

PILI ANNULATI

Also called *ringed hair*, pili annulati is characterized clinically by alternating light and dark bands of color along the hair shafts. The colors are reversed when the hairs are viewed by light microscopy. The banded appearance is obvious only in blond or lightly pigmented hair, which often has a sandy appearance (23). Banding can be present in the axillae, beard, and pubic areas, although most often it is discovered in scalp hair. Variability in phenotype can be seen, with only some hairs affected, as well as variable banding along affected shafts. The condition may be present at birth or appear during infancy. Hair growth is normal and in the majority of cases the hair is strong and sound, but there may be some degree of

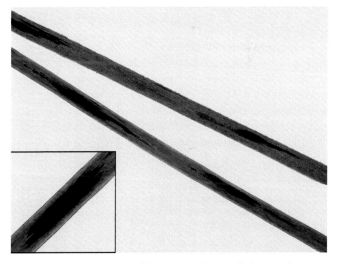

Figure 36.14 Pili annulati. Air-filled spaces within the shaft create dark areas when viewed with a light microscope. The air spaces alternate with normal cortex along the length of the shafts. The inset shows an air space filling most of the cortex.

shaft fragility. Trichorrhexis nodosa-like fractures may be produced in the dark bands. There are no other associated abnormalities and treatment is not required. The condition appears to be caused by a defect in hair cornification (24). The cortex of the abnormal bands contains clusters of air-filled spaces (Fig. 36.14), between cortical fibers and within cortical cells.

The air-filled spaces can be confined to the central portion of the shaft, or may involve the full thickness with associated cuticle disruption.

Pili annulati has been associated with alopecia areata on more than one occasion (25). It is not known whether or not this is pure coincidence. In one curious case, the condition improved after a temporary episode of alopecia totalis (26).

"BUBBLE HAIR"

This distinctive hair shaft abnormality is usually seen in young women with a localized area of uneven, fragile hairs (27). The involved hair is straighter and stiffer than normal. By light microcopy the hair shafts contain large, irregularly spaced bubbles that expand and thin the hair cortex (28) (Fig. 36.15). This same feature can also be seen with scanning electron microscopy (Fig. 36.16). Hair fractures occur at the site of larger bubbles.

The problem is caused by traumatic hair care techniques involving heat, as from a malfunctioning hair dryer (29,30). Once the damaged hair is trimmed, the condition resolves completely with gentle hair styling.

MONILETHRIX

Patients with monilethrix ("beaded hair") have extremely brittle, beaded hairs that emerge from keratotic, follicular papules. Hair shafts rarely grow more than 2–3 cm. The hairs fracture easily, usually resulting in severe alopecia. The course is variable and seasonal, and some patients may show improvement in adult life, while others seem to worsen. The condition usually appears in early childhood, predominantly on the occiput and nape, but it can affect the entire scalp. Occasionally the child is born bald, with beaded hairs appearing several months or years later. Facial and body hair is also involved in severe cases.

Monilethrix is usually inherited as an autosomal dominant trait with high penetrance but variable expressivity. Recessive phenotypes have also been described, as have sporadic cases. Monilethrix is associated with mutations in 3 type II hair cortex keratin genes, most commonly hHb6 but also hHb1 and hHb3 (31). Rare cases of the disease with nonvertical transmission have been found to overlap with localized autosomal recessive hypotrichosis, a disorder that shares the clinical features of monilethrix but lacks the characteristic beaded appearance of the hair shaft (31). The underlying gene, desmoglein 4 (DSG4), belongs to the desmosomal cadherin superfamily and is also expressed in the cortex of the hair shaft (32).

Hair shafts in patients with monilethrix show characteristic, evenly spaced, elliptical nodes that are 0.7–1 mm apart (Fig. 36.17). The nodes can easily be seen and the diagnosis established with a hand-held dermatoscope (33). The intervals between nodes will vary in different hairs from the same patient and hair follicles are not affected in a synchronized fashion (34). The segments of hair shaft between nodes are nonmedullated, tapered constrictions. Imbricated cuticular

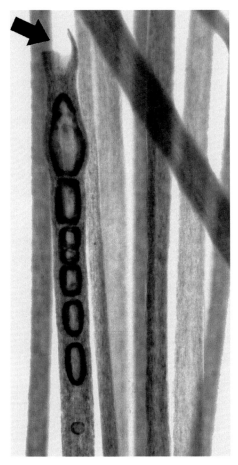

Figure 36.15 The "bubbles" of "bubble hair" expand and thin the cortex, resulting in hair fragility and fracture (*arrow*).

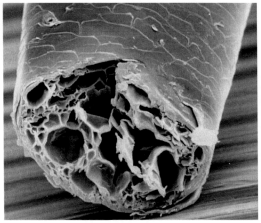
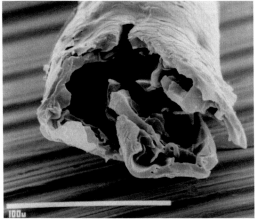

Figure 36.16 Scanning electron micrographs of the fracture point of two bubble hairs, clearly showing the vacuolated cortex.

scales are present on the nodes, whereas the internodes show abnormal longitudinal ridging and often absent scales. Scanning electron microscopy has demonstrated that the nodes correspond to the *normal* caliber of the hair and that the defective portion resides in the constrictions (35).

The hair roots have an architecture that conforms to the shaft abnormality, with alternating constrictions, so that the hair is deformed as it is being produced (36). Matrix cells destined to become cortical cells are particularly affected. This

seems to result in a decrease in the number of cortical cells and thinning of the hair shaft. The condition has been reported to temporarily improve with oral acetretin (37).

PILI TORTI

Pili torti is probably the most misdiagnosed structural hair shaft defect. It is often confused with monilethrix when studied with light microcopy. Hairs in pili torti are flattened and twisted on their longitudinal axes (Fig. 36.18). Each twist may be 90°, 180°, or up to 360°. Typically, runs of four or five closely set twists are found at irregular intervals along the hair shaft. Involved hairs are brittle, do not achieve normal length, and often have a spangled or beaded appearance. The fractured distal tip often shows longitudinal fraying (trichoptilosis). The hair follicles show no histological abnormalities other than some curvature and twisting.

Although it can be present at birth or emerge after puberty, pili torti typically appears in early childhood when normal scalp hairs are replaced by brittle, spangled hairs, especially in the occipital and temporal regions. The spangled appearance is due to unequal reflection of light from the twisted surface. The eyebrows and eyelashes may also be involved. There is a variable degree of hair fragility ranging from patchy alopecia with coarse stubble to hairs of 5 cm or more. Pili torti may improve after puberty or may persist throughout life.

It has been proposed that alterations of the inner root sheath (IRS) may lead to the abnormal molding and twisting of the hair shaft, and that these alterations may occur because of mitochondrial dysfunction (38).

Pili torti is also found in various syndromes, such as Menkes' kinky hair disease (39–41), Bjornstad syndrome (42), and Rapp–Hodgkin ectodermal dysplasia (43). The numerous other distinctive features of these syndromes allow for proper diagnosis, with pili torti offering an additional clue.

PILI MULTIGEMINI

This condition is typically found in the beard area, especially along the jaw, and sometimes presents as a localized folliculitis (Fig. 36.19) (44). Anywhere from two to eight hair matrices, each with its own papilla and separate IRS (Fig. 36.20), form clusters of shafts that emerge from a single follicular canal (44). Surrounding the cluster of hair bulbs is a common outer root sheath that separates to invest each ascending hair shaft. This can be seen by examining hairs that have been forcibly plucked

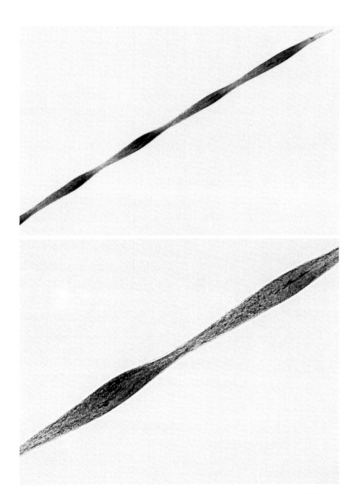

Figure 36.17 In monilethrix, the nodes correspond to the normal caliber of the hair and the defective portion resides in the constrictions. Original magnification ×40 (*upper panel*) and ×100 (*lower panel*). *Source*: Specimen courtesy of Antonelli Tosti, M.D.

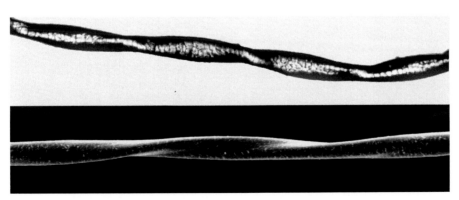

Figure 36.18 Pili torti, as viewed with the light microscope (*top*) and scanning electron microscope (*bottom*).

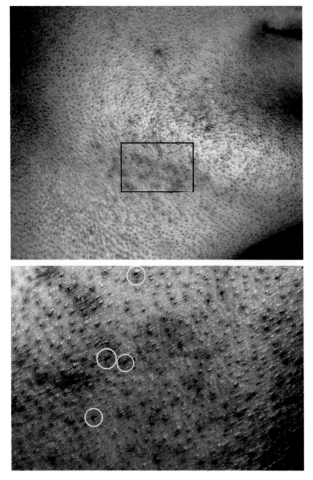

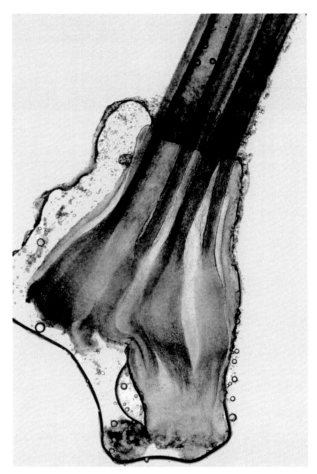

Figure 36.19 Typical case of pili multigemini. The *lower panel*, an enlarged view of the outlined zone seen in the *top panel*, shows some of the enlarged abnormal hairs (*circled*).

Figure 36.21 Forcibly plucked hair from a follicle demonstrating pili multigemini. A syncytium of outer root sheath envelops several separate matrices, each producing its own shaft.

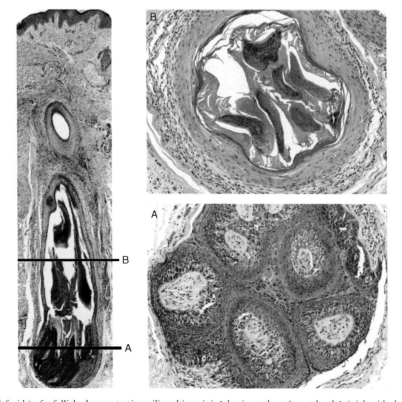

Figure 36.20 Vertical section (*left side*) of a follicle demonstrating pili multigemini. A horizontal section at level A (*right side, bottom*) shows a bulb with several "subpapillae," each with its own matrix and inner root sheath. A section through level B (*right side, top*) shows the compressed, misshapen shafts.

from the beard area (45) (Fig. 36.21). Reports in the medical literature have confused the condition with polytrichia (multiple separate follicles with shafts emerging from the same infundibulum) (46) and trichostasis spinulosa (47).

The shafts in pili multigemini have various shapes in cross-section (flat, ovoid, triangular, or grooved) (45), which probably results from the pressure between hairs in the same follicle (Fig. 36.20, *top right*). Usually the condition is totally benign, but it may be associated with perifollicular erythema resembling folliculitis (44). There is no specific treatment for pili multigemini, which tends to be persistent. The abnormal hairs will simply regrow after plucking. Electrolysis might be effective.

UNCOMBABLE HAIR SYNDROME (PILI TRIANGULI ET CANALICULI OR "SPUN GLASS" HAIR)

This condition was first described in 1973 as *cheveux incoiffables* (unstylable hair) (48). It has also been termed "spun glass hair" and *pili trianguli et canaliculi*. Many familial cases of uncombable hair have been reported, and in those instances an autosomal dominant pattern of inheritance appeared most likely (49). The typical clinical picture includes onset in infancy or early childhood; blonde to light brown hair; dry, frizzy, and spangled hair texture; and slow to normal growth rate. The hair is disorderly, stands out from the scalp, and cannot be combed flat. Some spontaneous improvement is often noted later in childhood (50).

The hair shafts in uncombable hair are usually triangular in cross-section, but can be kidney-shaped, flat, or irregular. Most of the hair shafts will demonstrate the triangular shape. Longitudinal grooves running along the entire shaft are common, hence the name *pili trianguli et canaliculi*. Although grooving of occasional hair shafts can be found on normal scalps, in the uncombable hair syndrome at least 50% of hair shafts demonstrate this abnormality. Grooves can often be seen with the light microscope (Fig. 36.22), although they are best visualized with the scanning electron microscope (51,52) (Fig. 36.23). Scalp biopsy reveals that the IRS has the same configuration as the shaft.

TAPERED HAIRS ("PENCIL POINT" HAIRS)

Tapered hairs that can be easily pulled from the scalp are always a pathological finding. Tapered hairs are found in all forms of *anagen arrest*. Anagen arrest is a pattern of hair loss caused by a sudden insult to the metabolic machinery of the hair follicle. As discussed in chapter 15, this phenomenon can occur in patients with rapidly progressive alopecia areata.

The classic and more familiar form of anagen arrest is seen when patients receive radiotherapy or systemic chemotherapy for the treatment of malignancy. The hair matrix is very sensitive to the toxic effects of X-irradiation and chemotherapy. Affected follicles produce shafts that become progressively smaller in volume and cross-sectional dimension. These hairs quickly taper down to a point, resulting in an extremely fragile constriction (Fig. 36.24). Hair shafts easily fracture at the constrictions, and "pencil point hairs" fall from the patient's scalp in great numbers (Fig. 36.25).

Several diseases cause hair loss with features of an anagen arrest. Severe, rapidly progressive alopecia areata (e.g., alopecia totalis in evolution) has a similar effect on the metabolic

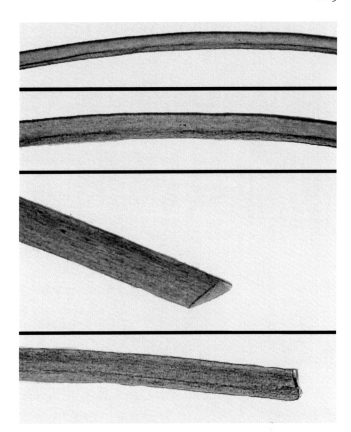

Figure 36.22 The prominent grooving and triangular cross-sectional shapes seen in the "uncombable hair syndrome" are visible even with light microscopy.

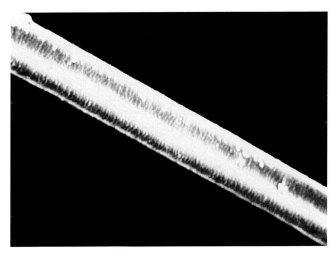

Figure 36.23 The grooving seen in the "uncombable hair syndrome" is best visualized with scanning electron microscopy.

machinery of hair follicles, and tapered hairs are often seen (Fig. 36.26). When patients with systemic lupus erythematosus and secondary syphilis experience rapid hair loss, it sometimes has features of an anagen arrest.

PERIPILAR CASTS ("PSEUDONITS" AND "HAIR CASTS")

Kligman (53) and Brunner (54) described this abnormality independently in 1957. Peripilar casts are often referred to as "hair casts," although the latter designation is imprecise (55).

Figure 36.24 In this patient with alopecia totalis in evolution, two hair shafts abruptly taper to a narrow point, at which the shaft fractures.

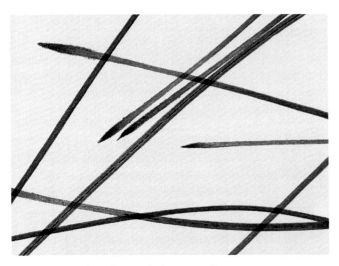

Figure 36.25 Gently pulling on the hair was sufficient to remove numerous "pencil point" hairs from a patient receiving systemic chemotherapy for a malignancy.

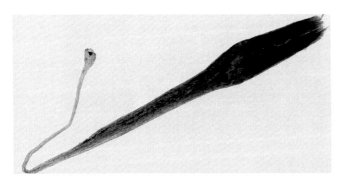

Figure 36.26 A tapered hair gently extracted from the scalp of a patient with rapidly worsening alopecia areata.

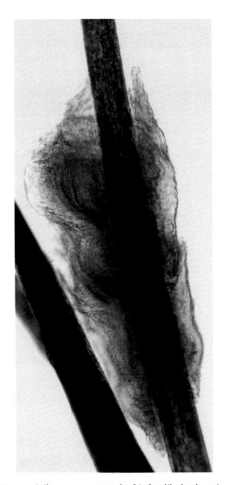

Figure 36.27 A peripilar cast composed of infundibular keratin. This is the most common kind of hair cast.

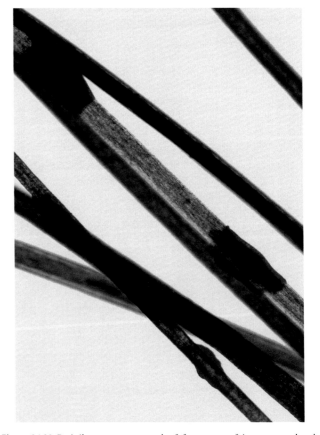

Figure 36.28 Peripilar casts composed of fragments of inner root sheath. These casts stain a dark blue with toluidine blue.

They are tubular masses of amorphous material that are perforated centrally by the hair shaft. Hair casts are conical proximally, and their distal end may taper or (in larger casts) may expand into a funnel shape. Some casts conform to the shape of the follicular canal and infundibulum. True ("classic") peripilar keratin casts are composed of cornified external root sheath (Fig. 36.27), rarely composed of internal root sheath

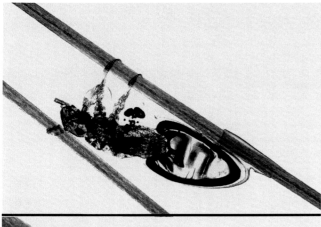

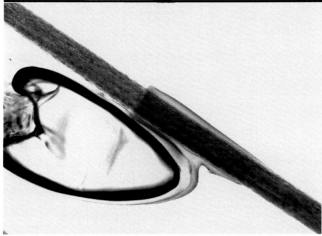

Figure 36.29 In the *top panel*, a juvenile louse is seen emerging from the egg casing. The enlarged view in the *lower panel* shows the attachment of the egg to the shaft.

(Fig. 36.28), and sometimes composed of both external and internal root sheaths. These types can be distinguished by staining with 4-dimethylaminocinnamaldehyde, which stains the IRS a reddish color, or with toluidine blue, which stains the IRS intensely blue (Fig. 36.28).

Peripilar casts should be easy to distinguish from true nits. A nit will have an ovoid egg casing that is attached to the side of the hair shaft by a thin coating of cement, which surrounds the shaft (Fig. 36.29).

REFERENCES

1. Chetty GN, Kamalam A, Thambiah AS. Acquired structural defects of the hair. Int J Dermatol 1981; 20: 119–21.
2. Dawber RP. An update of hair shaft disorders. Dermatol Clin 1996; 14: 753–72.
3. Itin PH, Fistarol SK. Hair shaft abnormalities--clues to diagnosis and treatment. Dermatology 2005; 211: 63–71.
4. Rogers M. Hair shaft abnormalities: Part I. Australas J Dermatol 1995; 36: 179–84; quiz 185–176.
5. Whiting DA. Structural abnormalities of the hair shaft. J Am Acad Dermatol 1987; 16(1 Pt 1): 1–25.
6. Mirmirani P, Huang KP, Price VH. A practical, algorithmic approach to diagnosing hair shaft disorders. Int J Dermatol; 50: 1–12.
7. Cheng AS, Bayliss SJ. The genetics of hair shaft disorders. J Am Acad Dermatol 2008; 59: 1–22; quiz 23–6.
8. de Berker D, Sinclair RD. The hair shaft: normality, abnormality, and genetics. Clin Dermatol 2001; 19: 129–34.
9. Mirmirani P. Ceramic flat irons: improper use leading to acquired trichorrhexis nodosa. J Am Acad Dermatol 2010; 62: 145–7.
10. Ghorpade A. Moustache twirler's trichorrhexis nodosa. J Eur Acad Dermatol Venereol 2001; 16: 296–7.
11. Rabut R. [Three cases of trichorrhexis nodosa circumscripta; role of scratching.]. Bull Soc Fr Dermatol Syphiligr 1951; 58: 563–4.
12. Camacho-Martinez F. Localized trichorrhexis nodosa. J Am Acad Dermatol 1989; 20: 696–7.
13. Scott DA. Disorders of the hair and scalp in blacks. Dermatol Clin 1988; 6: 387–95.
14. Liang C, Kraemer KH, Morris A, et al. Characterization of tiger-tail banding and hair shaft abnormalities in trichothiodystrophy. J Am Acad Dermatol 2005; 52: 224–32.
15. Fichtel JC, Richards JA, Davis LS. Trichorrhexis nodosa secondary to argininosuccinicaciduria. Pediatr Dermatol 2007; 24: 25–7.
16. Price VH, Odom RB, Ward WH, Jones FT. Trichothiodystrophy: sulfur-deficient brittle hair as a marker for a neuroectodermal symptom complex. Arch Dermatol 1980; 116: 1375–84.
17. Hashimoto S, Egly JM. Trichothiodystrophy view from the molecular basis of DNA repair/transcription factor TFIIH. Hum Mol Genet 2009; 18: 24–30.
18. Faghri S, Tamura D, Kraemer KH, Digiovanna JJ. Trichothiodystrophy: a systematic review of 112 published cases characterises a wide spectrum of clinical manifestations. J Med Genet 2008; 45: 609–21.
19. Sperling LC, DiGiovanna JJ. "Curly" wood and tiger tails: an explanation for light and dark banding with polarization in trichothiodystrophy. Arch Dermatol 2003; 139: 1189–92.
20. Netherton EW. A unique case of trichorrhexis nodosa: "bamboo hairs." Arch Dermatol 1958; 78: 483–7.
21. Bitoun E, Chavanas S, Irvine AD, et al. Netherton syndrome: disease expression and spectrum of SPINK5 mutations in 21 families. J Invest Dermatol 2002; 118: 352–61.
22. Powell J, Dawber RP, Ferguson DJ, Griffiths WA. Netherton's syndrome: increased likelihood of diagnosis by examining eyebrow hairs. Br J Dermatol 1999; 141: 544–6.
23. Rogers M. Hair shaft abnormalities: Part II. Australas J Dermatol 1996; 37: 1–11.
24. Giehl KA, Dean D, Dawber RP, et al. Cytokeratin expression in pili annulati hair follicles. Clin Exp Dermatol 2005; 30: 426–8.
25. Moffitt DL, Lear JT, de Berker DA, Peachey RD. Pili annulati coincident with alopecia areata. Pediatr Dermatol 1998; 15: 271–3.
26. Green J, Sinclair RD, de Berker D. Disappearance of pili annulati following an episode of alopecia areata. Clin Exp Dermatol 2002; 27: 458–60.
27. Brown VM, Crounse RG, Abele DC. An unusual new hair shaft abnormality: "bubble hair." J Am Acad Dermatol 1986; 15(5 Pt 2): 1113–7.
28. Elston DM, Bergfeld WF, Whiting DA, et al. Bubble hair. J Cutan Pathol 1992; 19: 439–44.
29. Detwiler SP, Carson JL, Woosley JT, Gambling TM, Briggaman RA. Bubble hair. Case caused by an overheating hair dryer and reproducibility in normal hair with heat. J Am Acad Dermatol 1994; 30: 54–60.
30. Gummer CL. Bubble hair: a cosmetic abnormality caused by brief, focal heating of damp hair fibres. Br J Dermatol 1994; 131: 901–3.
31. Zlotogorski A, Marek D, Horev L, et al. An autosomal recessive form of monilethrix is caused by mutations in DSG4: clinical overlap with localized autosomal recessive hypotrichosis. J Invest Dermatol 2006; 126: 1292–6.
32. Schweizer J. More than one gene involved in monilethrix: intracellular but also extracellular players. J Invest Dermatol 2006; 126: 1216–9.
33. Rakowska A, Slowinska M, Czuwara J, Olszewska M, Rudnicka L. Dermoscopy as a tool for rapid diagnosis of monilethrix. J Drugs Dermatol 2007; 6: 222–4.
34. de Berker D, Dawber RP. Variations in the beading configuration in monilethrix. Pediatr Dermatol 1992; 9: 19–21.
35. Ito M, Hashimoto K, Yorder FW. Monilethrix: an ultrastructural study. J Cutan Pathol 1984; 11: 513–21.
36. Tosti A. Dermoscopy of hair and scalp disorders with clinical and pathological correlations. London: Informa Healthcare, 2007.
37. Karincaoglu Y, Coskun BK, Seyhan ME, Bayram N. Monilethrix: improvement with acitretin. Am J Clin Dermatol 2005; 6: 407–10.
38. Mirmirani P, Samimi SS, Mostow E. Pili torti: clinical findings, associated disorders, and new insights into mechanisms of hair twisting. Cutis 2009; 84: 143–7.
39. Tumer Z, Moller LB. Menkes disease. Eur J Hum Genet 18: 511–8.
40. Bertini I, Rosato A. Menkes disease. Cell Mol Life Sci 2008; 65: 89–91.

41. Moore CM, Howell RR. Ectodermal manifestations in Menkes disease. Clin Genet 1985; 28: 532–40.

42. Hinson JT, Fantin VR, Schonberger J, et al. Missense mutations in the BCS1L gene as a cause of the Bjornstad syndrome. N Engl J Med 2007; 356: 809–19.

43. Silengo MC, Davi GF, Bianco R, et al. Distinctive hair changes (pili torti) in Rapp-Hodgkin ectodermal dysplasia syndrome. Clin Genet 1982; 21: 297–300.

44. Pinkus H. Multiple hairs (Flemming-Giovannini; report of two cases of pili multigemini and discussion of some other anomalies of the pilary complex. J Invest Dermatol 1951; 17:291–301.

45. Cambiaghi S, Barbareschi M, Cambiaghi G, Caputo R. Scanning electron microscopy in the diagnosis of pili multigemini. Acta Derm Venereol 1995; 75: 170–1.

46. Lester L, Venditti C. The prevalence of pili multigemini. Br J Dermatol 2007; 156: 1362–3.

47. Lee JS, Kim YC, Kang HY. The nevoid pili multigemini over the back. Eur J Dermatol 2005; 15: 99–101.

48. Dupre A, Bonafe JL, Litoux F, Victor M. [Uncombable hair syndrome. Pili trianguli et canaliculi (author's transl)]. Ann Dermatol Venereol 1978; 105: 627–30.

49. Calderon P, Otberg N, Shapiro J. Uncombable hair syndrome. J Am Acad Dermatol 2009; 61: 512–15.

50. Jarell AD, Hall MA, Sperling LC. Uncombable hair syndrome. Pediatr Dermatol 2007; 24: 436–8.

51. Hicks J, Metry DW, Barrish J, Levy M. Uncombable hair (cheveux incoiffables, pili trianguli et canaliculi) syndrome: brief review and role of scanning electron microscopy in diagnosis. Ultrastruct Pathol 2001; 25: 99–103.

52. McCullum N, Sperling LC, Vidmar D. The uncombable hair syndrome. Cutis 1990; 46: 479–83.

53. Kligman AM. Hair casts. Arch Dermatol 1957; 75: 509–11.

54. Brunner MJ, Facq LM. A pseudoparasite of the scalp hair. Arch Dermatol 1957; 75: 583.

55. Scott MJ Jr, Roenigk HH Jr. Hair casts: classification, staining characteristics, and differential diagnosis. J Am Acad Dermatol 1983; 8: 27–32.

Glossary

Anagen: Period of active hair shaft formation. Anagen follicles can be identified by the presence of a hair matrix (germinative epithelium) surrounding the hair papilla and by the presence of inner and outer root sheaths.

Anagen arrest: The abrupt cessation or diminution of hair shaft production that occurs with toxic insults to the anagen hair matrix such as chemotherapy or radiation therapy. The hair shaft will rapidly taper to a point and fall out (as "pencil-point hairs") while still in the anagen phase. The shedding phase is known as anagen effluvium (see below).

Anagen effluvium (or anagen defluvium): The shedding of hair shafts that have tapered to a point due to a toxic insult such as chemotherapy. The term is confusing because it suggests that anagen hairs fall out. They do not, only their shafts are shed while the follicles remain in the anagen phase. However, the forces that cause hair shaft tapering also tend to shift anagen hairs into the catagen/telogen phase. Therefore, an anagen effluvium is often associated with an increased percentage of telogen hairs.

Arao–Perkins body: A pad of elastic tissue that develops just deep to the follicular papilla. Sometimes vertical sections of follicular streamers will contain a series of Arao–Perkins bodies denoting the location of prior hair bulbs over successive, gradually shortening follicular cycles.

Biphasic alopecia: A term coined by Dr. Al Solomon to indicate conditions that behave as noncicatricial alopecia (no follicular loss) early in their course, but resemble a cicatricial alopecia (with permanent follicular loss) late in the disease. Examples are androgenetic alopecia, traction alopecia, and the hair loss associated with systemic lupus erythematosus.

Brocq's alopecia: Also known as *Pseudopelade of Brocq*. A clinical pattern of end-stage cicatricial alopecia characterized by irregularly shaped, smooth, pale patches or slightly depressed plaques. Most cases represent the end-stage of lichen planopilaris although the same pattern of hair loss can be caused by other inflammatory disorders.

Bulb (or hair bulb): The deepest portion of the hair follicle, usually located in the fat, comprising the basophilic germinative layer known as the hair *matrix*, and the hair *papilla*, a mesenchymal structure derived from the dermis.

Bulge (or bulge zone): The follicular epithelium adjacent to the attachment of the arrector pili muscle. This zone is believed to be the site of the stem cell population of the hair follicle.

Catagen phase: *Catagen* is a brief transitional phase between anagen and telogen, and lasts about 2–3 weeks. The epithelium of the lower portion of the follicle undergoes disintegration via cellular apoptosis, leaving an angiofibrotic strand or *streamer (stela)* indicating the former position of the anagen root. As these changes occur, the vitreous (or glassy) layer thickens markedly, becoming a prominent structure.

Catagen/telogen phase: As the brief catagen phase always leads to the much longer telogen phase, they can be conceptually linked together as the "catagen/telogen" phase.

Cicatricial alopecia: Synonymous with "scarring alopecia," cicatricial alopecia is the term favored by the North American Hair Research Society. The term implies that follicles have been selectively destroyed and replaced by connective tissue.

Club hair: Synonymous with *telogen hair* and indicating the formation of a club-like cornified structure within the hair bulb. See also "presumptive club hair."

Cornification: The term implies terminal differentiation of keratin-forming epithelium with loss of nuclei and organelles. In the final stages of cornification, cellular metabolism ceases and the cells are almost completely filled by keratin. Keratinization is a similar term sometimes used by other authors. In this text, they are used synonymously.

Crown: We use the term to describe the area surrounding the highest and most central portion of the top of the scalp (Fig. 1). Anterior to the crown is the frontal/anterior hairline zone; posterior to it is the vertex.

Cuticular layer: Surrounds the hair shaft and is the innermost layer of the three layers comprising the inner root sheath (IRS). It is immediately surrounded by Huxley's layer followed by Henle's layer.

Diffuse alopecia: A clinical pattern of alopecia with a uniform reduction in hair density over all portions of the scalp. This pattern is characteristically seen in telogen effluvium.

Doll's hairs: See "polytrichia."

Dysmorphic versus dystrophic hairs: The root "-morphic" is derived from the Greek word for "shape" or "form," and so dysmorphic refers to an abnormal shape or anatomic structure. The root "-trophic" is derived from the Greek word for food or nutrition, and so dystrophy implies abnormal growth. Therefore, hairs that are misshapen because of a physical insult are "dysmorphic" while those misshapen as the physiologic consequence of a disease state are "dystrophic." For example, hairs with incomplete anatomic features from forcible plucking are dysmorphic, whereas those that have miniaturized due to disease are dystrophic. This may seem to be a fine distinction, but an important one when clarity is at stake.

Dystrophic hairs: See "dysmorphic *vs* dystrophic hairs" above.

Ectothrix: Infection of the hair caused by fungal species that predominantly grow as spores on the surface of the hair shaft. This should not be confused with dermatophytes that are simply growing within the loose stratum corneum-like keratin that surrounds hairs in the follicular infundibulum.

Endothrix: Infection of the hair caused by fungal species that predominantly grow as spores (less often as hyphae) within the cortex of the hair shaft.

End-stage cicatricial alopecia: Alopecia histologically devoid or nearly devoid of any remaining hair follicles and demonstrating no specific features of any one cicatricial alopecia. This nonspecific diagnostic end point represents the culmination of all longstanding cicatricial alopecias.

Exclamation point hairs: Short hairs demonstrating a frayed, broken shaft that is narrowed and frequently hypopigmented proximally, terminating in a resting club.

Exogen: The phase following telogen, when the fully cornified telogen bulb and shaft are shed from the follicle.

Fibroplasia: The formation of fibrous tissue as a reparative or reactive process. Used interchangeably with fibrosis.

Fibrosis: The formation of fibrous tissue as a reparative or reactive process. Used interchangeably with fibroplasia.

Frontal scalp: The most anterior portion of the top of the scalp. This may also be referred to as the anterior hairline (Fig. 1). Posterior to the frontal scalp centrally is the crown. Posterolateral to the frontal scalp is the temporal scalp.

Glassy layer: See "vitreous layer."

Follicular phase: Refers to a phase of the hair cycle: anagen, catagen, telogen, or exogen.

Follicular scar: The column of connective tissue that replaces the hair follicle in any form of cicatricial alopecia.

Follicular unit: A roughly hexagonal grouping of follicles containing several terminal and vellus follicles with their associated sebaceous glands and arrector pili muscles. About 12 units are found in a section from a 4 mm punch biopsy from normal scalp, or approximately one per square millimeter.

Folliculitis decalvans: A highly inflammatory pattern seen in a number of cicatricial alopecias characterized by frequent perifollicular papules and pustules. It is almost always most severe on the vertex, likely because the most common underlying diagnosis is central, centrifugal cicatricial alopecia.

Forcible hair pluck: See "trichogram."

Hair bulb: Consists of the hair matrix and its nascent epithelial derivatives (root sheaths and shaft) that surround the mesenchymal papilla. Also, see "hair papilla."

Hair density: The number of viable hair follicles per unit area. For example, if a 4 mm diameter specimen (surface area = 12.6 mm²) contains 25 hairs, the hair density is 25 ÷ 12.6 = 2 hairs per square millimeter.

Hair papilla (also known as the mesenchymal or follicular papilla): The hair papilla contains specialized connective tissue cells, blood vessels, and nerve endings. It is surrounded by undifferentiated, actively dividing hair matrix cells.

Hair pull test: Gentle traction is exerted on a small lock of hairs (approximately 20) grasped between the thumb and index finger. This is repeated on several different areas of the scalp. For patients who shampoo regularly, we consider the upper limit of normal as 3 hairs per pull. If 4 or more telogen hairs are extracted with each pull, the pull test is considered positive (see note below). A pull test is frequently negative in androgenetic alopecia, but if positive, should only be so on the top of the scalp. A positive test in multiple scalp zones, including the occiput, is considered suggestive of telogen effluvium. A pull test that extracts anagen hairs may be used to assess for disease activity in inflammatory cicatricial alopecias, especially lichen planopilaris. A single anagen hair is also considered to be positive in such a case. Such active areas are the most fruitful sites to obtain a biopsy. [Note: Some authors feel that removal of more than six telogen hairs indicates a "positive" pull test. As this test has never been critically studied the optimal predictive value in various populations remains somewhat arbitrary.]

Hair stem: The portion of the hair follicle between the hair bulb and the isthmus. Also known as the suprabulbar zone.

Hair whorl: The spiral-patterned growth of hair (clockwise or counter clockwise) most commonly located at the vertex of

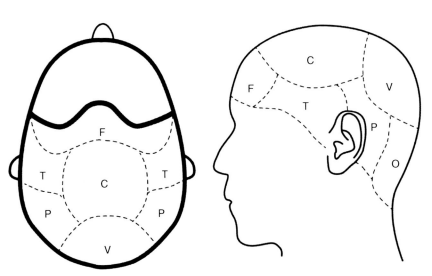

Figure 1 Zones of the scalp. *Abbreviations:* F, frontal; T, temporal; P, parietal; C, crown; V, vertex; O, occipital.

the scalp (Fig. 1). Whorls can occasionally be seen along the frontal hair line and in other locations within the scalp, and may be multiple.

Horizontal sections: See "transverse sections."

Henle's layer: The outermost of the three layers of the IRS. Henle's layer cornifies before the other layers of the IRS and is surrounded by the outer root sheath.

Huxley's layer: The middle of the three IRS layers, sandwiched between the cuticular layer and Henle's layer.

Indeterminate hairs: A "medium-sized" follicle, smaller than terminal and larger than vellus. Although the official definition is a follicle producing a shaft that is 0.03–0.06 mm in diameter, we use a comparison with the biggest shaft and the smallest shaft to help identify indeterminate hairs. See also "size of hairs" and "small terminal hairs."

Infundibulum: The most superficial portion of the hair follicle. The infundibulum is lined by epithelium with a granular layer and basket-weave stratum corneum, and is continuous with the epidermis. The hair shaft is not attached to the wall of the infundibulum allowing for freedom of movement.

Isthmus: The isthmus extends superficially from the arrector pili insertion (bulge area) to the entry of the sebaceous duct. The IRS falls apart (desquamates) and disappears within the isthmus, most often at its mid point.

Matrix: The germinative zone of the hair follicle epithelium, present only during the actively growing anagen phase of the hair cycle. The matrix is located in the hair bulb and surrounds the hair papilla. Daughter cells produced by the matrix form the hair shaft, IRS, and outer root sheath.

Medulla: A central structure that can be seen within some terminal hairs. It may be prominent or subtle, continuous or discontinuous. Animal hairs have much larger and more obvious medullary cavities.

Miniaturized hairs: Hairs that were large during early life but have become smaller (with thinner hair shafts) due to an acquired, physiological or pathological change. The fine cheek hairs of most children and women are vellus, but not miniaturized. Most of the "peach fuzz" hairs found in alopecia totalis are miniaturized. Despite this distinction, miniaturized hairs will often be used synonymously with vellus in various places in this text.

"Naked" hair shaft: A fragment of stranded hair shaft within the dermis or subcutis, often surrounded by mild granulomatous inflammation. This finding provides strong evidence for cicatricial alopecia.

Nanogen follicles (or nanogen hairs): A term coined by Dr. John T. Headington for the peculiar miniaturized hairs seen in alopecia areata. Our more specific definition is as follows: a miniaturized follicle producing little if any hair shaft, and often simultaneously exhibiting features of both the anagen and catagen/telogen phases. The presence of multiple nanogen hairs usually indicates that the patient has alopecia areata.

Occipital scalp: The inferior portion of the back of the scalp extending to the neckline (Fig. 1). It is bounded anterolaterally by the parietal scalp and superiorly by the vertex.

Papilla: See "hair papilla."

Parietal scalp: The posterolateral portion of the scalp in the vicinity of the ear (Fig. 1). It is bounded anteriorly by the temporal scalp, anterosuperiorly by the crown, posterosuperiorly by the vertex, and posteriorly by the occipital scalp.

Patterned alopecia: Clinical alopecia with a nonuniform reduction in hair density on the scalp. Patterned alopecia implies that the hair loss is confined to certain areas of the scalp, leaving other areas normal.

Perifolliculum: The specialized connective tissue stroma surrounding the pilosebaceous unit.

Pigment cast: Distorted residual pigmented matrix epithelium found within the follicular lumen at any level of the follicle. Pigment casts are most commonly seen in trichotillomania where forcible plucking has torn and displaced the matrix epithelium. Similar mechanical injury may underlie their presence in acute traction alopecia. They can also be seen in postoperative (pressure-induced) alopecia and in alopecia areata, where inflammation and/or rapid involution of the follicle can lead to amorphous collections of pigment from degenerating hair matrix cells.

Polytrichia: Also known as "tufting" and "doll's hairs," it can be recognized by the presence of numerous hair shafts exiting a single follicular ostium. Wide spacing is present between tufted ostia.

Presumptive club hair: In early telogen phase central cornification occurs in the deepest portion of the follicular epithelium, near the level of the attachment of the arrector pili muscle. This zone of cornifying epithelium gradually expands to form a bulbous mass known as the presumptive club. During exogen, this club-like structure and the overlying shaft falls from the scalp as a shed telogen hair (club hair).

Secondary hair germ: Irregularly shaped basaloid nipple of epithelium just deep to the bulb of a telogen hair and just superficial to the hair papilla, which remains after the involution of the catagen phase. It appears asterisk-shaped in horizontal sections. Once thought to be the site of hair regeneration, its function is currently unclear.

Size of hairs: The convention used in this text is to categorize the size of hairs based on the hair shaft diameter, not the overall diameter of the follicular epithelium. Thus a seemingly large follicle (based on epithelial diameter) with a very small shaft may be termed a *vellus* (or miniaturized) hair. A follicle with a large shaft diameter is called a *terminal* hair. One that is "borderline" in size is an *indeterminate* hair.

Small terminal hairs: Some authors call these *indeterminate hairs*. They are 0.03–0.06 mm in diameter. See also "Indeterminate hairs."

Stem of hair: See "hair stem."

Stela or stele (plural = stelae): The term stele was borrowed from the Greek word for a decorative pillar or stone column used for burial or commemorative purposes. Also known as a "follicular streamer" or "residual fibrous tract," it is a connective tissue column composed of collapsed fibrous root sheath marking the prior location of a miniaturized or regressed follicle. Follicular stelae in the lower dermis indicate overlying terminal catagen/telogen hairs or miniaturized vellus-like hairs. As catagen begins, the hair shaft and bulb start retracting upward, leaving behind an angiofibrotic streamer or stela linking the follicle to the site of the former anagen bulb.

Streamer: See "stela."

Suprabulbar zone: Referred to by some as the "stem" of the anagen follicle, this zone comprises the region just above the hair bulb and below the isthmus.

Telogen phase: In the telogen phase the hair bulb is situated at the bulge level where the arrector pili muscle inserts into the hair follicle. The telogen bulb contains a cornified club hair with a jagged surface, and lacks both pigment and an IRS. This club is surrounded by outer root sheath-type cells. At the base of this epithelial sheath is the *secondary hair germ* (see above).

Telogen count: The ratio of terminal telogen hairs to the total number of terminal hairs, usually expressed as a percentage. Vellus telogen hairs are not included in the telogen count. For example, if there are 20 terminal anagen hairs, 5 terminal catagen/telogen hairs, and 4 vellus hairs, the telogen count is $5/25 = 20\%$.

Telogen germ unit: After the club hair has been shed from the follicle the secondary hair germ (see above) is sometimes referred to as the telogen germ unit.

Terminal hairs: Terminal hairs are conspicuous and exceed 0.06 mm in diameter and 1 cm in length, and may be pigmented and contain a medulla. Some authors refer to small terminal hairs (0.03–0.06 mm) as indeterminate hairs. Terminal hairs are rooted in the subcutaneous tissue or deep dermis.

Terminal: vellus ratio: The cited average ratio of terminal to vellus hairs in normal scalp will vary from author to author, depending on how medium-sized hairs (indeterminate hairs) are counted. If all indeterminate hairs are assigned to the terminal hair total, then the terminal:vellus ratio will usually be higher than 4:1. If a portion of the indeterminate hairs are assigned to the vellus category the terminal:vellus ratio in normal scalp will be lower, but should still be greater than 2:1. We prefer to split the total number of indeterminate hairs evenly between the terminal and vellus counts. Please also refer to our definition of vellus, indeterminate and terminal hairs.

Transverse sections (synonymous with horizontal sections): Tissue sections cut parallel to the epidermal surface, thereby revealing hair follicles in cross-section. This is the authors' preferred way to evaluate alopecia biopsies.

Trichilemmal cornification (trichilemmal keratinization/outer root sheath cornification): The term implies cornification without the formation of trichohyaline or keratohyaline granules.

Trichoclasis: A longitudinal fracture of the hair shaft through the cortex but not completely severing the cuticle. This results in a break described as a "greenstick" fracture of the hair.

Trichogram: A small cluster of hairs that is forcibly plucked from the scalp. If enough hairs (50–70) are included in the pluck, it is a fairly reliable way to determine the telogen count.

Trichomalacia: This term describes hair shafts that are irregularly shaped, smaller than normal, and irregularly pigmented. It is found when hair shafts are physically damaged (as in trichotillomania) or when the metabolic machinery of shaft formation is severely affected (as in alopecia areata).

Trichoptilosis: A split of the hair shaft at the distal end creating a feathery appearance, colloquially known as "split ends."

Trichorrhexis nodosa: Breakage of hair shafts as the result of physical or chemical weathering that leads to focal cuticular damage and node-like bulging of cortical fibers. These findings may be seen in otherwise normal hair or as part of inherited hair fragility orders.

Trichoschisis: A narrow transverse fracture across the hair shaft through the cuticle and cortex resembling a "clean break."

Tufting: See "polytrichia."

Vellus hairs: Small hairs, typically with shafts that are 0.03 mm or thinner and often with adjacent IRSs as thick or thicker than the shaft. Primary (or true) vellus hairs are small from birth and have bulbs located in the mid-to-upper dermis (superficial to the isthmus of adjacent terminal hairs). In the healthy scalp there is usually only one true vellus hair per follicular unit. Secondary vellus hairs (or miniaturized hairs) have thicker outer root sheaths than primary vellus hairs. Their stelae (streamers), and sometimes even their bulbs, extend into the lower dermis or fat. They begin as larger (terminal) hairs and miniaturize over time.

Vertex: No standardized definition exists; the term is used in different ways by different authors. We use the term to describe the portion of the scalp surrounding the usual location of the "hair whorl" (Fig. 1). Anterior to the vertex is the crown; posterior and inferior is the occiput.

Vitreous layer: Also known as the *glassy layer*. This acellular zone just external to the outer root sheath represents the basement membrane zone of the follicular epithelium. The vitreous layer becomes markedly thickened during the catagen phase of the hair cycle.

Weathering: An all-encompassing term for the various physical and chemical forces (such as ultraviolet light, heating, brushing, bleaching, dyeing, relaxing, and so on) that damage hair shafts. This damage often manifests as a loss of hair luster and fractures of the shafts.

Zones of the scalp: The anatomic regions of the scalp referred to in this text are the frontal, temporal, crown, vertex, occipital, and parietal zones. These areas may be referred to in combination, as in "frontotemporal" zone. The exact definitions of these zones may vary between authors, but our concept is depicted in Fig. 1.

Index